AF695348

Vogl, Clauß, Li, Yeon (Eds.)

Computed Tomography

Springer
Berlin
Heidelberg
New York
Barcelona
Budapest
Hong Kong
London
Milan
Paris
Tokyo

T. J. Vogl, W. Clauß, G.-Z. Li, K. M. Yeon (Eds.)

Computed Tomography

State of the Art and Future Applications

With 233 Figures

Springer

Prof. Dr. Thomas J. Vogl
Universitätsklinikum Rudolf Virchow
Strahlenklinik und Poliklinik
Augustenburger Platz 1
13344 Berlin

Prof. Guo-Zhen Li
Beijing Hospital
No. 1 Da Hu Road, Dongdan
Beijing 100730
P.R. China

Dr. Wolfram Clauß
Schering AG
Klinische Entwicklung Diagnostika
Müllerstraße 170 – 178
13342 Berlin

Prof. Kyung Mo Yeon
Seoul National University Hospital
Diagnostic Radiology Department
28, Yunkeun-Dong, Jongro-Ku
110-799 Seoul, Korea

ISBN-13:978-3-642-79889-4

Library of Congress Cataloging-in-Publication Data.

Computed tomography : state of the art and future applications / T. J. Vogl ... (ed.). - Berlin ; Heidelberg ; New York ; Barcelona ; Budapest ; Hong Kong ; London ; Milan ; Paris ; Tokyo : Springer, 1995
ISBN-13:978-3-642-79889-4 e-ISBN-13:978-3-642-79887-0
DOI: 10.1007/978-3-642-79887-0
NE: Vogl, Thomas J. [Hrsg.]

This work is subject to copyright. All rights are reserved, whether the whole or part of the material is concerned, specifically the rights of translation, reprinting, reuse of illustrations, recitation, broadcasting, reproduction on microfilm or in other way, and storage in data banks. Duplication of this publication or parts thereof is permitted only unter the provisions of the German Copyright. Law of September 9, 1965, in its current version, and permission for use must always be obtained from Springer-Verlag. Violations are liable for prosecution under the German copyright law.

© Springer-Verlag Berlin Heidelberg 1996
Softcover reprint of the hardcover 1st edition 1996

The use of general descriptive names, registered names, trademarks, etc. in this publication does not imply, even in the absence of a specific statement, that such names are exempt from the relevant protective laws and regulations and therefore free for general use.

The publisher cannot assume any legal responsibility for given data, especially as far as directions for the use and the handling of chemicals are concerned. This information can be obtained from the instructions on safe laboratory practice and from the manufactures of chemical and laboratory equipment.

Typesetting: Fotosatz-Service, Köhler OHG, Würzburg;
SPIN: 10489638 21/3020-5 4 3 2 1 0 – Printed on acid-free paper

Preface

In the past 20 years, since its clinical introduction in 1975, computer tomography (CT) has been often praised and sometimes hotly debated. In the mid-1980s, due to continued developments in CT systems, especially reduced scanning times and increased scan frequency, CT was considered to be perhaps the most useful and powerful tool in the spectrum of diagnostic procedures. Soon afterwards, when magnetic resonance imaging (MRI) became available in most institutions, some of us thought this was the end of the CT era. However, the development of spiral CT, better contrast media, new scanners, and three-dimensional reconstruction algorithms assured the survival of CT and helped it to gain new credit.

In January 1995, 300 participants from Asia, USA, and Europe lively discussed "State of the Art and Future Aspects of CT" in Beijing, China. The workshop was designed to cover all essential aspects of modern CT imaging, including the historical development, different techniques, contrast agents, organ systems, and indications. The comparative evaluation of CT versus MRI and ultrasound was a central topic. Additionally, a special session was dedicated to "Angiography Tomorrow".

With the publication of the proceedings we aim to summarize the state of the art in both conventional and spiral CT imaging and to provide some suggestions as to the future role of the method. Hopefully, the book will be a guide for daily work with CT techniques for some time to come.

Berlin, July 1995

Thomas J. Vogl
on behalf of the Scientific Programme Committee

Contents

CHAPTER 1

Historical Development of X-Ray Contrast Media for Urography and Angiography

W. Clauss[1] and U. Speck[2]

This year 1995 we are celebrating the centenary of the discovery of X-rays. In 1895, W. C. Röntgen discovered the new rays and laid the foundation stone of X-ray diagnostics. Due to similar or even equal densities, many structures of the organism (e.g. vessels) could not be delineated and remained invisible. Therefore, the need for contrast media was soon recognized.

The systematic search for X-ray-absorbing materials began in 1896. Sehrwald [1] compared in vitro halogens (e.g. iodine and bromide) with different substances, e.g. metal salts and organic tissues (Fig. 1). In the same year, the first opacification of blood vessels was shown in an amputated hand (Fig. 2) by Haschek and Lindenthal [2]. The contrast medium used was Teichmann's paste, a mixture of mercury sulphide and lime and the exposure time was 57 min(!).

In the course of ongoing research work, different heavy metals proved to be effective contrast media. Due to the high toxicity of the free ions, they were admin-

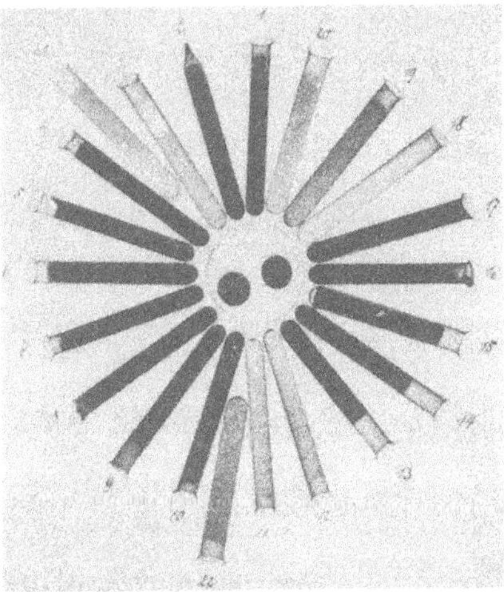

Fig. 1 Search for X-ray absorbing materials. *1*, iodine; *2*, bromine; *3*, chlorinated water 0,5%; *4*, potassium iodide; *5*, potassium bromide; *6*, potassium chloride; *7*, iodoform; *8*, bromoform; *9*, chloroform; *10*, airol; *11*, sponge; *12*, thyroiodine 3% + 97% lactose; *13*, fluorcalcium; *14*, potassium cyanide; *15*, silver nitrate; *16*, adhesive tape; *17*, lead plaster; *18*, empty glass; *19*, muscle of 1-year-old pig; *20*, thyroid gland of 1-year-old pig; *21*, muscle of 4-year-old ox; *22*, thyroid gland of 4-year-old ox. (from Sehrwald 1896)

[1] Clinical Development, Schering AG, Müllerstr. 178, 13342 Berlin, Germany.
[2] Research Laboratories, Schering AG, Müllerstr. 178, 13342 Berlin, Germany.

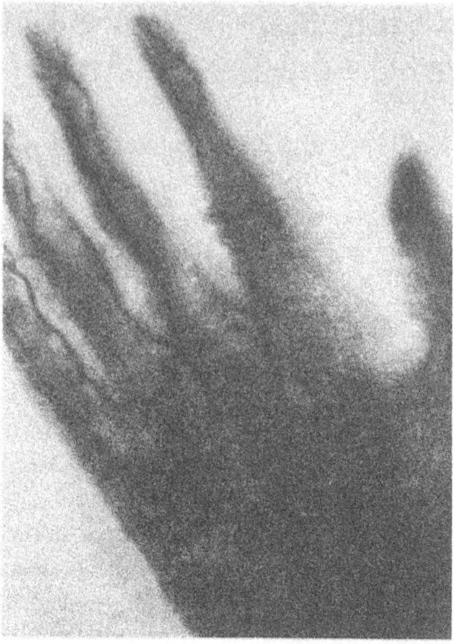

Fig. 2 Opacification of blood vessels in an amputated hand using Teichmann's paste (Haschek and Lindenthal 1896)

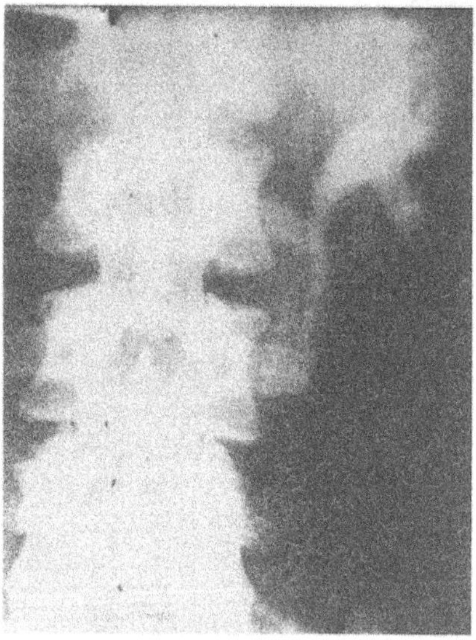

Fig. 3 Opacification of the renal pelvis after retrograde administration of thorium nitrate and sodium citrate (Burns 1915)

istered in the form of suspensions of insoluble oxides or salts. Nevertheless, poor tolerance restricted application to body cavities, such as the urinary tract or the gastrointestinal tract. In 1915, Burns [3] used 10% thorium nitrate and sodium citrate in water and obtained adequate opacification of the renal pelvis and ureter after retrograde administration (Fig. 3).

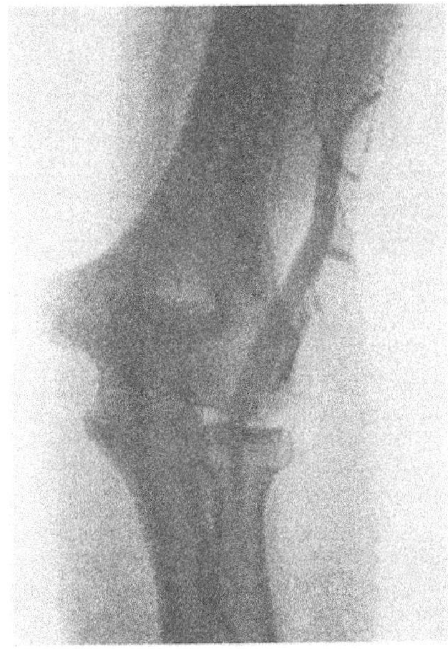

Fig. 4 Opacification of the vena basilica using strontium bromate (Berberich 1923)

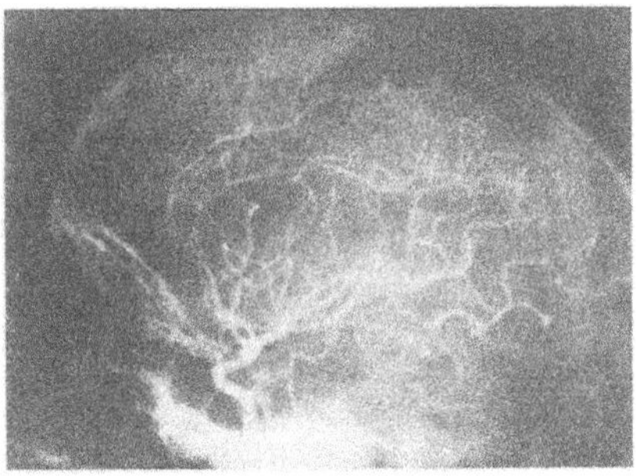

Fig. 5 Cerebral angiogram using thorium dioxide (Thorotrast) (Moniz 1931)

In 1923, Berberich [4] recommended 10%–20% aqueous strontium bromate for the visualization of vessels. Rapid dilution was prevented by mechanical interruption of the blood flow during the examination (Fig. 4).

From 1930 into the 1940s, a colloidal suspension of thorium dioxide appeared to be the ideal angiographic contrast medium. The contrast was excellent, as proved by the cerebral angiogram (Fig. 5) performed by the Portuguese neurologist Dr. Moniz [5]. The tolerance of this isotonic particulate preparation with the trade name Thorotrast seemed to be very good until its cancerogenic potential became obvious. The thorium particles were stored in the reticuloendothelial system and, due to their radioactivity, led to the formation of benign tumours, which became malignant in the course of time.

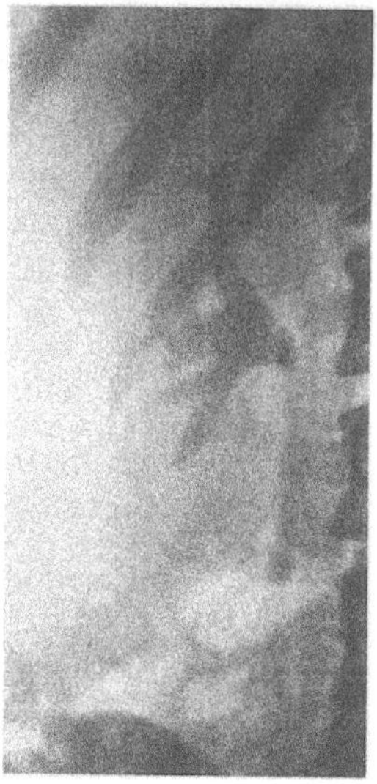

Fig. 6 Intravenous urogram using iodine bound to urea (Roseno 1929)

During the 1920s, salts of iodine were used more frequently but mostly with little success, due to low efficacy and severe side-effects. Only with very high doses could an intravenous urogram occasionally be detected, as was published by Roseno [6] in 1929 (Fig. 6).

However, the advantages of iodine, especially the high absorption of X-rays, the low toxicity and the fast and complete renal excretion, became more and more evident. It was bound to different organic molecules and some of them turned out to be suitable contrast media, such as Lipiodol for myelography.

In 1927 in Berlin, the chemists Binz and Rath, financially aided by Schering, synthesized the first contrast medium suitable for urography, Uroselectan. It was the American physician Swick who, in 1929, performed the initial clinical study at the Hedwig's hospital located close to Schering's research laboratory [7]. Head of the radiological department was von Lichtenberg, who erroneously received the credit for this scientific breakthrough [8].

The diagnostic results were so convincing that Schering started to manufacture and market Uroselectan in the same year (Figs. 7, 8). Uroselectan was supplied as a powder and had to be boiled before use. Chemically, it is a mono-iodinated pyridone derivative and belongs to the group of non-specific extracellular urographic contrast media (Fig. 9). Again, Binz and Rath succeeded in incorporating a second atom of iodine into the pyridone nucleus. This agent was called Uroselectan B and was marketed by Schering in 1932. Uroselectan B and the related agent diodrast (Diodone) dominated the world market for urographic contrast media for the next 20 years.

Based on the synthesis of the first tri-iodinated benzoic acid by Wallingford in 1951, Mallinckrodt developed acetrizoate (Urokon), while Schering and Winthrop developed the much safer contrast medium diatrizoate (Urografin and Hypaque

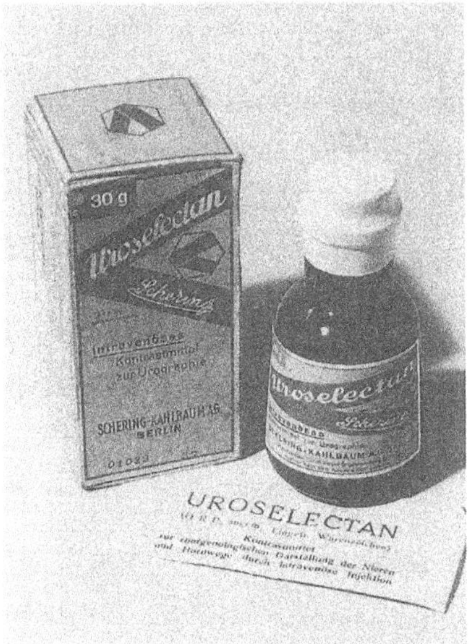

Fig. 7 Uroselectan for intravenous urography (Schering-Kahlbaum)

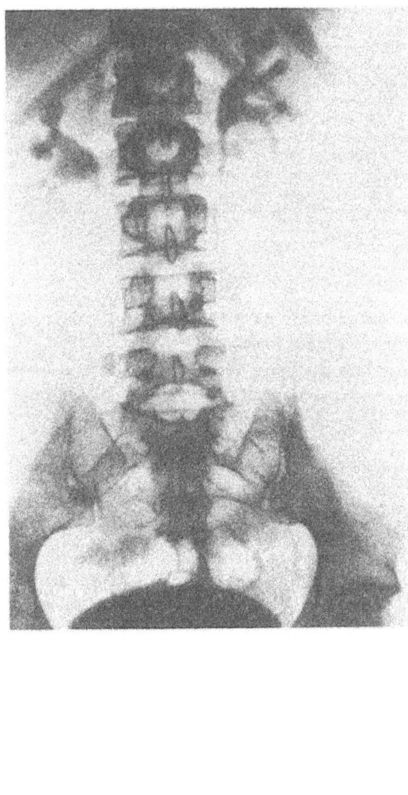

Fig. 8 Intravenous urogram using Uroselectan

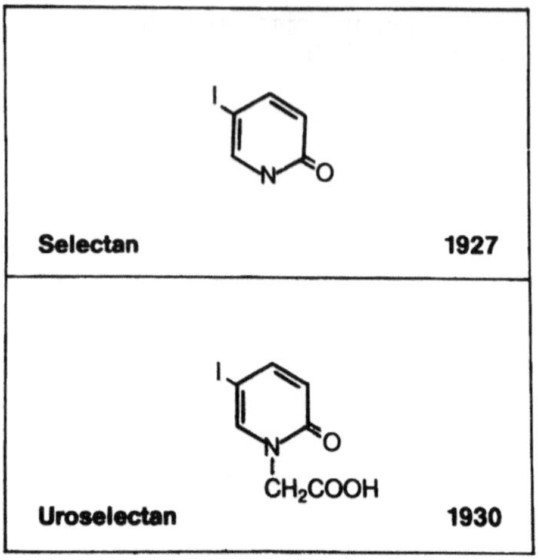

Fig. 9 Uroselectan: a mono-iodinated pyridone derivative

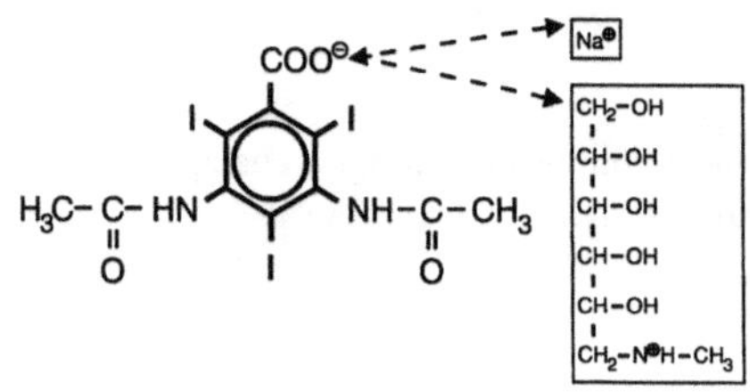

Fig. 10 Diatrizoate (Urografin): a tri-iodinated benzene derivate

Table 1 Ionic monomeric contrast media (one tri-iodobenzene ring with one carboxyl group)

Generic name	Trade name	Manufacturer	Year introduced
Diatrizoate	Urografin	Schering	1954
	Renografin	Squibb	1955
	Hypaque	Winthrop	1954
Iothalamate	Conray	Mallinckrodt	1962
Metrizoate	Isopaque	Nycomed	1962
Iodamide	Uromiro	Bracco	1965
Ioxithalamate	Telebrix	Guerbet	1973
Ioglicinate	Rayvist	Schering	1978

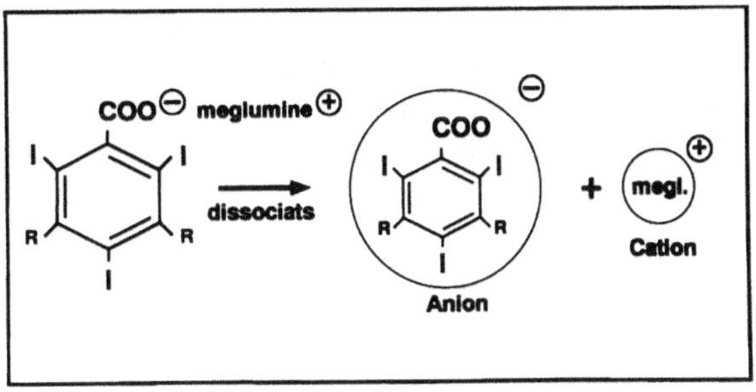

Fig. 11 Ionic monomeric contrast media dissociate in ions (anion and cation)

Table 2 Properties of ionic contrast media and their influence on tolerance

Property	Effect
Electrical Charge	Epileptogenicity
Hypertonicity	Damage of the Endothelium Transient Disturbance of the BBB Pain, Heat Thrombosis Hypervolaemia Vasodilatation Bradycardia Diuresis Arachnoiditis
Chemotoxicity	Neurotoxicity Organic psychic syndrome Dizziness Nausea Vomiting Anaphylactoid reactions (according to Lasser)

respectively) in 1954 (Fig. 10). Together with its derivates, such as iothalamate (Conray) and metrizoate (Isopaque, Triosil), this group has now been the standard contrast media for more than 30 years (Table 1). Due to the three iodine atoms per molecule, a high contrast efficacy was guaranteed. The side-chains in position 3 and 5 of the benzene ring are responsible for the low toxicity, the high hydrophilicity and the renal excretion. The ionic monomeric contrast media, characterized by one tri-iodobenzene ring with one carboxyl group, were almost universally used for urography, angiography and body cavities and for improved organ and tumour contrast.

With the increasing use of contrast media, some disadvantages became more obvious. Urografin-type contrast media dissociate into ions after intravascular injection (Fig. 11). The electrical charge of the particles can lead to epileptogenicity, and hypertonicity causes several side effects. In addition, the chemotoxicity, characterized in particular by the lipophilia or the lack of hydrophilia, causes some other undesirable effects (Table 2).

In 1969, the Swedish radiologist Almen [9] published concepts designed to reduce the hypertonicity of ionic contrast media:

- Particles
- Polymers, oligomers, dimers
- lodinated cations
- Non-ionic contrast media

All these concepts have since been tried out, with the first striking result being the development of non-ionic contrast media. In metrizamide (Amipaque), the ionic carboxyl group contained in the tri-iodinated benzoic molecule was replaced by a non-dissociating group which provided the required water solubility by several hydrophilic OH groups (Fig. 12). Several follow-up non-ionic products soon replaced the expensive metrizamide (Table 3). The low osmolality and the lack of electrical charge clearly improved the tolerability of the non-ionic monomeric contrast media [10].

Efforts to achieve similarly favourable results by using the ionic dimer ioxaglate (Hexabrix), characterized by two connected tri-iodobenzene rings with one carboxyl group (Fig. 13) were not successful [11]. The low osmolality leads to

Fig. 12 Non-ionic contrast medium metrizamide (Amipaque)

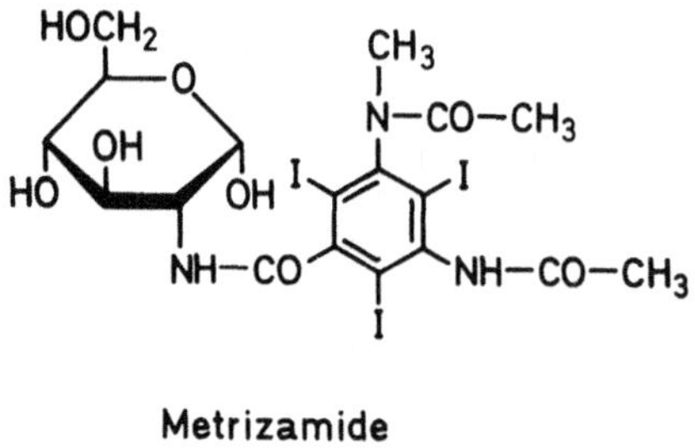

Table 3 Non-ionic monomeric contrast media (one tri-iodobenzene ring with several hydroxyl groups and no ionizing groups)

Generic name	Trade name	Manufacturer	Year introduced
Metrizamide	Amipaque	Nycomed	1977
Iohexol	Omnipaque	Nycomed	1982
Iopamidol	Iopamiron	Bracco	1981
Iopromide	Ultravist	Schering	1985
Ioversol	Optiray	Mallinckrodt	1988
Iopentol	Imagopaque	Nycomed	1991
Iomeprol	Iomeron	Bracco	1994
Iobitridol	Xenetix	Guerbet	1994

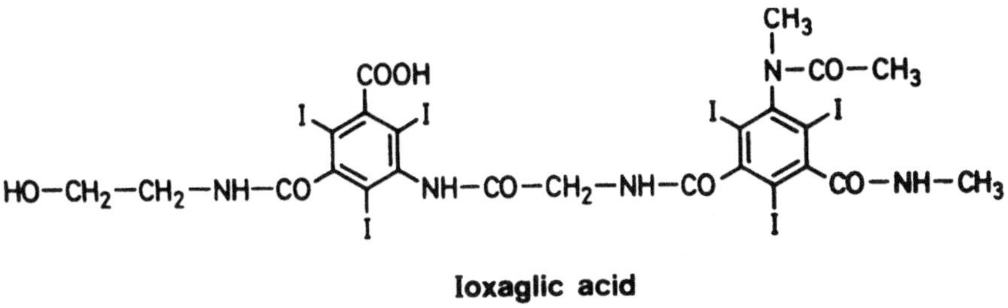

Fig. 13 Ionic dimer ioxaglate (Hexabrix)

a reduction of pain sensation and to less influence on the cardiovascular system, but the non-ionic media also show a very low incidence of typical contrast reactions, such as nausea, vomiting, allergy-like symptoms and less influence on kidney function. The largely improved neural tolerance of these products has been recognized since the introduction of Amipaque.

The synthesis of the hexa-iodinated non-ionic dimers iotrolan (Isovist) and iodixanol (Visipaque) represents the most recent advance in X-ray contrast media development [12]. The osmolality of iotrolan (Fig. 14) in all concentrations matches that of circulating blood and cerebrospinal fluid. The isotonicity and the extremely high hydrophilicity of iotrolan further reduce the side effects associated with myelography [13] as well as the pain and heat sensations associated with peripheral angiography [14]. Kidney function is less affected, as clinical trials have shown [15].

Non-ionic dimers meet almost all the requirements for ideal contrast media. It is unlikely that less toxic molecules will ever be synthesized. The intravenous median lethal dose (LD_{50}) of Iotrolan reaches 28 g iodine/kg body weight in rats. The comparable amount of contrast medium for a patient of 70 kg body weight would be about 7 l. Due to the limited distribution space, higher doses, in all probability, cannot be achieved even with the best-tolerated agents.

If the non-ionic dimers represent the logical end-point of 100 years of contrast media development, the question is now how to continue X-ray contrast media research?

The following approaches are now the main ones discussed:

- Replacement of the iodinated benzene ring by other chemical structures
- Search for metal chelates in view of the excellent tolerance of Magnevist in MRI
- Search for organ-specific contrast media. The uptake of liposomes by the reticuloendothelial system of the liver can be used to improve the contrast between healthy liver tissue and liver tumours or metastases

In conclusion, many attemps are being made on a worldwide scale to synthesize new X-ray contrast media with better tolerance and efficacy. Nevertheless, dimeric non-ionic contrast media such as Iotrolan will represent the state of the art for at least the next 10–20 years.

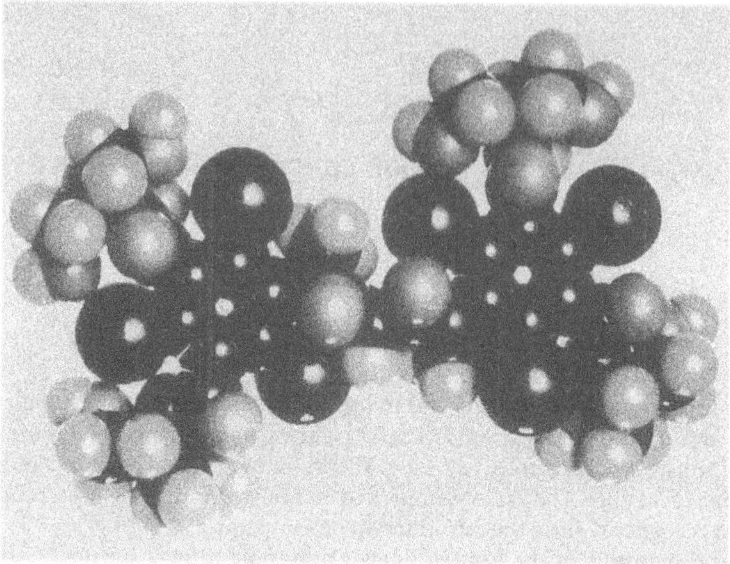

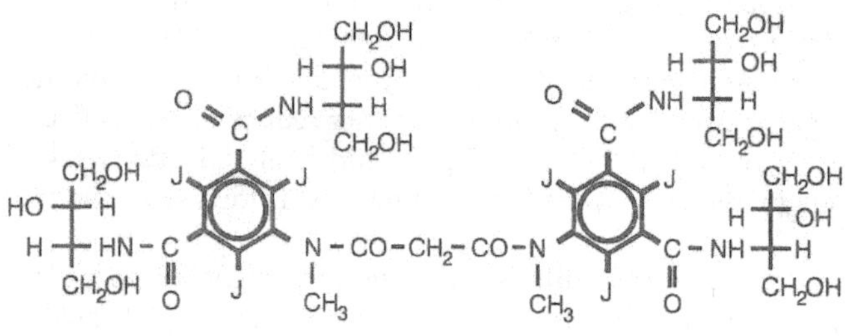

Fig. 14 Non-ionic dimer iotrolan (Isovist)

References

1. Sehrwald E (1886) Das Verhalten der Halogene gegen Röntgenstrahlen. Dtsch med Wschr 30:477–480
2. Haschek E, Lindenthal O Th (1886) Ein Beitrag zur praktischen Verwertung der Photographie nach Röntgen. Wien Klin Wschr 9:63–64
3. Burns JE (1915) Thorium – a new agent for pyelography. J AMA 26:2126–2127
4. Berberich J, Hirsch S (1923) Die röntgenographische Darstellung der Arterien und Venen am lebenden Menschen. Klin Wschr 49:2226–2228
5. Moniz E, Pinto A, Lima A (1931) Le Thorotrast dans l'encéphalographie artérielle. Rev Neurol 39:5
6. Roseno A (1929) Die intravenöse Pyelographie. Klin Wschr 25:1165–1170
7. Swick M (1929) Darstellung der Niere und Harnwege im Röntgenbild durch intravenöse Einbringung eines neuen Kontraststoffes: des Uroselectans. Klin Wschr 8:2087–2089
8. Grainger R G (1982) Intravascular contrast media – the past, the present and the future. Brit J of Radiol 55:1–18
9. Almén T (1969) Contrast agent design. Some aspects of the synthesis of water-soluble contrast agents of low osmolality. J Theoretical Biol 24:216–226

10. Katayama H, Yamaguchi K, Kozuka T, Takashima T, Seez P, Matsuura K (1990) Adverse reactions to ionic and non-ionic contrast media. Radiology 175:621–628
11. Farero CD, Rossini G, Martegani A (1993) A comparison of iopamidol and ioxaglate in CT enhancement. Eur Radiol 3:77–82
12. Dawson P, Howell M (1986) The non-ionic dimers: a new class of contrast agents. Brit J Radiol 59:987–991
13 Ringel K, Klotz E, Wenzel-Hora BI (1989) Iotrolan versus Iopamidol: A controlled, multicenter, double-blind study of lumbar and direct cervical myelograpy. Fortschr Röntgenstr und Nukl: Supplement Vol. 128:153–157
14. Gmeinwieser JK, Wenzel-Hora BI (1993) Arteriography of extremities and penis with iotrolan 280 versus non-ionic monomers: Clinical phase II and III trials. Presentation at RSNA
15. Clauß W, Dinger J, Meißner C (1995) Renal tolerance of iotrolan 280 – a meta-analysis of 14 double-blind studies. In: Proceedings of the Isovist symposium: Monte Carlo, Monaco, April 29–30, Eur. Radiol 5:79–84

CHAPTER 2

China's Diagnostic Radiology

Geng-Nian Liu[1]

This year is the centenary of the discovery of roentgen rays by Roentgen, the great German scientist. As in various countries of the world, China's diagnostic radiology has made very spectacular progress in the past 10 years. China currently has 2500 computed tomography scanners (CT) and 250 magnetic resonance imaging (MRI) machines. The China Radiology society has more than 5000 members (not including ultrasonic and nuclear medical staff). There are 11 journals related to clinical radiology (Table 3). There are various academic activities conducted by the society each year (including activities conducted in the various branch societies), and it has become one of the most active societies among the dozens of societies affiliated to the Chinese Medical Association.

Looking back on its history, the development of China's diagnostic radiology has traversed a long and tortuous road. When I was a medical student at the Medical School of Beijing University in the 1940s, there were only two radiology professors in the whole of Beijing: Professor Zhi-Guang Xie (C.K. Hsieh) of Peking Union Medical College and Professor Liang Duo of the Medical School of Beijing University. There were few hospitals equipped with radiological equipment. In 1947, while I was working in the People's Hospital (formerly the Chung Ho Hospital), the radiological department was equipped with only an open-wire X-ray machine for fluoroscopy. During fluoroscopy, high-tension cables gave off sparks, the room was filled with the smell of oxygen, and one had a headache after long hours of work. Once I nearly died when my hand carelessly came into contact with the bare high-tension cable. The X-ray tube of another X-ray machine used in general radiography consisted of cooled water which boiled after taking a few X-ray films. In order to continue work, we had to wait until it cooled. In gastrointestinal barium examination, it was very hard to take an X-ray picture, because there was no spot film device. It was not until 1950 that the hospital bought an X-ray machine with a spot film device manufactured by Siemens. I used that machine for more than 10 years. Later on, my interest was aroused in the field of radiological diagnosis of the digestive system.

[1] Department of Radiology, Third Hospital, Beijing Medical University, Beijing, China.

Chinese Society of Radiology

Prior to 1949, there was no radiological society, neither were there any national academic activities. In 1952, the first National Committee of the Chinese Society of Radiology was set up in Beijing, with Professor Wang Shao-Xun as the Chairman of the Committee and Professor Liang Duo as the vice chairman.

Since 1981, a nationwide academic conference has regularly convened once every 4 years; a national committee was re-elected concurrently.

For the chairman of the national committee as well as the time and location of the conferences held, see Table 1.

Subsocieties of the Chinese Society of Radiology

Since the beginning of the 1980s, as a result of the fast development of the various branches of radiological sciences, the Society has organized academic activities, together with subsocieties. More than 20 subsociety conferences have been held in the past 10 years. The various subsocieties have set up, committees and elected committee chairmen and members. There are seven subsocieties in all, concerned with musculo-skeletal radiology, thoraco-cardiovascular radiology, abdominal radiology, interventional radiology, neuroradiology, radiological technology, and pediatric radiology. For the establishment of the various subsocieties and the names of the committee directors, see Table 2.

Table 1 The Development of the Chinese Society of Radiology (CSR)

1952	Establishment of 1st National Committee of the CSR in Beijing (Chairman: Wang Shao Xun)
1956	1st National Meeting of the CSR, Beijing 2nd National Committee of the CSR was elected (Chairman: Wang Shao Xun)
1963	3rd National Committee of the CSR was elected in Shanghai (Chairman: Wang Shao Xun) 2nd National Meeting of the CSR, Shanghai
1981	4th National Committee of the CSR was elected in Zheng Zhou (Chairman: Wang Shao Xun) 3rd National Meeting of the CSR in Zheng Zhou
1985	5th National Committee of the CSR was elected in Hang Zhou (Chairman: Liu Geng Nian) 4th National Meeting of the CSR in Hang Zhou
1989	6th National Committee of the CSR was elected in Wu Han (Chairman: Liu Yu Qing) 5th National Meeting of the CSR in Wu Han
1993	7th National Committee of the CSR was elected in Beijing (Chairman: Liu Geng Nian) 6th National Meeting of the CSR in Beijing

Table 2 Establishment of subsocieties of the Chinese Society of Radiology (**CSR**)

A.	Establishment of Subsociety Committee; 1st National Meeting of Neuroradiology, Beijing, 1987 (Chairman: Wu En Hui)
B.	Establishment of Subsociety of Thoracic Cardiovascular Radiology: 1st Meeting, September 1983, Gui Yang (Gui Zhou) 1st Committee established, 1990, Kai Feng (He Nan) Chairman: Liu Yu Qing)
C.	Establishment of Subsociety of Abdominal Radiology: 1st National Meeting, 1983, Fu Zhou (Fu Jian) 1st Committee established, 1991, Beijing (Chairman: Liu Geng Nian)
D.	Establishment of Subsociety of Muscular Skeletal Radiology: 1st National Meeting, 1982, Jiu Jiang (Jiang Xi) 1st Committee established, 1991, Qing Dao (Shan Dong) (Chairman: Wang Yun Zhao)
E.	Establishment of Subsociety of Pediatric Radiology: 1st National Meeting, 1990, Shanghai 1st Committee established, 1990, Shanghai (Chairman: Yao Qing Hua)
F.	Establishment of Subsociety of Interventional Radiology: 1st National Meeting, 1986, Wei Fang (Shan Dong) 1st Committee established, 1990, Hang Zhou (Zhe Jiang) (Chairman: Lin Gui)
G.	Subsociety of Radiological Technologists: 1st National Meeting, 1987, Wu Hang (Hu Bei) 1st Committee established, 1989, Da Tong (Shan Xi) (Chairman: Fan Yan)

Medical Staff in Diagnostic Radiology

From the 1930s to the 1940s, China had only a few radiologists working in big hospitals. Since the 1950s, hospitals have trained a great number of radiologists and technicians. Up until now, all medium and small city hospitals have set up radiology departments with doctors and technicians.

There are already more than 5000 members of the Radiological Society acting as visiting physicians.

Imaging Equipment in China

In the past 10 years, China's imaging equipment has undergone a great development, which has accelerated the progress of the various branches of learning. This progress uncludes:

1. Conventional X-ray machines: 200–500 mA X-ray machines made in China have been installed in local hospitals, about 50000 machines.

Table 3 Chinese journals of radiology

1.	Chinese Journal of Radiology (Beijing), established 40 years ago
2.	Journal of Clinical Radiology (Hu Bei)
3.	Journal of Practical Radiology (Shaan Xi)
4.	Journal of Clinical Medical Imaging (Shen Yang)
5.	Chinese Journal of Techniques of Medical Imaging (Beijing)
6.	Roentgen Praxis (Wu Hang)
7.	Journal of Foreign Medicine: Clinical Radiology (Tian Jin)
8.	Chinese Medical Abstract, Radiological Diagnosis (Wu Han)
9.	Chinese Journal of Medical Imaging (Beijing)
10.	Journal of Interventional Radiology (Shanghai)
11.	Journal of Computed Imaging (Shanghai)

2. CT scanners: 2500 sets of CT have been installed throughout the country, a small portion of which are the products of joint ventures.
3. MRI equipment: there are altogether 250 sets in the whole country, a small portion of which are the products of joint ventures in China.

Radiology Periodicals

Due to the need for scientific exchange, more than 11 medical imaging periodicals have been published; some of them are monthly distributed reaching 25000 copies each issue. For the names of the periodicals, see Table 3. This large-scale distribution has played an important role in the training of the large number of staff at the grass-roots level.

Training of Radiology Staff

Graduates from medical colleges and schools wishing to become radiologists train for 5 years after graduation. Those who pass the examination are promoted to chief physician. In teaching hospitals, they should undergo training in order to specialize in a particular area.

Students who have spent 3 years training in intermediary medical schools are assigned to local hospitals after graduation. After working for a period, some will be selected for 1 year of advanced studies at teaching hospitals and will return to their original hospitals after this period. In general, conventional X-ray diagnosis will be their major subject of study and work. Branches of the Radiological Society will continue to do a great deal of education work.

New Progress in the Technique of Imaging Diagnosis

During the past 10 years, imaging diagnosis techniques have undergone great development; national periodicals and journals have published many articles. Here I quote a few examples:

1. CT techniques have gradually been popularized throughout the country; some larger hospitals have already mastered CT Angiography, CTA technique by spiral CT. Conventional CT techniques have played an important role in improving the quality of clinical medical care and research. It is now planned to popularize use in middle and small hospitals provided with such facilities.
2. Since 1990, more MRI equipment has been imported. Some large hospitals have already mastered the technique, as well as undertaking.
3. The technique of interventional radiology has made spectacular progress in the last few years, e.g., the use of expandable metallic stents for the treatment of portal hypertension and massive bleeding with good results. National statistics have been published with about 500 cases. Several hundreds of plastic mitral valves have been treated by nonoperative methods with very good results.

Problems. The extent to which hospitals have mastered the technique of imaging diagnosis varies, and further training is necessary. The installation of imaging equipment is still uncommon; however the situation will gradually improve with technical progress and the advancement of the national economy.

CHAPTER 3

Technical Foundations of Spiral Computed Tomography*

Willi A. Kalender[1]

Introduction

The Introduction of continuously rotating computed tomography (CT) measurements systems provided the technological basis for spiral CT. Slip rings are used to transfer the necessary electrical energy to the rotating gantry and to transmit the measured data from the rotating part to the computer system; the cables that were used traditionally in CT scanners and which limited scanning to single 360° turns (alternating in clockwise and counterclockwise directions) have been replaced. The first slip-ring scanners became available in 1987 (Somatom Plus, Siemens Medical Systems, Erlangen, Germany, and TCT 900S, Toshiba Medical Systems, Tokyo, Japan). These systems were designed primarily for fast dynamic scanning. Scan times of 1 s became routinely available for the first time; repeated scanning of a single slice with zero interscan delay, allowing for the study of the dynamics of contrast media inflow or physiological phenomena, was another feature of these systems. However, spiral scanning had not yet been conceived when these systems were introduced. Although dynamic CT was well established and the need for the shortest possible scan time was evident, volume scanning had not yet been considered.

Physical performance measurements and clinical studies with spiral CT were presented for the first time at the 1989 Radiological Society of North America annual meeting. These reports were well received, and the practical advantages of a scan mode covering complete anatomic regions in a single exposure were immediately apparent. However, there was concern that image quality might be compromised in spiral CT scanning, and the limitations of the first experimental implementation were still obvious. It was not until 1990 that the first scanner with a spiral CT product option became available (Somatom Plus, Siemens Medical Systems): it took until 1992 for general acceptance of spiral scanning to be reached.

---

* This chapter has been published previously by Saunders, Philadelphia, in Seminars in Ultrasound, CT, and MRI, vol. 5, no. 2, pp. 81–89, 1994.

[1] Institute for Medical Physics, University of Erlangen, Krankenhausstr. 12, 91054 Erlangen, Germany.

Technical Principles and Parameters of Data Acquisition

X-ray computed tomography sonsists of measuring attenuation profiles of a transverse slice of a patient or object from a multitude of angular positions. For this purpose, an X-ray tube is used, with its beam collimated to a fan defining the image plane, in conjunction with a detector array traveling on a circular path around the patient. Typically, 360° are covered to collect a complete set of data. Thereafter, the respective image is reconstructed and the patient is shifted a small distance through the gantry for the measurement of the next transverse section. This procedure is repeated slice by slice. To receive images of high quality, it is important that the patient does not move during the data acquisition process to avoid unsharpness (similar to that in classical radiography) and motion artifacts (inherent to image reconstruction in CT when inconsistent data are given). Short scan times are desirable to limit such motion effects in single scans. Short total examination times also are desirable to limit motion between scans because movement can cause omission of anatomic levels and discontinuities in multiplanar or three-dimensional (3D) displays. These effects often are a significant drawback to conventional CT. (We refer to "conventional CT" in this article whenever scans are acquired successively, slice-by-slice.)

In contrast, spiral CT is a volume scanning procedure in which the patient is shifted continuously through the gantry. The scanning principle is illustrated schematically in Fig. 1.

Whereas the radiographic tube and detector system rotates around the patient with data acquired continuously, the patient travels typically at a speed of one slice thickness per 360° rotation. In practice, this means values of 1–10 mm/s. Relative to the patient, the focus of the X-ray tube describes a spiral or helical path, which led to the different names given to this scanning procedure.

The selection of scan parameters in spiral CT is very similar to that in conventional CT (Table 1). Scan times and tube currents must be limited to avoid excessive heating of the X-ray tube: total scan times of 20–60 s (which are now available) are sufficient to cover most applications, however. The only additional parameter to be selected in spiral CT is the table feed distance (d) in millimeters per 360° rotation. (On most current scanners, which operate at 1 s per single 360°

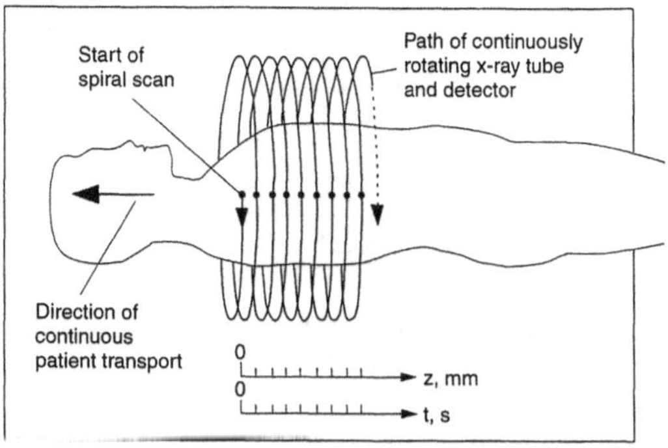

Fig. 1 Scan principle in spiral CT. (Reprinted, with permission, from [5])

Table 1 Scan parameters in spiral CT

Variable	Typical value
Tube voltage	80–140 kVp
Tube current	100–300 mA
Scan time	20–60 s
Slice thickness	1–10 mm
Table feed	1–20 mm per 360°
Data processing algorithms	360° and 180° slice interpolation
Image reconstruction algorithms	Same as in conventional CT

scan, the value of *d* corresponds directly to the speed in millimeters per s. That distance usually equals the thickness of a single slice or a multiple of up to twice that thickness (see below). Image reconstruction is the same, in principle, as in conventional CT, and the same algorithms and reconstruction kernels are available. However, an additional step of data processing, the so-called slice or section interpolation, is necessary before image reconstruction can be started.

Principles of Image Reconstruction

In spiral CT, a single data set is obtained that represents the volume covered in the given number of spiral turns. Directly reconstructing any 360° spiral segment would result in images corrupted by motion artifacts, equal in appearance to those obtained in conventional CT when the patient moves (Fig. 2a). It was because of such effects and related negative expectations that spiral CT was accepted rather slowly initially. To correct the effect of moving the patient continuously during the scan it is necessary to first calculate a planar data set from the vomule data set for each image to be reconstructed (Fig. 2b). The simplest approach is to interpolate the data for every angular position from the two projections measured in the same angular position just before and after the table position z_0 (Fig. 2c). This intermediate calculation step demands appreciable computational efforts, but it provides a significant advantage inherent to volume scanning. Images can be reconstructed at any position within the scanned volume, with arbitrarily fine spacing and in an overlapping fashion if desired (Fig. 2d). The choise is independent of the scan pattern and can be made retrospectively. For multiplanar or 3D reconstructions, e.g., in which overlapping images are preferred for high-quality displays, images can be provided by one spiral scan without the need for additional scanning [7–9]. In some cases, even submillimeter spacing of images is requested, as in inner ear studies [10]. These requirements can be fulfilled easily by spiral scans.

A variety of interpolation algorithms is available to calculate planar data sets from volume scans. The procedure described above uses data points measured 360° apart: the literature often refers to this class as 360° algorithms. They are easy to implement and robust with respect to image quality, but they tend to broaden slice sensitivity profiles strongly (see below). Therefore, a different class of algo-

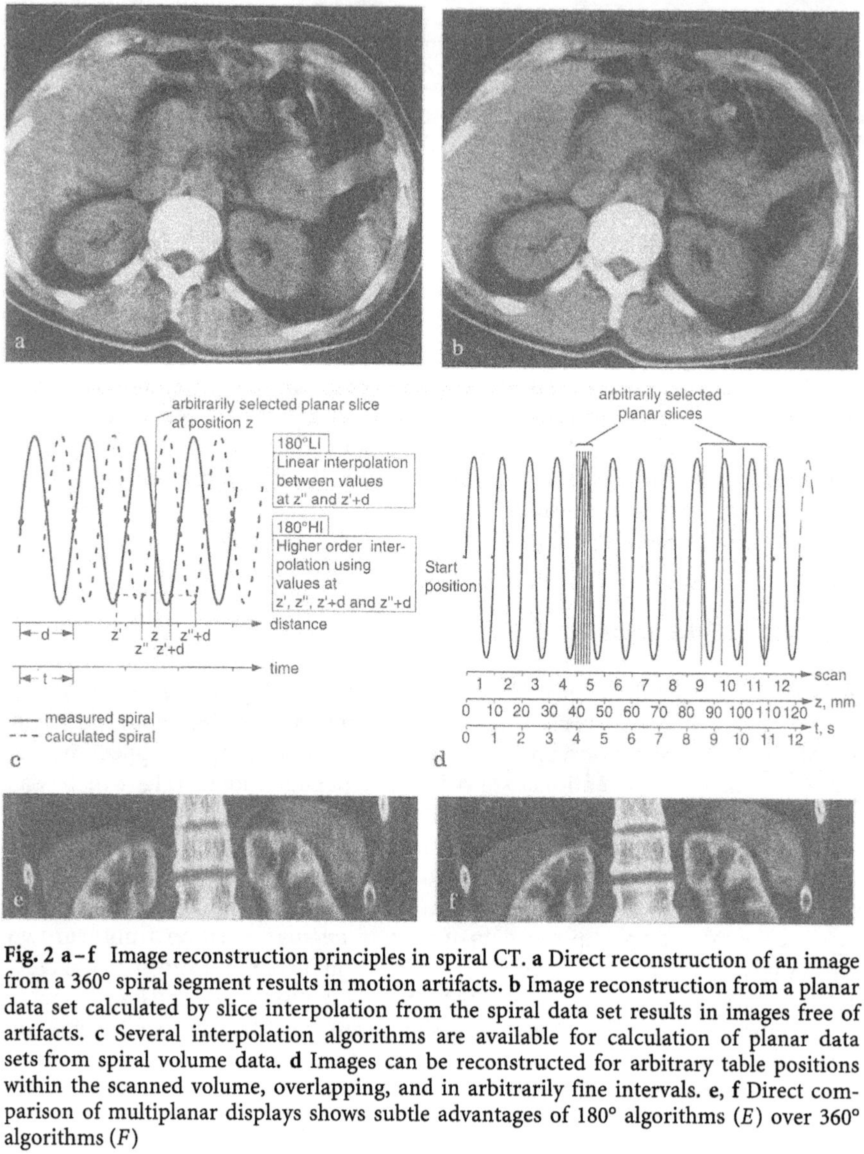

Fig. 2 a–f Image reconstruction principles in spiral CT. **a** Direct reconstruction of an image from a 360° spiral segment results in motion artifacts. **b** Image reconstruction from a planar data set calculated by slice interpolation from the spiral data set results in images free of artifacts. **c** Several interpolation algorithms are available for calculation of planar data sets from spiral volume data. **d** Images can be reconstructed for arbitrary table positions within the scanned volume, overlapping, and in arbitrarily fine intervals. **e, f** Direct comparison of multiplanar displays shows subtle advantages of 180° algorithms (*E*) over 360° algorithms (*F*)

rithms has been developed that uses data points for interpolation that are only 180° apart (Fig. 2c). They take advantage of the fact that all object details are viewed from two opposing directions (e.g., anterior-posterior und posterior-anterior) in a 360° rotation. This redundancy in data is used to calculate a second spiral, which is offset from the measured spiral by 180°; data 180° apart can thus be made available for interpolation. Such algorithms are referred to as

180° algorithms, e.g., 180° LI when linear interpolation (LI) is used [11]. They offer the advantage of improved slice sensitivity profiles and, thus, can provide improved spatial resolution in the longitudinal direction (compare Fig. 2e and Fig. 2f).

Image Quality in Spiral CT

Only a few differences in image quality are to be expected between conventional CT and spiral CT because the complete measurement system and most scan parameters are identical. Spatial resolution in the image plane, for example, should be the same if the same reconstruction parameters are chosen; these can be verified easily by measurements (Fig. 3). Regardless, the quality of the radiographic spectra is independent of the type of scanning procedure. Correspondingly, CT values of arbitrary objects should be the same in both cases, i.e., contrast is unchanged.There may be differences in the contrast measured for small objects: see below. Similar considerations apply to other imagequality parameters, such as field homogeneity and artifact behavior. Differences should be expected only with respect to pixel noise and slice sensitivity profiles, and as a direct consequence, for resolution along the *z* axis, the body's longitudinal direction.

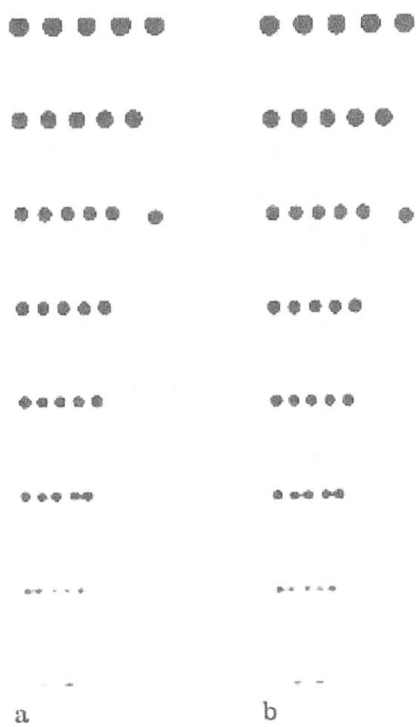

Fig. 3 a, b Comparison of spatial resolution in the scan plane. **a** Conventional CT. **b** Spiral CT Performance is identical (reconstrucion with standard body kernel in both cases)

Image Pixel Noise

In addition to its dependence on the usual scan parameters, pixel noise in spiral CT also depends on the slice interpolation algorithm. For a direct comparison with conventional CT scans it is assumed that slice thickness, voltage, tube current, and reconstruction parameters are the same. Under these conditions the noise level in spiral CT images can be evaluated easily. The situation is theoretically well understood.

For 360° LI, in which a total range of 2 × 360° of data is used, a reduction in pixel noise has to be expected when compared with conventional CT. We were able to show that the theoretical value of $\sqrt{2/3}$ agreed precisely with measurements [12]. For 180° algorithms, which use a smaller data range, noise should increase by a factor of approximately $\sqrt{2}$ compared with 360° LI [11]. Here also, excellent agreement is given between prediction and experiment. Respective results are assembled in Table 2, which shows noise values for spiral CT relative to noise measured in conventional CT.

Table 2 Image pixel noise in spiral CT

Interpolation algorithm	Theoretical value	Measured value
360° LI	0,82	0,83
180° LI	1,13	1,12

LI, linear interpolation

Slice Sensitivity Profiles

Slice-sensitivity profiles (SSP) describe the thickness of an imaged section and the extent to which details within the section contribute to the signal. The ideal shape of an SSP is the rectangle, in which all points within the slice contribute equally and points outside of the slice do not contribute to the image at all. In real CT systems, the rectangular shape is approximated to a satisfactory degree for single-slice acquisition (Fig. 4a). In spiral CT, with the object moving during acquisition, a certain degree of broadening of the SSP results (depending on the table speed and on the slice interpolation algorithm). The underlying phenomena have been analyzed and are well understood; a full derivation has been given in the literature for both 360° LI [12] an 180° [11].

The SSPs in spiral CT result from a convolution of the original profile with the so-called motion function, a triangle of unity area with a base width of 2 d for 360° LI; d is the table feed in mm/360° rotation (Fig. 4a). The larger the feed value d, the more the resulting profile broadens at its base. This can be verified easily for arbitrary combinations of scan parameters. In all cases, there was excellent agree-

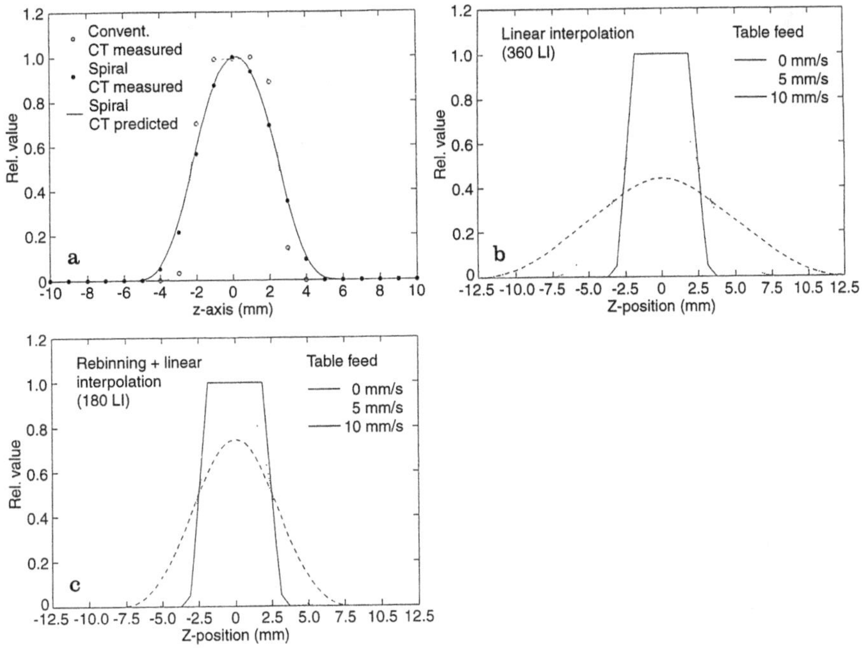

Fig. 4 a–c Slice sensitivity in spiral CT. **a** Spiral CT profiles result from a convolution of the original profile with the motion function. There is excellent agreement between calculated (–) and measured profiles (•) for spiral CT. **b, c** Profiles are broadened with increasing table feed values for 360 LI (*B*) and 180 LI (*C*)

ment between experimental results and theoretical predictions (Fig. 4b). The SSPs for 180° LI can be similarly predicted. The motion function has a base width of d only narrower than in the case of 360° LI (Fig. 4c). A point of particular interest in spiral CT is the possibility to choose table feed values greater than the slice thickness. The ratio of feed value d to slice thickness S, a dimensionless quantity, is called the pitch. Theoretically, the pitch can be increased up to a value of 2 without suffering significant image quality problems. In routine practice, pitch values from 1.0 to 1.7 are chosen. Typical examples are table feed values of 3 mm/s for a 2-mm slice thickness (pitch, 1.5) for orthopedic examinations or 6–8 mm/s with a 5-mm slice thickness (pitch, 1.2–1.6) for examinations of the abdomen. The exact choice of pitch is often adapted to the volume to be covered, e.g., if a 5-mm slice thickness and 40-s scan time are desired and a range of 24 cm has to be covered, then 240 mm/40 s = 6 mm/s is chosen, corresponding to a pitch of 1.2 (6 mm per 360° rotation divided by 5-mm slice thickness).

Contrast and Spatial Resolution in the Longitudinal Direction

Broadening of slice sensitivity profiles is undesirable in any case because of its implications on image quality. Above all, slight blurring of structures that are changing along the z axis must be considered. Brink et al. [13] described respective effects in the *x*/*y* image plane for abdominal studies with 360° LI reconstructions. These effects are reduced by using 180° algorithms, but in principle some negative effects are always present when wider slices are used or when profiles are broadened. Spatial resolution along the *z* axis is similarly influenced. There is a second aspect, however, that must be considered and that dominates performance: sampling in the *z* direction.

To explain the respective differences between conventional CT and spiral CT, consider the search for focal lesions. These occur naturally at random sites not known at the beginning of the diagnostic procedure. How well they are imaged three-dimensionally with conventional CT depends on how well the chosen scan pattern fits the random positions of the lesions. In the best possible case, slices are chosen such that the center of the slice and the center of the lesion coincide: in this case, maximum contrast is reached. With the same probability the center of the lesion can also coincide with the border of two adjacent slices, ie, the contrast is halved for lesions with a diameter equal to the slice thickness or less. In spiral CT, the situation is completely different because many images can be reconstructed arbitrarily in an overlapping fashion for the measured volume. An image with maximal contrast is always available.

These principle considerations are illustrated in Fig. 5a in which a sphere of 5-mm parameter is imaged with 5-mm slice thickness. Analogous considerations apply to the case of two lesions of equal diameter that are imaged separately (Fig. 5b). The performance in conventional CT always depends on the random relation of scan pattern and lesion position. In spiral CT, maximal performance can be ensured when a sufficient number of images are reconstructed. Thus, spiral CT offers significant advantages with respect to image quality despite the slight degradation of SSP. These differences in performance have been confirmed in detail by simulations, experiments (Fig. 5c, d), and specimen studies [14]. They also are evident in 3D clinical studies (Fig. 6). A completely new CT application, CT angiography [15–17], is based on this performance.

Fig. 5 a–d Comparison of contrast and spatial resolution along the *z*-axis. **a, b** Dependence on sampling both in conventional CT and in spiral CT. Performance in conventional CT varies with the random relationship of scan pattern and lesion localation. Phantom experiments verified that contrast and spatial separation of spheres are significantly better in spiral CT. (Reprinted, with permission, from [14])

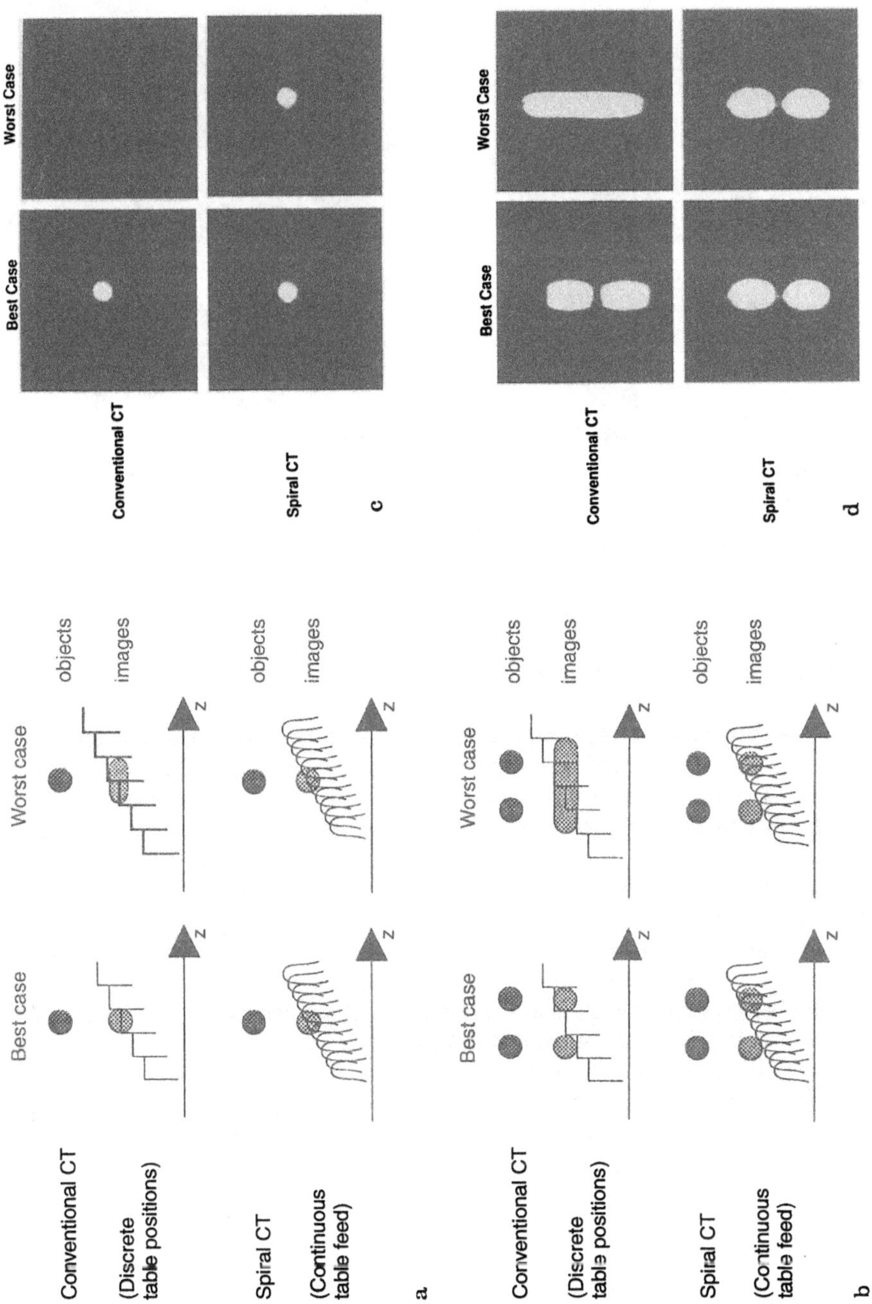
Conventional CT
(Discrete table positions)
Spiral CT
(Continuous table feed)
Best case
Worst case
objects
images
z
a
b
Best Case
Worst Case
Conventional CT
Spiral CT
c
d

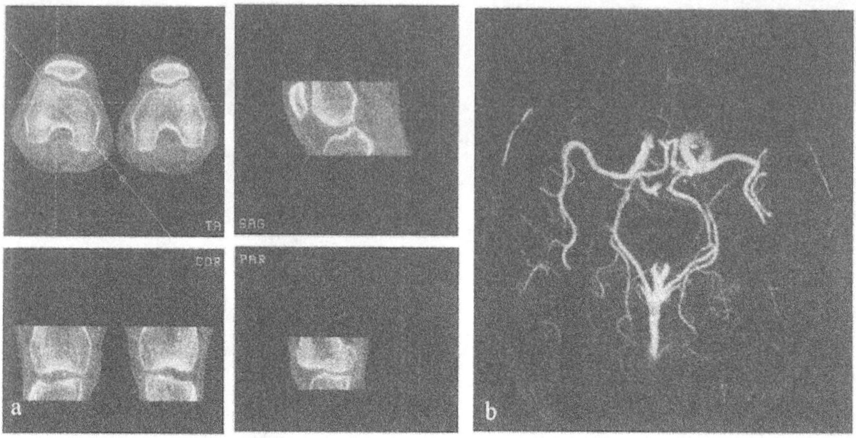

Fig. 6 a, b Clinical examples showing the high spatial resolution offered by spiral CT in all directions. **a** Muliplanar display of spiral CT axamination of the knee (2-mm slice thickness, 3-mm table feed per s. **b** CT angiography: maximum intensity projection display of the intracranial arterial circulation

Patient Dose Considerations

Concern about patient dose in radiographic procedures has always been great and is increasing as alternative imaging modalities such as MRI and ultrasound, which do not use ionizing radiation, improve steadily in performance. The advent of volume scanning met with some reservations, particularly that exposing the patient to a complete volume would lead to higher doses than exposing single slices only. Rather, the following shows that spiral CT can be considered a low-dose CT procedure.

There are few principle differences between spiral CT and conventional CT with respect to dose. This had to be expected for reasons similar to those given in the discussion on image quality. In both cases, dose increases with tube current, tube voltage, scan time, and slice thickness. The same conversion factors from milliampere seconds (mAs) product to dose apply in both cases. Also, for comparison purposes it is assumed that the same anatomic range is investigated, whether by one volume scan or by many contiguous single slices only a few representative slices are required. Therefore, there is no indication for spiral scanning.

There are several practical reasons why the dose imparted to the patient is less in spiral CT than in conventional CT: (a) tube currents in spiral CT are set to lower values than in conventional CT because of the technical limitations discussed; (b) the need to retake single scans that sometimes results from a lack of patient cooperation is largely eliminated in spiral CT; (c) the practice of taking overlapping scans in conventional CT for high-quality 3D displays is replaced by the ability to arbitrarily calculate many overlapping images from one spiral scan without renewed exposure; (d) the possibility of using pitch values greater than 1 leads to an immediate reduction in dose compared with con-tiguous scanning.

Table 3 Dose values in some typical spiral CT examinations

Anatomic region	Head	Chest	Abdomen	Pelvis
Scan range (cm)	16	32	30	16
Slice width (mm)	5	10	5	3
Scan time (s)	32	32	40	40
Tube current (mA)	210	210	165	165
Organ of interest	Eye lens	Lung	Liver	Bladder
Organ dose (mSv)	28,1	23,3	12,9	13,3
Effective dose (mSv)	1,1	6,7	4,3	2,7

Thus, spiral CT may help to limit patient dose in CT examinations. Information seems to be the best strategy to address the public concerns about dose exposure. Dose values must be specified, both for organs of interest and for the whole body as an effective dose [18]. Respective values are compiled in Table 3 for some typical examinations in a normal male, using a kerma in air value of 14,6 mSv/100 mAs specified for the Somatom Plus at 120 kVp. It is understood that these dose values vary widely with the selection of scan parameters and type of scanner used. They indicate the orders of magnitude involved, however, and follow for a crude comparison with other exposures and risks. The natural background radiation level of about 2,4 mSv per year offers one point of orientation.

Conclusions

Spiral CT offers a number of significant advantages for clinical CT examinations. The short total scan times make it the method of choice for many contrast-medium studies, and for pediatric and trauma examinations. Spiral CT offers continuous sampling in the z direction providing improved contrast and spatial resolution [14]. Similar performance is not available with conventional CT under practical conditions because a large number of overlapping single scans would be required at the expense of longer study times and increased patient exposure. These advantages result in a significantly improved performance of spiral CT in some clinical tasks, e.g., in lesion detection [19–21] or CT angiography [15–17].

The broadening of slice sensitive profiles with 360° algorithms was one point of concern that has been relieved by providing 180° algorithms. Limited tube currents are another point of concern preventing the use of spiral CT in those applications in which high dose and low pixel noise are required. Although developmental efforts in X-ray tube and generator technology received greater attention with the advent of volume scanning, milliampere values for longer scan times are always less than those for short scans. Whenever patient dose is of particular concern, this limitation also can be seen as an advantage. Spiral CT may be a means of reducing effective dose. The ability to choose pitch values greater than 1 also contributes to dose reduction.

Scanning in spiral mode can be considered a mature technology. There will be further improvements in technical scanning parameters, above all further increases in X-ray power and refinements in the data processing algorithms aimed at higher *z* axis resolution. These will bring further slight improvements. The important step – from slice imaging to volume imaging – has already been successful.

References

1. Vock P, Jung H, Kalender WA (1989) Single-breathhold volumetric CT of the hepatobiliary system. Radiology 173 (P): 377
2. Vock P, Jung H, Kalender WA (1989) Single-breathhold spiral volumetric CT of the lung. Radiology 173 (P): 400
3. Kalender WA, Seissler W, Vock P (1989) Single-breath-hold spiral volumetric CT by continuous patient translation and scanner rotation. Radiology 173 (P): 414
4. Oudkerk M, Kalender WA (1989) CT of hilar adenopathy with 1-second and subsecond scan times. Radiology 173 (P): 452
5. Kalender WA, Seissler W, Klotz E et al. (1990) Spiral volumetric CT with single-breathhold technique, continuous transport, and continuous scanner rotation. Radiology 176: 181–183
6. Vock P, Soucek M, Daepp M et al. (1990) Lung: Spiral volumetric CT with single-breathhold technique. Radiology 176: 864–867
7. Hirschfelder H, Weber P (1992) Spiral CT – A valuable tool for orthopedic examinations. In: Felic R, Langer M (eds) Advances in CT H. Berlin Heidelberg: Springer Verlag, pp 63–68
8. Ney D, Fishman E, Kawashima A et al. (1992) Comparison of helical and serial CT with regard to three-dimensional imaging of musculoskeletal anatomy. Radiology 185: 865–869
9. Fishman E, Wyatt S, Ney D et al. (1992) Spiral CT of the pancreas with muliplanar display AJR Am J Roentgenol 159: 1209–1215
10. Esselman G, Coticchia J, Wippold F. et al. (1994) Test titting an implantable hearing aid using three dimensional CT scans of the temporal bone. Amer J Otol (in press)
11. Polacin A, Kalender WA, Marchal G (1992) Evaluation of section sensitivity profiles and image noise in spiral CT. Radiology 185: 29–35
12. Kalender W, Polacin A (1991) Physical performance characteristics of spiral CT scanning. Med Phys 18: 910–915
13. Brink JA, Heiken JP, Balfe DM et al. (1992) Spiral CT: Decreased spatial resolution in vivo due to broadening of section-sensitivity profile. Radiology 185: 469–474
14. Kalender W, Polacin A, Suess C (1994) A comparison of conventional and spiral CT with regard to contrast and spatial resolution: An experimental study on the detection of spherical lesions. JCAT 18: (in press)
15 Napel SA, Marks MA, Rubin GD et al. (1992) CT angiography with spiral CT and maximum intensity projection. Radiology 185: 607–610
16. Rubin G, Dake M, Napel S et al. (1993) Three-dimensional spiral CT angiography of the abdomen: Initial clinical experience. Radiology 186: 147–152
17. Mistretta C (1993) Relative properties of MR angiography and competing vascular modalities. JMRI 3: 685–698
18. Kalender W (1993) Calculation of effective dose in CT: Radiology, (in press)
19. Costello P, Anderson W, Blume D (1991) Pulmonary nodule: Evaluation with spiral volumetric CT. Radiology 179: 875–876
20. Heywang-Koebrunner S, Lommatzsch B, Fink U et al. (1992) Comparison of spiral and conventional CT in the detection of pulmonary nodules. Radiology 185 (P) 131
21. Remy-Jardin M, Remy J, Giraud F et al. (1993) Pulmonary nodules: Detection with thick-section spiral CT versus conventional CT. Radiology 187: 513–520

CHAPTER 4

Contrast Media Research and Development

W. Krause[1]

As early as 1929 the first water-soluble ready-to-use contrast medium for urography was introduced in the market. Since that time the chemical structures of the molecules and therefore their characteristics have changed considerably. The desirable features of an optimal contrast agent include chemical stability, maximal contrast enhancement, biological inertness and complete elimination from the body. Accordingly, optimization of compounds followed two major directions, first, increasing the iodine content of the molecule and thereby improving the "potency" as an imaging agent, and, second, reducing osmolality and thereby improving tolerability. The three major steps forward in the development of contrast agents were the discovery of the triiodinated benzene ring resulting in the classical ionic monomers (optimization of contrast quality and reduction of osmolality to one third), the synthesis of nonionic compounds (elimination of electric charge) and the recent introduction of the nonionic dimers (achievement of isotonicity). In the following, the progress in contrast media research and development will be reviewed. X-ray technology – and especially contrast agents for use in computed tomography – will cover the broadest area.

Since its first clinical application in 1971 computed tomography (CT) has made very rapid progress. Two major objectives have been followed during this developmental process, first, improving the resolution and, second, shortening scanning and evaluation times. While scan times of the first generation CT machines were in the order of minutes and reconstitution of images took additional time, today only 1–2 s are necessary (fast CT). Volumetric scanning allows for three-dimensional images. The next generation offering scan times in the millisecond range (ultrafast CT) is already available. This reduction of scan times not only improves patient comfort but also and – even more importantly – gives better images of the abdomen due to excluding breathing artefacts and opens up new possibilities, for example, in cardiovascular diagnostics.

Except for images of the skeletal system, in most cases CT is used in combination with a contrast medium in order to improve the diagnostic potential. One of the major applications is the search for primary tumors or metastases of the liver which shall be more closely covered later. For this indication contrast media play a major role. I will therefore start with some pharmacokinetic considerations.

Following intravenous injection, the contrast agent is rapidly distributed within the intravascular space volume. In the aorta, which can be considered as a

[1] Research Laboratories of Schering AG, Müllerstr. 170, 13342 Berlin, Germany.

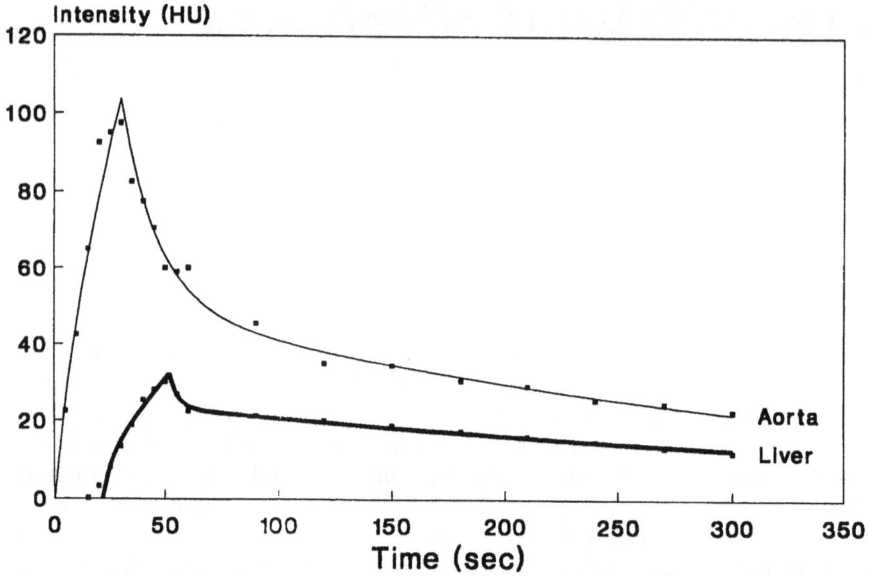

Fig. 1 Time-density curves in aorta and liver after intravenous injection of 300 mg iodine/kg diatrizoate (60%) at a rate of 2 ml/s (means of N = 6). Data are taken from the literature [1]. Curve-fitting was performed using the computer program TOPFIT [6]

measure of this compartment, following injection at a rate of 2 ml/s, maximal concentrations and therefore highest density values are observed after approximately 30 s [1]. Thereafter, concentrations decline biphasically with half-lives of approx. 10 s and 230 s (Fig. 1). The two phases can be explained by the processes of distribution of the contrast agent and extravasation into the extracellular space volume of well and less well perfused tissues and by renal elimination. If we consider the liver parenchyma as an example of extracellular space, we find a maximum concentration after approximately 40 s. This means that the rate of extravasation is extremely high.

This rapid rate of extravasation hampers the detection of liver tumors or metastases. In CT, tumorous tissue can be differentiated from normal liver tissue by its vascularization. Hyper- or hypovascularized tumors can be distinguished from healthy liver tissue by increased or decreased density after contrast media injection. For tumors with identical vascularization relative to the surrounding parenchyma differentiation is not possible, since both types of tissue are isodense. The localization of tumors is optimal during the short time period in which the contrast agent has not yet extravasated. Otherwise the differences in density are equilibrating. Another prerequisite is, of course, a rapid scanning sequence. Protracted or multi-phase injection schemes are therefore less suitable. Figure 2 shows the effect of increasing the injection rate on the CT density in the aorta. An example of the density in the aorta and liver following a biphasic infusion scheme is given in Fig. 3. The issue of injection regimens has attracted considerable interest recently and a large number of different recommendations has been offered

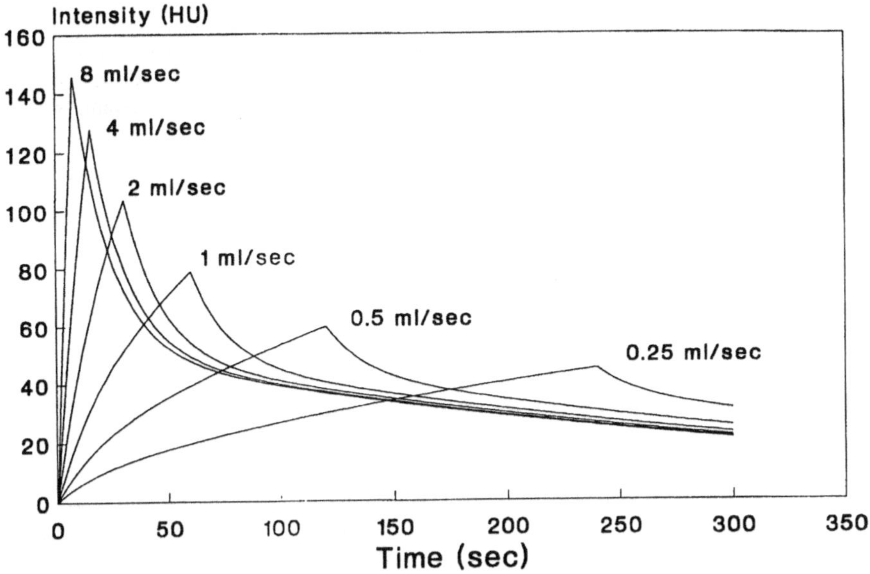

Fig. 2 Time-density curves in the aorta after intravenous injection of 300 mg iodine/kg diatrizoate (60%) at different rates. Data for 2 ml/s were taken from the literature [1]. Simulation for the other rates was performed using the computer program TOPFIT [6]

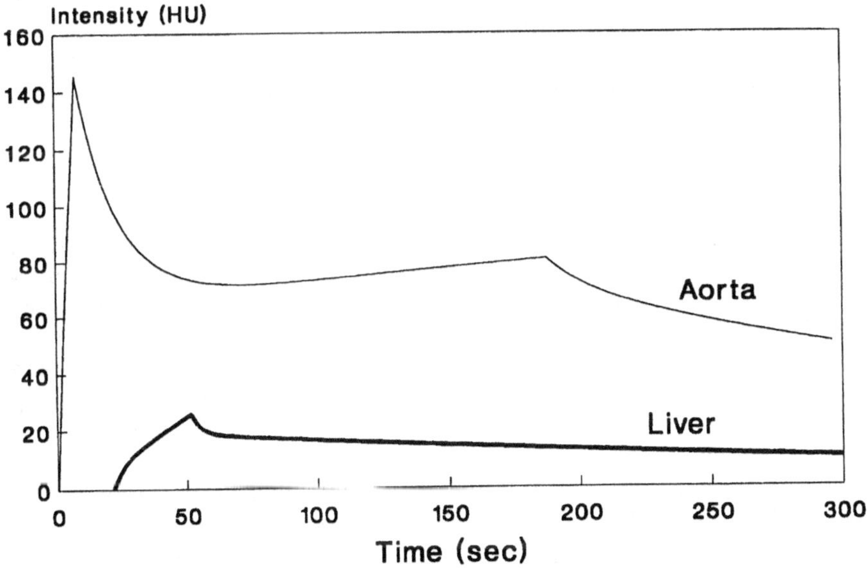

Fig. 3 Time-density curves in the aorta and liver after a biphasic intravenous injection of diatrizoate (60%). Phase I: 300 mg iodine/kg at 8 ml/s and 300 mg iodine/kg at 0.33 ml/sec. Data for 2 ml/s were taken from the literature [1]. Simulation for the other rates was performed using the computer program TOPFIT [6]

Table 1 Characteristics of contrast media suitable for rapid intravenous injection

Issue	Consequence
High iodine content	Greater density difference
No electrical charge	Improved tolerability
Low osmolality	Less side-effects
Low viscosity	Easily injectable
Balanced hydrophilicity	Good solubility

[2–5]. According to our own calculations using a computer program [6], very rapid monophasic injections should offer the greatest difference in density between vessels and the liver parenchyma for a relatively long time period. Rapid injection on the other hand requires a short scanning time and that the contrast media are very well tolerated. Table 1 gives a summary of characteristics which make compounds suitable for rapid intravenous injection.

All presently available compounds are exclusively synthesized out of the chemical class of triiodinated benzoic acid derivatives. To date, four different groups of compounds are on the market: ionic, high-osmolar agents of the diatrizoate type, non-ionic, low-osmolar compounds of the iopromide type, the ionic, low-osmolar dimeric product, ioxaglate and the two nonionic dimers, iotrolan and iodixanol (Fig. 4).

Ionic compounds fulfill the following primary requirements: high hydrophilicity, negligible protein binding and sufficient water solubility. However, because half of the ions in the aqueous phase – sodium or meglumine ions – do not contribute to imaging, the osmotic pressure and all osmolality-related side-effects are necessarily very high. Calcium binding by the carboxylic acid group and, for the pure sodium salts, a simultaneously very high sodium load induce a negative inotropic effect. High osmolality may result in bradycardia. Other side-effects such as nausea, vomiting and severe allergy-like events (urticaria, bronchospasm, drastic blood pressure decrease and unconsciousness) have been shown to have a much higher incidence compared to non-ionic, low-osmolar compounds [7–9]. Other adverse reactions include hemodynamic effects [10]. In addition to these clinically observed differences between ionic and nonionic contrast agents, numerous preclinical invitro and invivo studies such as damage to the blood-brain barrier [11] have clearly demonstrated that electric charge and high osmolality are the two main factors for the lower tolerability of ionic compounds. Table 2 gives a summary of the preclinical studies which are usually performed before starting phase I trials in humans and, additionally, tries to allocate the observed interactions with the test paradigm to five possible mechanisms. These are electric charge, osmolality, ions present in the preparation, lipophilicity/hydrophilicity and, finally, remaining factors of unknown origin which are designated as chemotoxicity. Table 2 clearly shows that charge and osmolality are in most cases the dominating factors to elicit adverse effects.

The presently available low-osmolar nonionic monomers (see Table 3) are well-tolerated and highly efficient contrast agents. Investigations on the molecular structure of X-ray contrast agents have shown a correlation between the

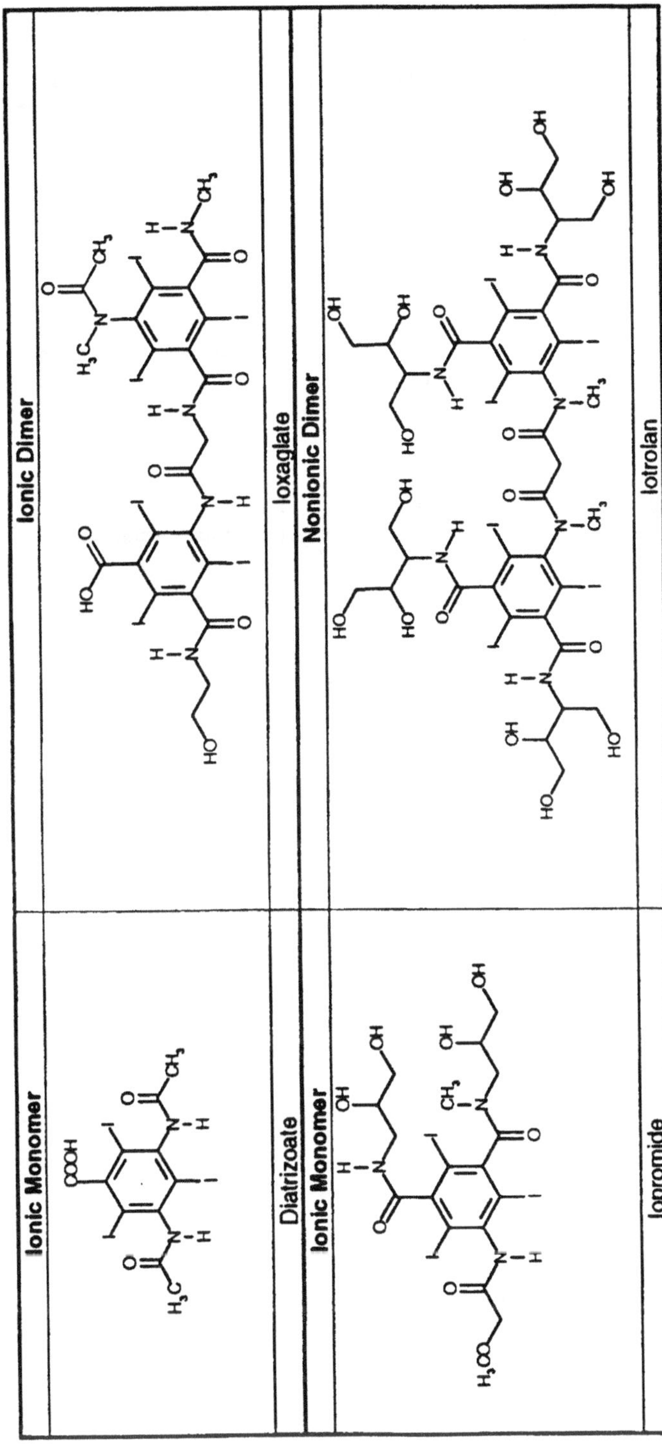

Fig. 4 Structural formulae of representative contrast agents from the four different classes

Table 2 Preclinical examination of contrast agents and the mechanisms responsible for side-effects

Issue	Result/mechanism
Physicochemistry	
Osmolality (mOsm/kg)	1500^{a}, $580-680^{b}$, 580^{c}, 300^{d}
Viscosity (mPas)	$4.5\text{-}6.5^{a-c}$, $>8^{d}$
Partition coefficient	$0.04-0.05^{a}$, $0.04-0.1^{b}$, 0.1^{c}, $0.005-0.01^{d}$
Invitro Pharmacology	
Protein binding (%)	low (< 10)
Complement	*activation* dependent on charge, osmolality, chemotoxicity
Lysozyme	*inhibition* dependent on charge, chemotoxicity
Histamine	*release* dependent on *charge*, osmolality, chemotoxicity
Hemolysis	*inhibition* dependent on charge, chemotoxicity
Erythrocyte morphology	*damage* dependent on *charge*, *chemotoxicity*, osmolality
General Toxicity	
LD_{50} (g iodine/kg)	$5-10^{a}$, $10-15^{b}$, $>20^{d}$
Neural Toxicity	Effects dependent upon:
Intracisternal	*Charge*, *osmolality*, lipophilicity, chemotoxicity
Intracerebral	*Charge*, *osmolality*, lipophilicity, chemotoxicity
Special Toxicity	Effects dependent upon:
Vessel pain	*Osmolality*, chemotoxicity
Kidney	? (Nonionics probably more favorable)
Proteinuria	Charge, osmolality, chemotoxicity
Cardiovascular	*Charge*, *osmolality*, *ions*, chemotoxicity
Blood-brain barrier damage	*Osmolality*, chemotoxicity, ions
Endothelial damage	*Osmolality*, charge
Local tolerance	Charge, osmolality, chemotoxicity
Pharmacokinetics	
Blood level	$t_{1/2}$(terminal) approximately 2 h
Excretion	Glomerular filtration
Tissue distribution	Extracellular
Diagnostic Potential	Depending on iodine concentration, osmolality (osmodilution) and viscosity (diffusion)

a Ionic monomers
b Nonionic monomers
c Ionic dimer
d Nonionic dimers

Table 3 Contrast agents available on the market

Ionic monomers	Nonionic monomers	Ionic dimer	Nonionic dimers
Diatrizoate	Iohexol	Ioxaglate	Iodixanol
	Iopamidol		Iotrolan
	Iopromide		
	Ioversol		

molecular weight and osmolality/viscosity. The higher the molecular weight, the higher are both osmolality and viscosity and the lower is their iodine content. Molecular iodine contents range from 45.6% for iopentol to 49% for iopamidol.

The development of a new contrast agent takes approximately 6–12 years. The major portion of this period is clinical development, which takes 3–6 years. Preclinical research has to be estimated at 2–3 years and chemical synthesis of the compound at 1–3 years. The individual steps which have to be considered in this process are summarized in Table 4. Time can be saved by taking the risk of parallel actions in the preclinical and clinical areas. However, a certain number of pharmacological and toxicological tests is always the prerequisite for trials in humans.

As an example for a nonionic monomer, more detailed data shall be given for iopromide (Ultravist, Schering AG). Iopromide has an osmolality of 586 mosm/kg at a concentration of 300 mg iodine/ml [12]. This is at the lower end of osmolality compared with other monomers. The most obvious osmolality-related side-effect is vessel pain. In this test, iopromide showed a tolerability superior to that of iopamidol, a contrast medium with a slightly higher osmolality. In additional studies the effects of osmolality have been studied in a number of test models including rabbit endothelium [13], subcutaneous injection into rat hind feet [14], invivo microcirculation experiments [15, 16], and blood-brain barrier damage in rabbits [17, 18]. In all these studies the good tolerance of iopromide could be demonstrated. In the other pharmacological test systems iopromide again exhibited a good tolerability, similar or superior to that of the other contrast media. These data are in good agreement with results reported in the literature, such as

Table 4 Stages of the development of contrast agents. Parallel processes are marked by identical numbers

Chemistry	Stage	Preclinical development	Stage	Clinical development	Stage
Search for lead compound	1	Establishment of test models	1	Phase I: healthy volunteers	4
Synthesis of derivatives	2	Screening of compounds	2	Phase II: dose-finding in patients	5
Upscaling of synthesis	3	Extensive pharmacological and toxicological characterization	3	Phase III: verification of dose, extensive testing	6
Large-scale production	4	Development of formulation	3–4	Preparation/submission of New Drug Application (NDA)	7
		Establishment/validation of analytical procedures	3–6		
		Stability testing: drug substance, preparation	3–6		
1–3 years		*2–3 years*		*3–6 years*	

studies on histamine release [19–21] and changes in blood cell morphology. Iopromide prolonged the bleeding time in rats in contrary to diatrizoate. This result was unexpected since it is general opinion that nonionic compounds do not influence clotting parameters to the same extent as ionic substances do. Regarding the prolongation of the thromboplastin time, iopromide was less active than diatrizoate (at higher concentration) and more active than other nonionic monomers. In a platelet aggregation test, iopromide also showed a higher potency than other nonionic monomers. The extensive toxicological examination of iopromide reported in the literature demonstrated the good tolerance of this contrast agent [22–24].

The pharmacokinetic parameters of iopromide are practically identical to that of other urographic contrast agents. This means that the pharmacokinetics are characterized by rapid extracellular distribution followed by renal elimination. Within the dose ranges for clinical use there is no dose-dependence of half-lives or clearance rates [25].

Further improvements in contrast agents have been seen after lowering the osmolality to values identical to that of blood (300 mOsm/kg). This is of advantage not only for the local tolerance resulting in further reduction of pain but also for patients with cardiac insufficiency who have to tolerate an increase in blood volume of up to 1000 ml within several minutes, if high doses of a conventional ionic contrast medium are injected. As an example for an isotonic compound, details of iotrolan (Isovist, Schering AG) are summarized in the following paragraph [26–30].

Due to its dimeric, nonionic character and its six iodine atoms per molecule, iotrolan is isotonic to blood at the concentrations used for angiography and CT (280 and 320 mg iodine/ml). Additives are therefore not necessary. Iotrolan is extremely hydrophilic exhibiting a butanol/water partition coefficient of 0.005 [12]. This is approximately one order of magnitude greater than that of the most hydrophilic monomer. The viscosity of dimers generally is greater than that of monomers. As a consequence of the slightly higher viscosity and the isotonicity, dilution in the vessel system and the kidney is slower than that observed for monomeric compounds. The imaging window is accordingly somewhat greater. Biochemical tests of iotrolan in comparison with monomeric substances have shown the higher inertness of this molecule. Protein binding and the inhibition of enzyme systems such as acetylcholinesterase, collagenase or urokinase are extremely low. The interaction with cell membranes of the endothelium, blood particles or the complement system is also negligible. Due to isotonicity, osmolality-related side-effects of iotrolan are considerably less frequently observed than for monomeric non-isotonic compounds. The reduced adverse events include heat and pain during injection and hemodilution with its consequences on hematocrit and hemodynamic stability. The cardiovascular tolerance of iotrolan, in particular, has been studied extensively and its superiority over monomeric contrast agents has been reported. The studies included investigations of the effects on the microcirculation [31] and hemodynamic parameters such as blood pressure, heart rate, cardiac output and peripheral resistance [32].

Modifications of the presently available contrast media formulations by adding different ions [33] or oxygen [34] are considered helpful by some investigators. In animal experiments, it could be shown that ventricular fibrillation, induced by high doses of nonionic contrast agents, could be avoided by adding 3–70 mmol sodium to the preparation. An additional improvement was seen regarding the negative inotropic effect of some nonionic compounds when the formulation was saturated with oxygen before use.

An alternative approach has been followed by looking for additives which improve the tolerance of the contrast agents. The prostacyclin analogue iloprost (Fig. 5), has been tested for this purpose [35]. The microcirculation is considerably disturbed by high-osmolar contrast agents. However, low-osmolar compounds still have a significant negative effect. The addition of iloprost totally prevented this disturbance.

Future chemical synthesis in the area of X-ray technology might concentrate on the search for less viscous dimeric nonionic compounds or, alternatively, leaving the area of iodine altogether and replacing it by metal ions such as gadolinium. Metal complexes have been reconsidered for X-ray technology since the advent of MRI. Metal salts or oxides such as $SrBr_2$ or ThO_2 (Thorotrast) have long ago been studied as X-ray contrast agents. However, high toxicity and incomplete excretion have usually caused the discontinuation of their use. The exceptionally high tolerability of Gd-DTPA, however, might cause a change in this attitude. Compounds other than triiodinated benzoic acid derivatives possibly show some of the typical side-effects at a reduced frequency. Further advantages are the greater absorptivity of X-rays by metals compared to iodine and the possibility of using radiation with a higher energy which will reduce radiation exposure of the patients. Future research has to be directed towards the synthesis of such compounds with an increased number of metal atoms per molecule.

The presently available contrast agents based on the triiodobenzene ring and possible compounds based on metal complexes are of the same type regarding the "efficiency" of imaging. They are substances with an extracellular distribution and renal elimination. Except for the biliary contrast agents – which will not be reviewed in this chapter – no tissue specificity has been achieved so far. Research, therefore, has been directed towards the search for tissue-specific substances. The most accessible target organ is the liver.

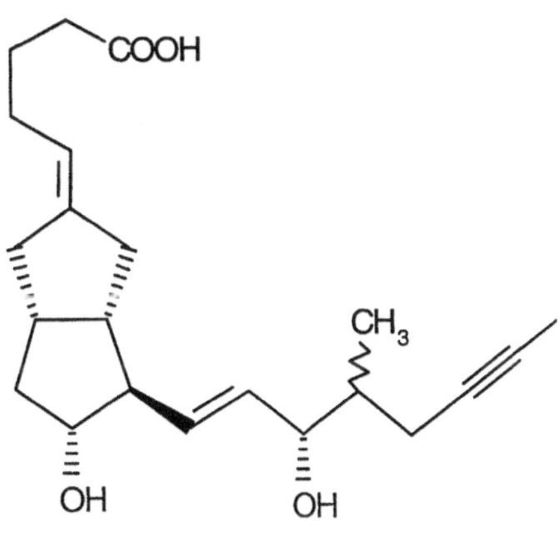

Fig. 5 Structural formula of iloprost

So far all attempts to achieve sufficiently high concentrations of water soluble contrast agents in the liver have failed. Emulsions of iodinated oils caused unacceptable side effects, whereas emulsions of perfluorooctylbromide display unsatisfactory efficacy which can only be compensated by very high and, accordingly, not very tolerable doses.

A totally different route has been chosen by the encapsulation of angiographic/urographic contrast agents into liposomes. The entrapped compounds are taken up by the reticuloendothelial system (RES) of the liver, the spleen or the bone marrow and allow for imaging of the liver or the spleen. Several approaches are currently in the early research stage [36, 37]. In the following, data will be presented on iopromide encapsulated into liposomes. The tolerability and imaging efficacy of this preparation was tested in a number of invitro and invivo models [38–41].

Multilamellar iopromide-carrying liposomes (Fig. 6) were prepared from phosphatidylcholine, cholesterol and stearic acid (4:5:1) by the ethanol-evaporation technique. The freeze-dried liposomes are reconstituted before use by adding 135 m*M* mannitol solution. Mean size after resuspension was approximately 0.5 μm and the osmolality of the preparation was 600 mOsm/kg. The median lethal dose (LD_{50}) in mouse and rat was approximately 3 g iodine/kg. The pharmacokinetics in rat and rabbit were dose dependent. Increasing the dose considerably resulted in lower total clearance and longer terminal half-life. Elimination of iodine was complete and the main route of excretion was via the kidneys. The iopromide-containing liposomes are taken up by the reticuloendothelial system of the liver and the spleen. Figure 7 shows the tissue distribution of iopromide in the rat after intravenous injection of iopromide-carrying liposomes at a dose of 200 mg iodine/kg. After entering the cells, the liposomes are degraded and the iopromide is released. It will leave the cell either by a diffusional process or by active transport and – once back in the blood – it is eliminated via the kidney. A clinically relevant CT enhancement of the liver (increase of 30 HU) was reached after a dose of approximately 200 mg iodine/kg in rat and 150 mg iodine/kg in rabbit [38–41]. The time window for imaging starts immediately

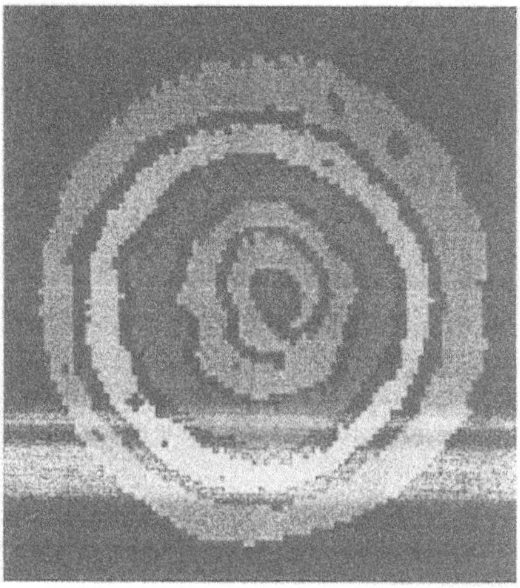

Fig. 6 Microscopic view of an iopromide-carrying liposome

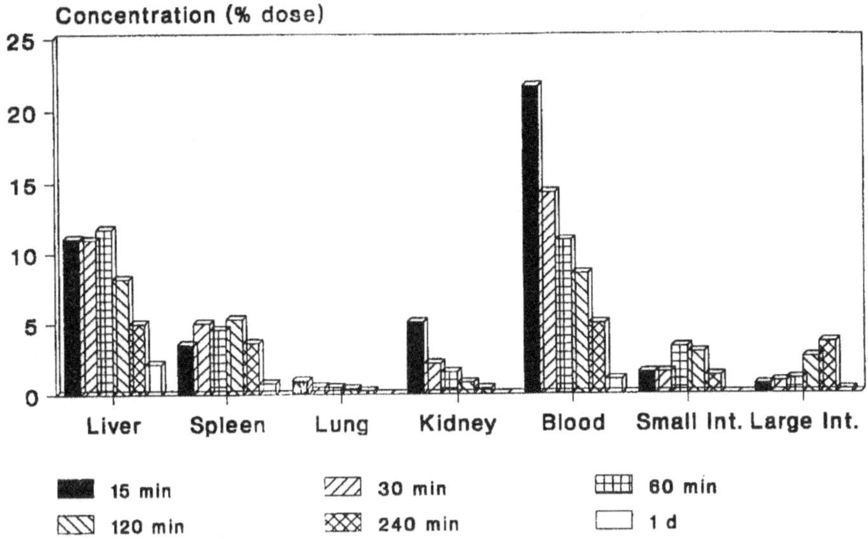

Fig. 7 Tissue distribution of iopromide in mice (means of N = 5) after intravenous injection of iopromide-carrying liposomes at a dose of 250 mg iodine/kg

after injection and lasts for several hours. Since tumor tissue or metastases do not contain RES cells, they are not able to accumulate iopromide and can therefore easily be distinguished from healthy tissue as hypodense structures. Blood vessels can be distinguished from lesions since immediately after injection their density is increased due the unencapsulated portion of iopromide (approximately 60% of the dose) which is not removed from the preparation. Lesions down to a size of 2–3 mm can be distinguished using iopromide-carrying liposomes.

In summary, the use of iodine-carrying liposomes in X-ray technology, seems to be a valuable tool for imaging the upper abdomen, especially the liver. Since "alternative" contrast agents such as other iodine-containing particles or emulsions have so far been shown to be either not sufficiently effective or to exhibit non-tolerable side-effects, liposomes are at present the only class of agents with a promising profile. Alternative indications for liposomally encapsulated iopromide might be their use in indirect lymphography.

A further possible approach to visualize lesions in the liver would be the injection of contrast agents which do not extravasate. These "blood-pool agents" have been investigated extensively [42–47]. Two principal approaches have been selected, first, the synthesis of macromolecular contrast agents and, second, the use of emulsions or suspensions of either water-insoluble compounds or particles. However, to date, no agent has reached clinical trials. The principle of synthesizing a macromolecular substance which will remain within the intravascular space volume seems to be simple: iodination of a suitable high-molecular "carrier" or attachment of a triiodinated moiety to this carrier. The critical factor is molecular size. The resultant compound should be large enough to stay within the vessel system and small enough to be eliminated via the kidney. However, whether this is possible at all, has not yet been elucidated. A molecular weight of more than

20000 does result in longer residence times in the intravascular space. The problem which everybody involved in this area of research has encountered, however, is that suitable carriers, preferably of a definite molecular weight, are not available. Since the excretability of the macromolecular compound depends on its filterability by the kidney, any high-molecular components will be retained in the body.

One way to overcome this problem would be the use of biodegradable carriers. In this case the starting molecular weight would lose its importance. Biodegradability can be achieved by different means. One possibility is through the attack of enzymes. However, these enzymes have to be present in the blood, since this is the only body compartment which can be reached by non-extravasating substances. In blood, esterases are available which can be utilized for the purpose of biodegradation of iodine-carrying polymers. Although polymers which are biodegradable per se are available such as starch or polyesters, they are usually no longer degraded after derivatization with iodine. The reason is most probably steric hindrance of the enzyme systems involved. Although the need for blood-pool agents is very high possible applications are summarized in Table 5 the successful identification of a suitable development candidate has not yet been reported.

In summary, future directions of research will cover new nonionic dimers, possibly iodine-free extracellular contrast agents, blood-pool compounds and tissue-specific substances. Table 6 illustrates application needs for these contrast agents. The future will show whether the high expectations of the radiological community will be met.

Table 5 Indications for blood-pool contrast agents

Region of interest	Indication	Detection mechanism
Vessel system	Occlusion, aneurysm	Vessel shape
Liver	Lesion detection	Vascularization
Heart	Ischemia, infarct, occlusion, reperfusion, collateral formation	Perfusion intensity and kinetics
Lungs	Tumor	Vascularization
	Inflammation	Abnormal capillary permeability (extravasation)
Soft tissue	Relative blood volume	Quantitation of intravascular space
	Tumors	Enrichment of contrast medium
Lymphatic tissue	Tumors, metastases	Reticulo endothelial system uptake?

Table 6 Future directions in contrast agent research

Type of contrast agent	Improvement/new indications
Nonionic dimers	Lower viscosity
Iodine-free extracellular compounds	No iodine-related side-effects
Blood-pool contrast agents	Intravascular distribution
RES-specific substances	Liver and spleen imaging

References

1. Clausen C, Lochner B (1983) Dynamische Computertomographie. Springer, Berlin, Tokyo, p 39
2. Costello P, Dupuy DE, Ecker CP, Tello R (1992) Spiral CT of the thorax with reduced volume of contrast material: a comparative study. Radiology 183:663–6
3. Baron RL (1994) Understanding and optimizing use of contrast material for CT of the liver. AJR 163:323–331
4. Small WC, Nelson RC, Bernadino ME, Brummer LT (1994) Contrast-enhanced spiral CT of the liver: effect of different amounts and injection rates of contrast material on early contrast enhancement. AJR 163:87–92
5. Chambers TP, Baron RL, Lush RM, Dodd III GD, Miller WJ (1994) Hepatic enhancement: comparison of ionic and nonionic contrast agents in the same patients. Radiology 190:721–5
6. Heinzel G, Woloszczak R, Thomann P (1993) TOPFIT 2.0 Pharmacokinetic and pharmacodynamic data analysis system for the PC. Gustav Fischer, Stuttgart, Jena, New York
7. Schrott KM et al. (1986) Iohexol in der Ausscheidungsurographie. Fortschr d Medizin 7:153–156
8. Katayama H, Yamaguchi K, Kozuka T, Takashima T, Seez P, Matsuura K (1990) Adverse reactions to ionic and nonionic contrast media. Radiology 175:621–628
9. Palmer FJ (1988) The RACR survey of intravenous contrast media reactions final report. Australasian Radiology 32:426–428
10. Schräder R, Baller D, Hoeft A, Korb H, Wolpers HG, Hellige G (1983) Reduced side-effects of low osmolality non-ionic contrast media in coronary arteriography – comparative experimental study in dogs. In Taenzer V, Zeitler E (eds) Contrast Media in Urography, Angiography and Computerized Tomography, Thieme Verlag, Stuttgart, p 67–77
11. Miyazawa T, Nakagawa H, Oshino N (1989) Role of red blood cell deformation in toxicity of contrast media in cerebral angiography. Invest Radiol 24:383–389
12. Krause W, Miklautz H, Kollenkirchen U, Heimann G (1994) Physicochemical parameters of X-ray contrast media. Invest Radiol 29:72–80
13. Thiesen B, Mützel W (1990) Effects of angiographic contrast media on venous endothelium of rabbits. Invest Radiol 25:121–126
14. Kim SH, Park JH, Kim YI, Kim CW, Han MC (1990) Experimental tissue damage after subcutaneous injection of water soluble contrast media. Invest Radiol 25:678–685
15. Klopp R, Niemer W, Schippel W, Münster W (1989) Tierexperimentelle Untersuchungen zur Mikrozirkulation ionischer und nichtionischer Röntgenkontrastmittel. Radiol Diagn 30:324–8
16. Klopp R, Niemer W, Schippel W (1991) Kontrastmittelwirkungen auf die Fließbedingungen der Mikrozirkulation (tierexperimentelle Studie). In: Peters PE, Zeitler E (eds) Röntgenkontrastmittel, Nebenwirkungen, Prophylaxe, Therapie, Springer-Verlag, Berlin, p 52–64
17. Wilcox J, Evill CA, Sage MR (1986) Effects of intracarotid ionic and non-ionic contrast material on the blood-brain barrier in a rabbit model. Neuroradiology 28:271–274
18. Wilson A, Wilcox J, Evill C, Sage M (1989) The effect of contrast medium viscosity on the blood-brain barrier after intracarotid injection in the rabbit. AJNR 10:129–133
19. Amon EU, Ennis M, Lorenz W, Schnabel M, Schneider C (1990) Histamine release induced by radiographic contrast media. Comparison between pulmonary and peritoneal mast cells derived from normotensive and spontaneously hypertensive rats. Int Arch Allergy Appl Immunol 92:203–208
20. Ennis M, Amon EU, Lorenz W (1989) Histamine release from canine lung and liver mast cells induced by radiographic contrast media. Agents and Actions 27: 1/2: 101–103
21. Ennis M, Lorenz W, Nehring E, Schneider C (1991) In vitro and in vivo studies of radiographic contrast media-induced histamine release in pigs. Agents and Actions 33: 1/2:26–9

22. Günzel P (1992) Arzneimitteltoxikologie: Diagnostika (Röntgen- u a Kontrastmittel). In: Hess R (ed) Arzneimitteltoxikologie: Anforderungen – Verfahren – Bedeutung, Thieme Verlag, Stuttgart, p 397–404
23. Bhargava AS, Hofmeister R, Siegmund F, Schöbel C, Günzel P (1990) Effect of three nonionic contrast media on rats and rabbits with regard to renal changes. Arzneim Forsch 40:822–829
24. W Krause, C Schöbel, WR Press (1994) Preclinical testing of iopromide. II Toxicological evaluation, Arzneim Forsch, 44 (11):1275–9
25. W Krause, G Schuhmann-Giampieri, Th Staks, J Kaufmann (1994) Dose proportionality of iopromide pharmacokinetics and tolerability after iv injection in healthy volunteers. Eur J Clin Pharmacol 46 (4):339–43
26. Sovak M, Ranganathan R, Speck U (1982) Nonionic dimer: development and initial testing of an intrathecal contrast agent. Radiology 142:115–8
27. Mützel W, Press WR, Weinmann HJ (1989) Physicochemical properties and general pharmacology of the nonionic dimer iotrolan. In: Recent developments in nonionic contrast media, Taenzer V, Wende S (eds.), Thieme, Stuttgart, p 28–32
28. Speck U, Mützel W, Mannesmann G, Pfeiffer H, Siefert HM (1980) Pharmacology of nonionic dimers. Invest Radiol 15:317–322
29. Press WR, Mützel W, Schöbel C (1989) Tolerance of iotrolan after subarachnoid injection in animals. In: Recent developments in nonionic contrast media, Taenzer V, Wende S (eds), Thieme, Stuttgart, p 126–133
30. Nauert C, Mützel W (1989) Experimental urography in dogs: diagnostic quality and pharmacokinetic behaviour of iotrolan in comparison to nonionic and ionic, monomeric contrast media. In: Recent developments in nonionic contrast media, Taenzer V, Wende S (eds), Thieme, Stuttgart, p 211–4
31. Klopp R, Niemer W, Schippel W, Krause W (1994) Changes in the microcirculation of the intact rat heart after iodinated and Gd-containing contrast media. Cardiovascular and Interventional Radiology 17:S123
32. Muschick P, Wehrmann D, Schuhmann-Giampieri G, Krause W (1994) Cardiac and haemodynamic tolerability of different X-ray contrast media in the anaesthetized rat. Cardiovascular and Interventional Radiology 17:S125
33. Baath L (1990) Sodium addition and/or oxygen saturation of iohexol during normal and reduced perfusion pressure. Effects on contractile force and risk of ventricular fibrillation in the isolated heart. rabbit Acta Radiologica 31:525–530
34. Baath L, Almén T, Öksendal A (1990) Oxygen saturation of the low osmolar contrast media iohexol, ioxaglate and iodixanol. Effects on contractile force and frequency of ventricular fibrillation in the isolated rabbit heart. Acta Radiologica 31:519–523
35. Krause W, Klopp R, Niemer W, Schippel W Elimination of the diatrizoate-induced effects on the microcirculation by the prostacyclin derivative, iloprost. Invest Radiol (in press)
36. Corot RD, Carrillon Y, Dandis G, Eloy R, Amiel M (1990) Ioxaglate-carrying liposomes. Computed tomography study as hepato-splenic contrast agent in rabbits. Invest Radiol 25:S95–S97
37. Passariello R, Pavone P, Patrizio G, di Renzi P, Mastantuono M Giuliani S (1990) Liposomes loaded with nonionic contrast media. Hepatosplenic computed tomographic enhancement. Invest Radiol 25:S92–S94
38. Krause W, Sachse A, Wagner S, Kollenkirchen U and Rößling G (1991) Preclinical characterization of iopromide-carrying liposomes. Invest Radiol 26:S172–S174
39. Krause W, Leike J, Sachse A and Schuhmann-Giampieri G (1993) Characterization of iopromide liposomes. Invest Radiol 28:1028–1032
40. Sachse A, Leike J, Rößling G, Wagner S and Krause (1993) W Preparation and evaluation of lyophilized iopromide-carrying liposomes for liver-tumor detection. Invest Radiol 28:838–844
41. Schuhmann-Giampieri G, Leike J, Sachse A, Krause W (1994) Characterization of iopromide-carrying liposomes. J Liposome Res 4 (1):239–53

42. Mattrey RF (1991) Blood-pool agents are the ideal agents for computed tomography. Invest Radiol 26: S55–6
43. Doucet D, Meyer D, Chambon C, Bonnemain B (1991) Blood-pool X-ray contrast agents. Evaluation of a new iodinated polymer. Invest Radiol 26: S53–4
44. Revel D, Chambon C, Havard P, Dandis G, Canet E, Corot C, Amiel M (1991) Iodinated polymer as blood-pool contrast agents. Computed tomography evaluation in rabbits. Invest Radiol 26: S57–8
45. Lautrou J, Paris D, Schaefer M, Meyer D, Chambon C, Doucet D (1990) Iodinated polymers. Pharmacokinetics of blood-pool imaging products. Invest Radiol 25: S109–10
46. Cassel DM, Young SW, Brody WR, Muller HH, Hall AL (1982) Radiographic blood pool contrast agents for vascular and tumor imaging with projection radiography and computed tomography. J Comput Assist Tomogr 6: 141–6
47. Sako M, Okuda K, Shimizu T, Hasegawa M, Hase M, Murakami T, Hirota S, Kono M (1987) Iodinated starch as a new potential blood pool contrast agent: Preliminary report. In: Advance and Future Trends of Contrast Media: Proceedings of the International Symposium on Contrast Media, Tokyo, Nov 6–7, Japan Convention Services Inc

Computed Tomography of the Brain: A Brief Oberview from a University Hospital in Taiwan

Chin-Yin Yu[1]

X-ray computed tomography (CT) was the modality of choice for demonstrating intracranial pathology in both routine and emergency conditions before the development of magnetic resonance imaging (MRI), and it remains an important imaging tool, especially for critical patients. In our hospital, the average number of cases of CT examination is 650 per month; of these more than 350 are of the brain and neck. The categories of intracranial disorders include trauma, cerebral vascular disease (CVA), inflammatory process (encephalitis, meningitis, and brain abscess), neoplasm (primary and secondary tumors), and congenital and metabolic disorders. Trauma is a major problem in Taiwan (especially from motorcycle accidents). Common findings in cases of head injury are subdural and epidural hematomas, subarachnoid hemorrhage, contusion hemorrhage, brain edema and skull fractures. More than half of the brain CTs performed in our hospital are either brain injury or CVA. The hemorrhagic type of the CVA represents a difference between Taiwan and Western countries, as it accounts for 40% of CVA in Taiwan [1].

The routine protocol of brain CT in our hospital is prallel to supra-orbito-meatal (SOM) line to reduce the radiation dose to the lens. We use a 10 mm slice thickness for the supratentorial part and a 5-mm thickness for the posterior fossa without any skip region. The pre- and post-contrast medium study have the exact same level, unless the patient moves during the examination. The contrast medium we routinely use is an ionic form, at doses of 100 ml for patients over 50 kg and 2 ml per kg for those less than 50 kg. Non-ionic contrast media will only be paid for by the health insurance under specific conditions. We use a fast drip (pressure pump) and start to scan after half of the dose is in the patients IV line. For the study of lymph nodes in the neck region, double doses may be necessary and good bolus effect is helpful.

In our hospital, the X-ray energy used in a routine brain scan is 120 Kvp, 120 mA over a 2 s-scan. For a temporal bone study, high energy and thin slices (1.5 mm or less) are mandatory for both axial and coronal section. The disadvantage of CT study of the brain and neck is that the coronal scan is very uncomfortable for the patient, and not everyone can tolerate the position long enough.

The development of computer systems has helped to improve the speed of scanning and reconstruction. The slip ring design is helpful in reducing the time

[1] Department of Diagnostik Radiology, National Cheng Kung University Hospital Tainan, Taiwan.

needed for the scanning cycle. For spiral CT, the scan time of an axial scan is routinely 1 s and this helps to reduce possible motion artifacts. The spiral sequence is good for dynamic studies (arterial versus venous phase) and CT angiography and provides a large data file for three-dimensional reconstruction of vertebrae and facial bones [2,3] in trauma or congenital anomaly.

References

1. Yu CY, Huang KM, Hsu CY (1983) CT in cerebral vascular disease. Chinese J Radiol 8:302–18
2. Heiken JP, Brink JA, Vannier MW (1993) Spiral (Helical) CT. Radiology 189:647–56
3. Schwartz RB (1994) Neuroradiological applications of spiral CT. Seminars in Ultrasound, CT & MRI 15:139–47

CHAPTER 6

Clinical Application of Computed Tomography in Discography

Tae-Sub Chung[1]

Introduction

Discography, the injection of contrast media into the nucleus pulposus, is a diagnostic technique used to evaluate cases of lower back pain, in which the results of other imaging studies are normal or conflicting. The diagnostic merits and applications of lumbar discography have always been controversial and this position is unchanged, even with the advent of computed tomography and magnetic resonance imaging [1–3]. Initially, many believed that MR imaging would eliminate the need for discography; however, with the recognition of multisegmental disc disease on MRI studies and the increased use of spinal fusion procedures, the need for this provocative and morphologic test has grown. Discography, by means of induced pain, is the only neuroradiological examination that presently allows a pathologic disc to be ascertained; it is a precious element in the identification of disc or discs causing the clinical symptoms. Induced pain is not to be confused with the pain provoked by discal distention with consequent stretching of nerve terminals: the latter presents the distinguishing feature of being dull, essentially mechanical and slight in magnitude [4].

CT discography is effected by exploiting the contrast injected directly into the disc during discography and successively performing a delayed CT scan. CT discography allows extremely precise anatomico-neuroradiological investigation of the disc, unequivocally demonstrating disc pathologies that are difficult to interpret with plain CT scans and sometimes even with MRI [4].

Indications

Uses of CT discography include the following: diagnosing a lateral disc herniation [5, 6]; differential diagnosis between fibrosis and recurrent herniation after surgery [7]; additional evidence in the case of erroneous intradiscal puncture

[1] Department of Diagnostic Radiology, Yonsei University Medical College, YongDong Severance Hospital, 146–92, Dogok-Dong, Kangnam-Ku, Seoul 135–270, Korea.

(annulography) [8]; further diagnostic investigation in the case of discrepancy between clinical findings and neuroradiological examinations [4]; revealing internal disc interruption[8]; and determining the type of disc lesion as protrusion, extrusion, or sequestration [1].

It has been suggested that MRI may make lumbar discography obsolete [9]. This would be true if a normal T2-weighted image shows that the disc is normal by all discography parameters. However, discography remains the only pain-provocative test in situations of multiple level disc abnormalities or in instances of equivocal MRI imagings [10].

Technique

A mild analgesic is given to hospitalized patients, but no premedication is used when discography is performed as an outpatient procedure. With the patient in the lateral decubitus position, a posterolateral extradural approach from the asymptomatic or less symptomatic side is used. An 18-gauge Hustead needle is then positioned under fluoroscopic control until it rests against the posterolateral annulus. A 22-gauge Chiba needle is then passed through the Hustead needle into the center of the disc. After satisfactory needle placement, normal saline is injected into the disc for the test.

After the saline injection, water soluble contrast medium is injected into the disc. The volume, resistance, pain response, and radiographic appearance are noted. Usually 1.0 cc contrast medium is injected, attentively assessing the presence of pain response. The CT examination utilizing the intradiscal contrast injection is performed within 2 h after discography, to attenuate the elevated opacification of the contrast itself and allow for homogeneous diffusion inside the disc. Three or four thin slice scans are usually taken at the center of disc to avoid the artifacts due to partial volume effect. In the eventuality of herniated migration, contiguous slices may be performed pedicle to pedicle with sagittal and coronal reconstruction images. Use is made of both wide-window images, to study the diffusion of contrast in the canal and bony structures, and narrow-window images, to study the thecal sac and nonopaque scarring.

CT Discography Findings

CT discography findings can be classified as follows:

1. Normal CT-discography: rounded centrodiscal opacity (Fig. 1a–d).
2. Degeneration: entire disc is irregularly opacified by contrast media (Fig. 2a–d).
3. Annulography: contrast opacifies the fibers of annulus.
4. Herniated disc: direct visualization of the herniated pathway is evidenced by a more or less regular, linear contrast leak, with opacification of the herniated area (Fig. 3a–d).
   a) Intraforaminal and extraforaminal herniated disc: diagnostic accuracy is 93.8%, as opposed to 50% on direct CT scan [5].
   b) Postoperative scar tissue: contrast does not diffuse in the epidural space [11].

Discussion

Discography is purely a diagnostic test, the interpretation and significance of which have evolved during the past few decades. Currently, the most important feature of this test is reproduction of the patient's pain [12, 13]. Holt [14] performed discography on asymptomatic volunteers and showed a high false-positive rate (26%).

Walsh et al. [13] reported 100% specificity with no false positive results on lumbar discography. The study by Walsh et al. had the following strengths: (a) a more sophisticated evaluation of response to pain; (b) expert needle placement (2% poor or invalid placement, compared with 25% in Holt's study); and (c) use of less-irritating, nonionic contrast media. During the past two decades, discography has been used to assess proper needle placement before chemonucleolysis [15].

Fig. 1a–d A 40-year-old woman with normal lumbar disc at L4-L5. **a** Among the multileves of discography in lumbar spine, discography at L4-L5 shows a normal pattern of bilocular appearance and hypertransparent horizontal septum. **b** Axial magnetic resonance imaging with gradient echo technique shows normal L4-L5 intervertebral disc. **c** T2WI sagittal image of L spine shows normal bright signal intensity of L4-L5 intervertebral disc. However, slightly decreased signal intensity of L3-L4 and L5-S1 intervertebral discs may suggest mild degenerative changes. **d** Round centrodiscal opacified contrast media is noted on CT discography at L4-L5. Small amount of contrast leak through oblique needle puncture site at Rt posterolateral direction

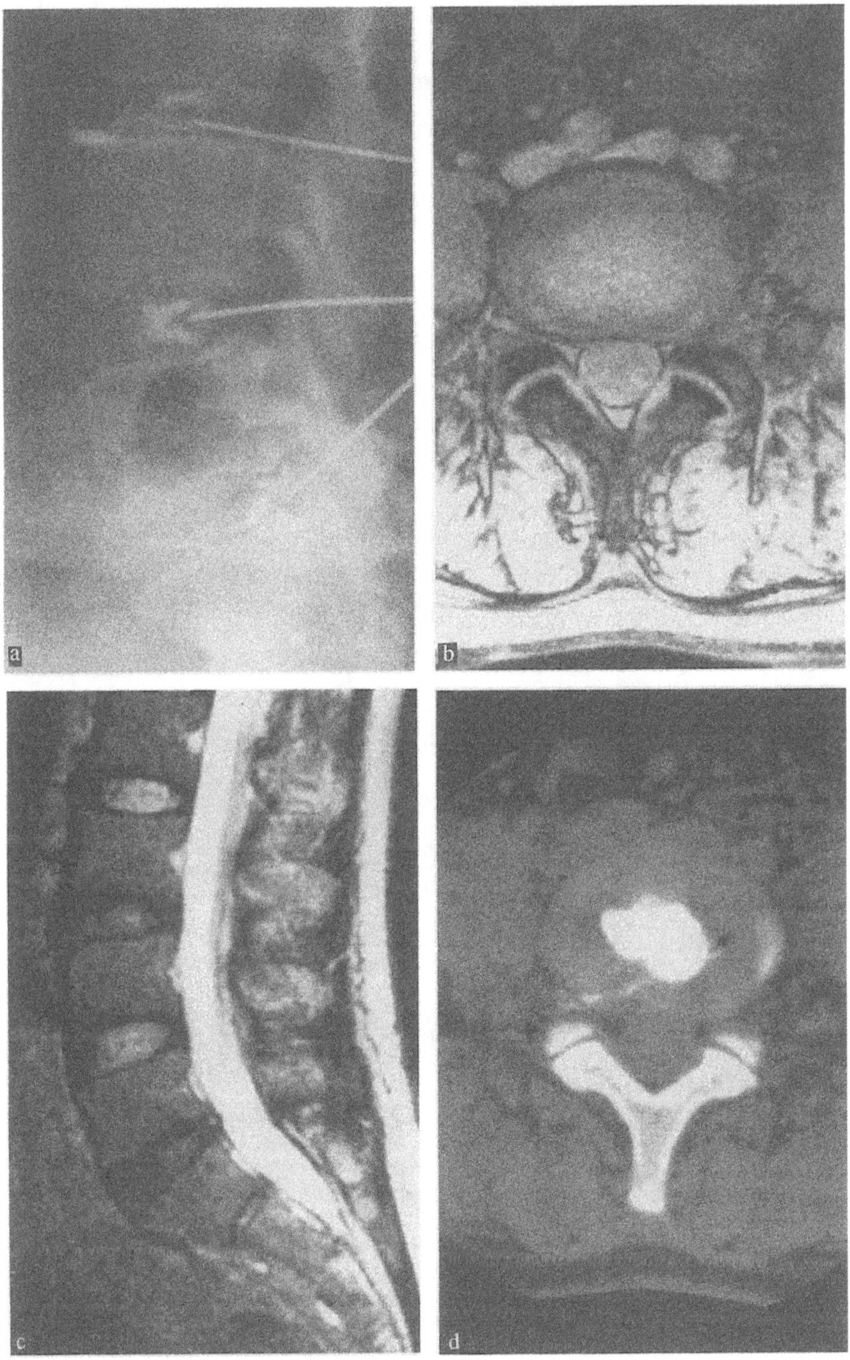
a
b
c
d

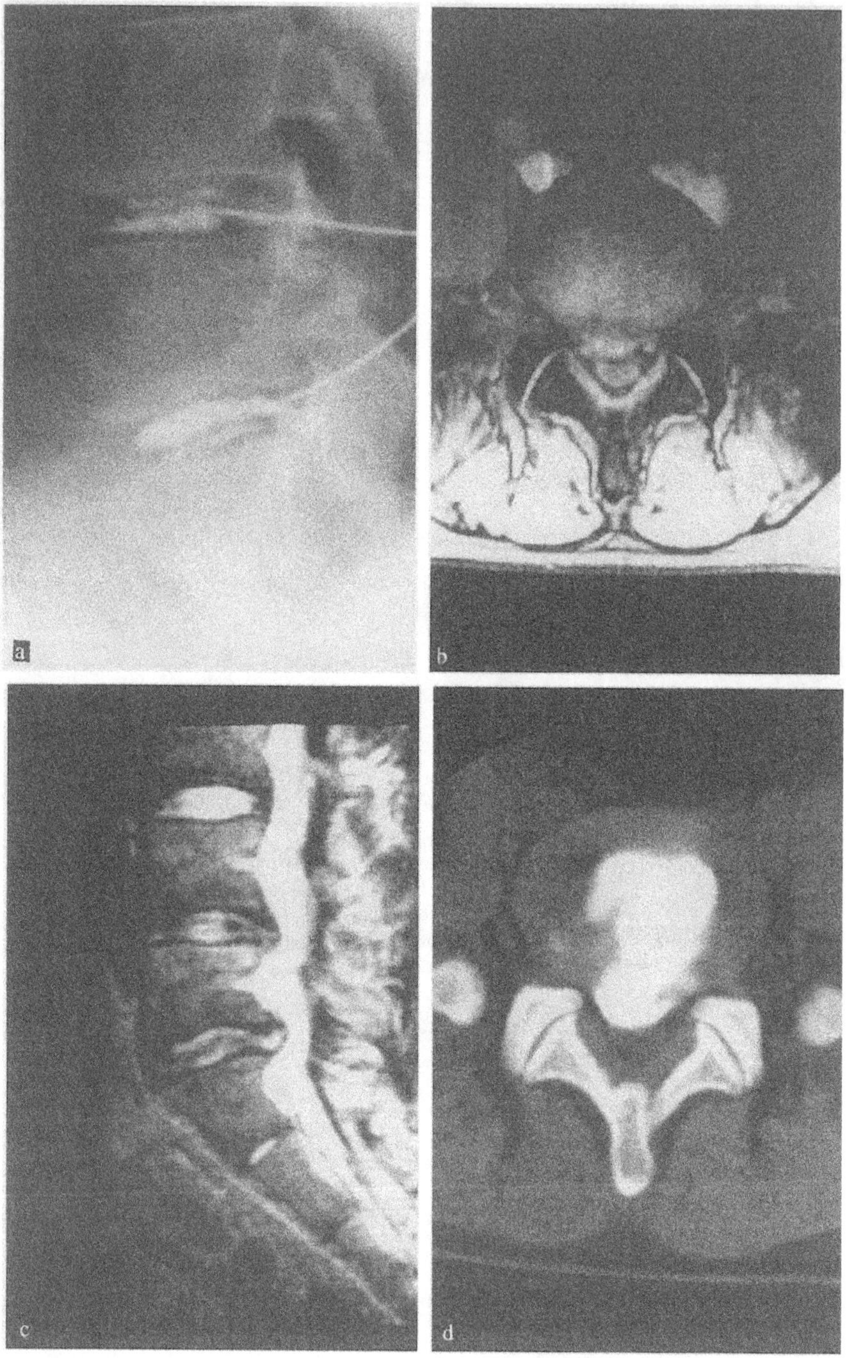
a
b
c
d

The indications for discography have changed since the introduction of CT and MRI, which show disc herniation and degeneration noninvasively [16]. In Bernard's series [3] of 190 discs for which MRI and discographic findings were available, the two tests agreed in 89% of the cases. Bernard explains the discrepancy on the basis of early disc degeneration; in such early degeneration, the sensitivity of discography exceeds that of MRI. However, others compared discography with MRI and found no advantages to be gained by performing discography [10, 17]. These kinds of controversies over discography have raged for more than 40 years.

MRI, because of its noninvasiveness and elevated anatomical definition, seems to be certainly a significant means of investigation in the postoperative lumbar discal hernia patient. However, CT discography defines the type of disc herniation and is useful in evaluating the previously operated spine [3]. Sometimes, this information is of more value to the surgeon than to the radiologist, since it influences the selection of treatment options [3]. Discography remains the only pain provocative challenge of the lumbar disc, and CT discography is, in fact, the only examination that allows the direct visualization of the nucleus pulposus, whether intradiscal or herniated, differentiating it from the annulus and any scarring [4].

Fig. 2 a–d 23-year-old man. **a** Contained and subligamentously collected contrast medium is noted at L4-L5 and L5-S1 on lateral projection of discography. Good opacification of herniated areas is noted (*arrows*). **b** Axial gradient echo image through the L5-S1 disc shows impingement on the thecal sac and effacement on the epidural fat by herniated disc (*arrow*). **c** The disc herniation at L5–S1 has identical signal intensity with original nucleus pulposus on sagittal T2WI. Posterior longitudinal ligament is intact on the another proton density image. **d** CT discography at L5-S1 reveals good visualization of ruptured area of annulus with contrast opacification of the herniated nucleus pulposus area. However, there is no remarkable epidural leak of contrast medium

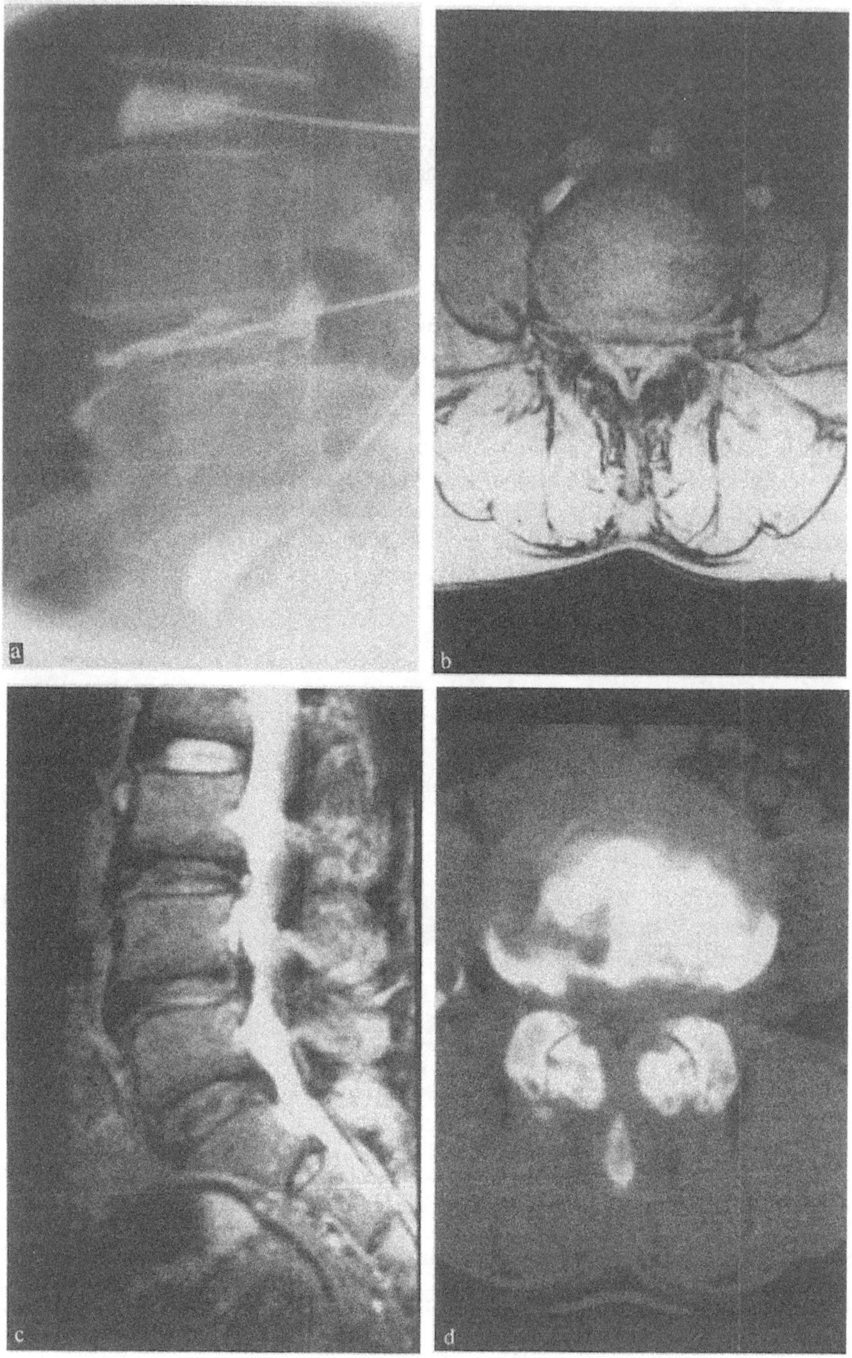

References

1. Bernard TN Jr., Kirkaldy-Willis WH (1987) Recognizing specific characteristics of non-specific low back pain. Clin Orthop 217:266–280
2. Bosacco SJ (1986) Lumbar discography: redefining its role with intradiscal therapy. Orthopedics 9:399–401
3. Bernard TN Jr. (1990) Lumbar discography followed by computed tomography: refining the diagnosis of low-back pain. Spine 15:690–707
4. Fabris G, Lavaroni A, Leonardi M (1991) Discography. 1st ed Udine: Centauro, 11–26
5. Jackson PR, Glah JJ (1987) Foraminal and extraforaminal lumbar disc herniation: diagnosis and treatment. Spine 12:577–585
6. Kornberg M (1987) Extreme lateral lumbar disc herniations. clinical syndrome and computed tomography recognition. Spine 12:586–589
7. McFadden JW (1986) The stress lumbar discogram. Spine 13:931–933
8. Kornberg M (1987) Computed tomography of the lumbar spine following discography: clinical application in selective cases. Spine 12:823–825
9. Gibson MJ, Szypryt EP, Buckley JH, Worthington BS, Mulholland RC (1987) Magnetic resonance imaging of adolescent disc herniation. J Bone Joint Surg 69-B:699–703
10. Schneiderman G, Flannigan B, Kingston S, Thomas J, Dillin WH, Watkins RG (1987) Magnetic resonance imaging in the diagnosis of disc degeneration: correlation with discography. Spine 12:276–281
11. Grenier N, Vital JM, Greselle JF, et al. (1988) CT-discography in the evaluation of the postoperative lumbar spine. Neuroradiology 30:232–238
12. Millette PC, Melanson D (1982) A reappraisal of lumbar discography. J Can Assoc Radiol 33:176–182
13. Walsh TR, Weistein JN, Spratt KF, Lehmann TR, Aprill C, Sayre H (1990) Lumbar discography in normal subjects: a controlled, prospective study. J Bone Joint Surg[Am] 72-A:1081–1088
14. Holt EP (1968) The question of lumbar discography. J Bone Joint Surg[Am] 50-A:720–725
15. Sachs BL, Spivey MA, Vanharanta H, et al. (1989) Techniques for lumbar discography and CT/discography in clinical practice. Appl Radiol 18:28–30
16. El-Khoury GY, Renfrew DL (1991) Percutaneous procedure for the diagnosis and treatment of lower back pain: discography, facet-joint injection, and epidural injection. AJR 157:685–691
17. Gibson MJ, Buckley J, Mawhinney R, Mulholland RC, Worthington BS (1986) Magnetic resonance imaging and discography in the diagnosis of disc degeneration. J Bone Joint Surg [Br] 68-B:369–373

Fig. 3 a–d 53-year-old woman with neurologic intermittent claudication. **a** Discography at L4-L5 reveals significant degeneration of the disc, which appears flattened with fuzzy margins. Contrast medium diffuses towards the periphery and leaks into regional epidural space through fissure. **b** Axial gradient echo image through L4-L5 disc level reveals extrinsic compressed dural sac from diffusely expanded disc. L4-L5 disc shows indistinct signal intensity between nucleus pulposus and annulus fibrosus. **c** Sagittal T2WI of L spine reveals diffusely decreased signal intensity of nucleus pulposus at L4-L5 disc level with mild posterior herniated nucleus pulposus through fissure of annulus fibrosus. **d** CT discography at L4-L5 shows irregular opacification of disc by contrast medium from disc degeneration

Chapter 7

Future Role of Computed Tomography in Neuroradiology

W.J. Huk[1]

Introduction

Computered tomography (CT) was the first major revolution in diagnostic imaging since the detection of X-rays by Conrad Röntgen in 1895, the 100th anniversary of which is celebrated by the radiological community this year. It opened a new era by the fact that it was the first technique to present direct information on the intracranial anatomy. Only those who know from their own experience about the problems and the insufficiency of previous methods to obtain only indirect data from inside the head can realize the impact of this new technique on neurosciences.

CT was also the first imaging method to produce digitalized pictures of tranaxial sections. The basis for this new development was provided by modern computers which enabled the instant reconstruction of images from a large amount of data. With this tool, it was only logical to look for other physical phenomena which could be utilized for diagnostic imaging to obtain more or different diagnostic information with perhaps better quality. The results of these efforts are magnetic resonance imaging (MRI), positron emission tomography (PET), and single photon emission tomography (SPECT). After a period of clinical evaluation of these new modalities in comparison with CT, a competitive situation has emerged, where users under the pressure of shrinking budgets have to decide between CT and MRI. PET and SPECT, as functional techniques with a much reduced spatial resolution of anatomical detail, both represent a different group of diagnostic modalities which cannot be compared directly to CT and MRI.

In order to decide which technique, CT or MRI, is superior for which purpose, one has to look at the requirements neuroradiology has to fullfill in the evaluation of central nervous system (CNS) diseases.

[1] Department of Neuroradiology, Neurosurgical Hospital of the University of Erlangen-Nürnberg, Schwabachanlage 6, 91054 Erlangen, Germany.

CNS Disease

CNS diseases include the following:

- CNS trauma
- Tumors
- Vascular diseases
- Inflammatory diseases
- Degenerative and metabolic disease
- Malformations
- Diseases of the spine and spinal cord (common diagnostic problems)

CNS Trauma

In the acute phase, CNS trauma includes:

- Intracranial (extra-/intracerebral) hemorrhage
- Concussion/contusion/laceration
- Open/closed fractures

In the post-acute/chronic phase, it includes:

- Subacute/chronic hematoma
- Ventricular dilatation
- Ischemia/infarction
- Infection
- Cerebrospinal fluid fistula
- Seizures

In the acute phase the immediate, accurate and safe analysis of the intercranial situation, while maintining vital functions, is mandatory in order to decide whether or not surgery is necessary and, if so, where, what and how should be operated. In this phase CT is the method of choice because of its reliable demonstration of intercranial hemorrhage within less than 5 min. In the subacute and chronic phase, however, MRI is superior to CT because of its high soft tissue contrast, its lack of bone hardening artifacts, and the detection of hemosiderin deposits. This allows the evaluation of brain stem concussions, CSF fistulas, and seizures from superficial cortical injuries (Figs. 1, 2).

1 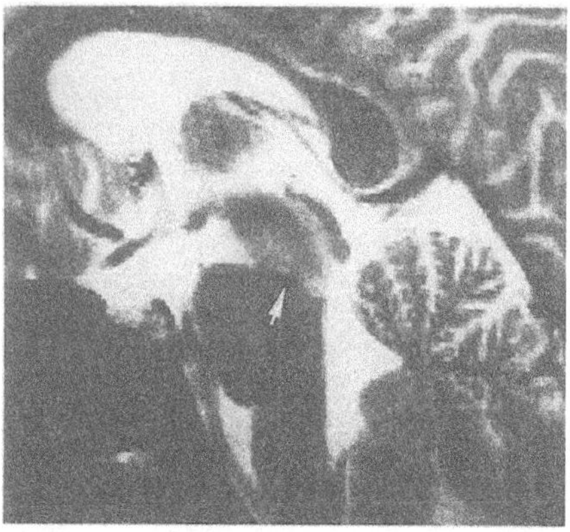

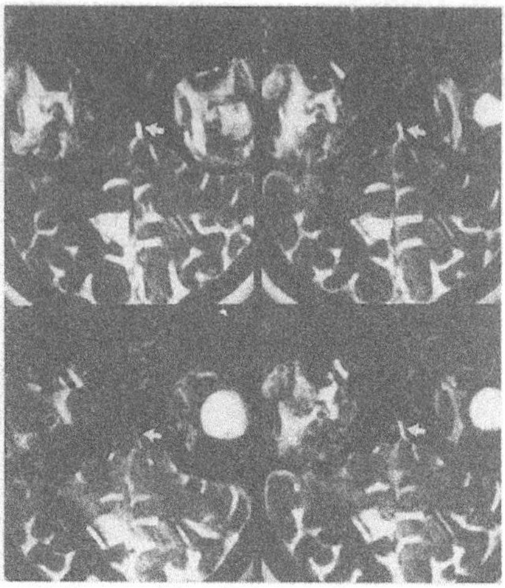 2

Fig. 1 Hemosiderin deposits (*arrow*) at the pontomesencephalic junction after hemorrhagic contusion of the brain stem causing internuclear ophthalmoplegia. T2 weighted midsaggital section

Fig. 2 Post-traumatic right frontobasal cerebrospinal fluid (CSF) fistula (*arrows*) not seen on CT cisternography with intrathecal contrast medium. Heavily T2 weighted three-dimensional sequence; coronal sections

Intracranial Tumors

Intracranial tumors include:

- Intra-axial tumors
- Extra-axial tumors
- tumors of the meninges and related tissues
- Metastases
- tumors of adjacent tissues (i.e., paranasal sinuses)

For the diagnosis of intracranial tumors, MRI is superior to CT when the early and detailed demonstration of the site, size, shape, and structure of a tumor has to be visualized, especially adjacent to bony structures (Fig. 3). However, when the calcification of tumor tissue or the invasion and destruction of bone is suspected, CT will be required to provide this complementary information.

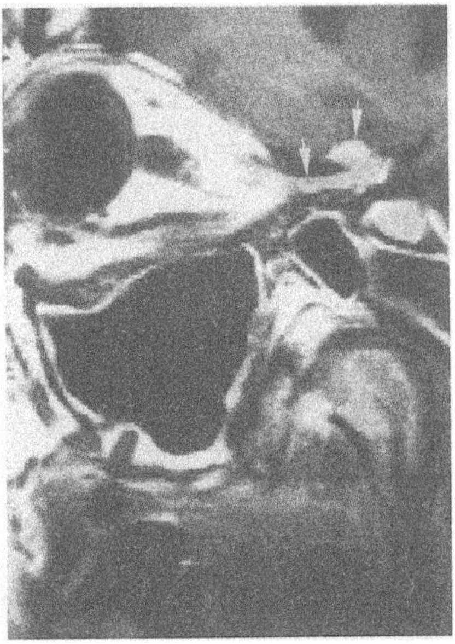

Fig. 3 Small meningioma at the entrance of the optic canal (*arrows*). Parasagittal T1 weighted section of 3-mm slice thickness after intravenous application of Gadolinium DTPA

Vascular Diseases

Vascular diseases include:

- Ischemia / stroke
- hemorrhage
- Intracranial aneurysms
- Vascular malformation (AVM, dural-AVM, cavernoma, venous anomaly)

For the demonstration of the sequelae of vascular disease in the early and late phase of the disease, MRI is superior to CT because of its increased potential to demonstrate early ischemic edema (Fig. 4) and the possibility of evaluating tissue perfusion and diffusion.

When the vascular tree and its pathological changes have to be evaluated, however, angiography is still the gold standard. On a noninvasive basis, however, MRI will give some information on the intravascular flow, which in the diagnosis of intracranial vascular thrombosis has already become part of the clinical routine. For the anlysis of the shape of intracranial aneurysms, MRI and CT with three-dimensional data acquisition and reconstruction are able to visualize details which are not demonstrated well enough on the projection images of conventional angiography (Fig. 5). Modern spiral CT is able to depict small intramural calcifications of sclerotic vascular stenosis, which is of major importance for the preoperative planning of endovascular balloon dilatatation (PTA-Fig. 6).

Fig. 4 Ischemic infarction of the right pons (*arrow*). T2 weighted axial section

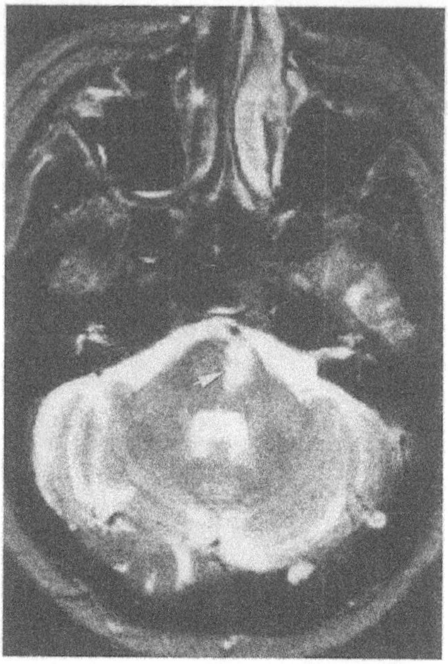

5 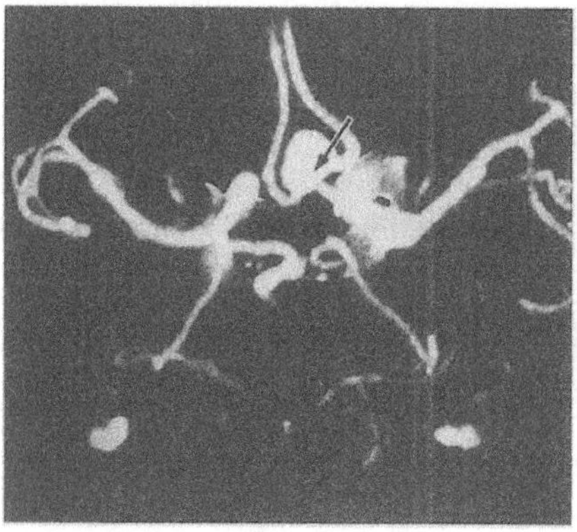

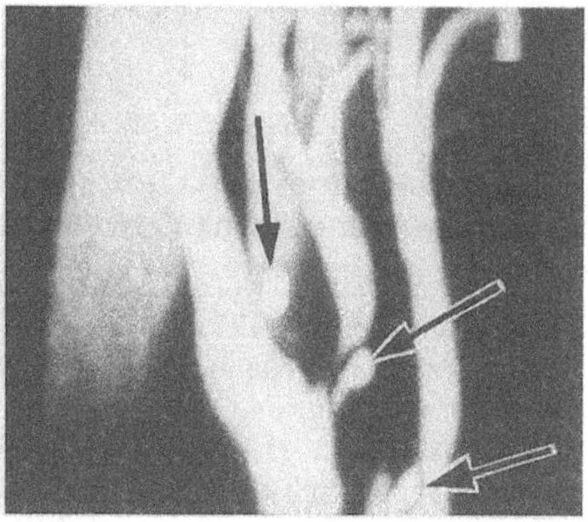 6

Fig. 5 Aneurysm of the left anterior communication artery (*arrow*) with wide neck excluding it from endovascular coil embolization. Three-dimensional maximum intensity projection (MIP) (spiral CT) after intravenous bolus injection of contrast medium

Fig. 6 Intramural calcifications (*arrows*) of a stenotic carotid bifurcation. Three-dimensional maximum intensity projection (MIP) (spiral CT) after the intravenous bolus injection of contrast medium

Inflammatory Disease

Inflammatory diseases include:

- Infection of the brain (bacterial, viral)
- Infections of the meninges (bacterial, viral)
- Parasitic infections
- Fungal infections

In this group of diseases, again, MRI is the method of choice because of its high soft tissue contrast, which enables an early detection of inflammatory edema; inflammatory changes of the dura adjacent to the bone are also more clearly seen because of the lack of bone-hardening artifacts. Associated calcifications can be identified more reliably with CT (Fig. 7a, b).

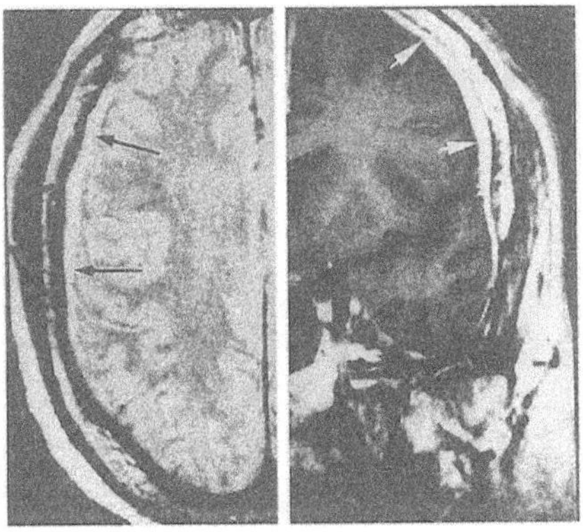

Fig. 7 a, b Lymphocytic infiltration of the dura in chronic meningitis. **a** PDW axial section without contrast medium. **b** T1 weighted coronal section after i.v. gadolinium-DTPA

Degenerative and Metabolic Diseases

Degenerative and metabolic diseases (inherited/acquired) include disorders:

- Of myelination
- Affecting primarily white matter (leukodystrophies, multiple sclerosis, intoxications)
- Affecting primarily gray matter (storage diseases, dementias, systemic degeneration, etc.)
- Affecting gray/white matter
- Affecting primarily basal ganglia

MRI again is the method of choice to analyze the pathological details of brain structures with a high resolution of contrast and space (Fig. 8).

8 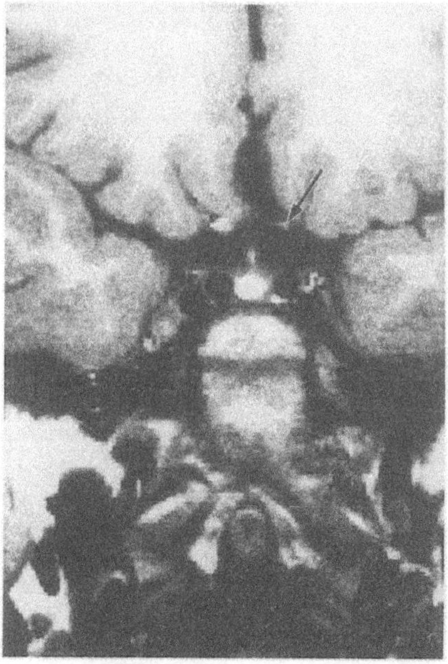

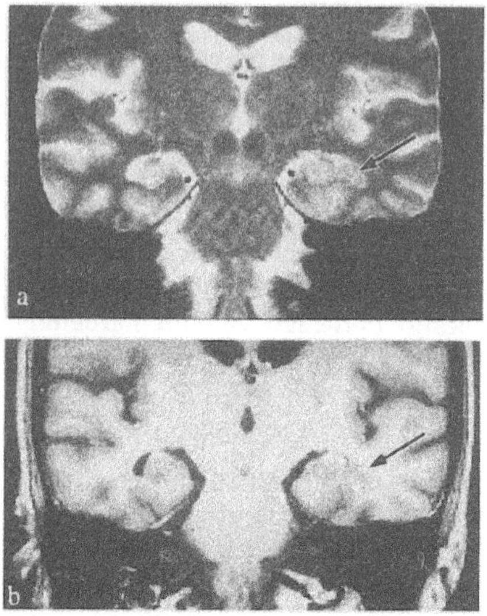

9

Fig. 8 Unilateral atrophy of the left optic nerve (*arrow*). T1 weighted coronal section

Fig. 9a, b Heterotopic gray matter (*arrows*) in the left temporal horn. Coronal sections. **a** T2 weighted. **b** T1 weighted without contrast medium

Congenital Malformations

Congenital malformations include:

- disorders of neural tube closure (e.g., Chiari I–III, cephaloceles), commissures and midline structures (e.g., holopresencephaly, aplasia of the corpus callosum), and, cell migration (e.g., ectopias, cortical dysplasias; Fig. 9a, b)
- Destructive anomalies (e.g., hydranencephaly, porencephaly, schizencephaly, etc.)
- Neuroectodermal dysplasias (e.g., neurofibromatosis, tuberous sclerosis, Sturge-Weber disease, etc.
- Miscellaneous anomalies (e.g., cysts, congenital hydrocephalus, macro-/microcephalus, etc.)

In congenital malformations a high spatial and contrast analysis of anatomical details in all three dimensions is needed, which is better provided by MRI than CT (Fig. 9a, b). Additional information about calcifications and/or details of associated changes of bone structures may require a CT examination.

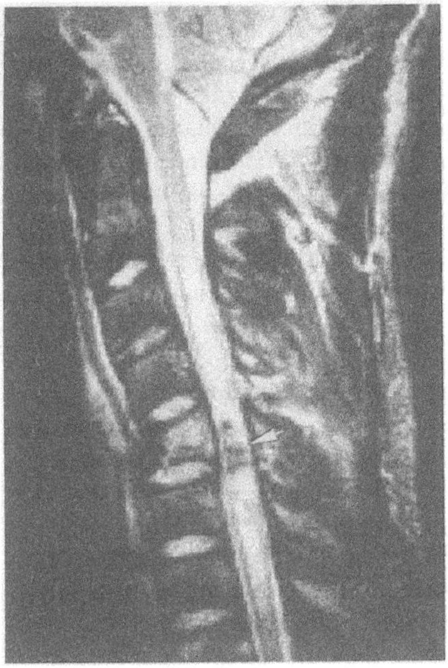
10

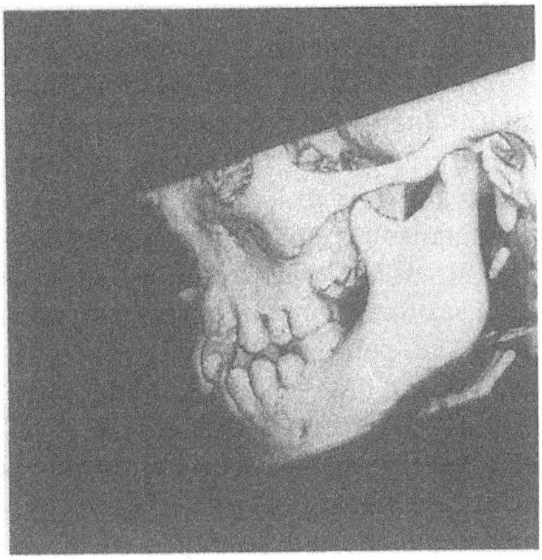
11

Fig. 10 Hemorrhagic contusion (*arrow*) and post-traumatic edema of the cervical cord; edema of the bone marrow of the fractured vertebra C5. T2 weighted midsagittal section

Fig. 11 Spiral CT of the skull. Three-dimensionl reconstruction of the facial bones

Spine and Spinal Cord

The same is true for all groups of diseases of the spine and spinal cord, where CT is limited to axial sections and is subject to bone artifacts. Whereas the bony structures of the vertebrae and also pathological changes of the vertebral disks can be evaluated by CT quite well, information about disorders of the spinal cord is not sufficient in most cases (Fig. 10).

Conclusion

When summarizing, it becomes obvious that the majority of diagnostic questions in diseases of the CNS can be answered by MRI. Thus MRI has replaced CT as the screening method of choice in patients with suspected neurological disease. CT is reduced to a few diagnostic situations where MRI is inferior to CT, such as acute head injury and the analysis of minute bony structures or three-dimensional reconstructions of the skull and spine (Fig. 11).

As far as the future of CT in neuroradiology is concerned, we must consider possible future developments of CT technology. Recent advances in CT were achieved with the spiral technique, which provides major advantages in the visualization of moving structures such as the heart, vessels, and abdominal organs and with the help of improved and fast three-dimensional reconstruction of vascular and bony structures. The high speed of spiral CT and the advanced manipulation of image data, however, have not yet produced a higher spatial and density resolution. The lack of true additional information is the reason why there are almost no publications to be found in the recent literature about the progress of CT in CNS disease.

Nevertheless, the high speed of spiral CT can be utilized for dynamic studies such as quantitative measurements of brain perfusion, and CT angiography offers further insight into vascular anatomy, which is helpful in the analysis of aneurysms or extracranial stenosis associated with coil embolization and PTA (percutaneous transluminal angioplasty), respectively (Figs. 5, 6).

MRI, on the other hand, will also advance to achieve faster image creation, open scanners with free access for patients and operators, MRI-guided interventions and perhaps intraoperative MRI, MRI flow studies (perfusion and diffusion), and functional MRI. Finally, image fusion is the merging of image data of MRI, digital subtraction angiography (DSA), magnetoencephalography (MEG), PET, SPECT – and perhaps more in the future – for the multidimensional analysis of the morphology and function of the diseased brain, thus enabling function-guided therapy and surgery.

In my opinion, the future of neuroimaging belongs to MRI if we compare the diagnostic potential of CT and MRI without economic limitations. However, besides these theoretical aspects, strong practical and economic factors will influence the fate of CT positively. For quite some time to come, CT will still be faster, much cheaper, and easier to handle than MRI; above all, it will remain the technique of choice in acute head injury. It is the best and only alternative to MRI to bring the benefits of modern imaging to a large number of patients in a short time at reasonable costs.

CT technology seems to be limited by the fact that its only parameter for creating tissue contrast is based on differences of radiodensity, which cannot be extended indefinitely. MRI is superior because it is able to utilize several physical phenomena for the improved visualization of the brain's morphology and function.

CHAPTER 8

Computed Tomography of the Head and Neck

Thomas J. Vogl, Wolfgang Steger, and Nico Hidajat[1]

Introduction

In clinical evaluation in the head and neck should start with clinical investigations, such as inspection and palpation. Imaging modalities include conventional X-ray, ultrasound, magnetic resonance tomography, computed tomography and digital substraction angiography as diagnostic and interventional methods. Pathological lesions that may need radiological methods for the evaluation of the exact diagnosis, are subdivided into congenital deformities, tumorous lesions, inflammatory disease, vascular disorders and traumatic lesions. This article is proposed to discuss the value of computed tomography in the evaluation of lesions in the head and neck.

Technical Parameters

In our institution CT examinations are performed using a Somatom Plus S scanner (Siemens, Germany). The tube voltage lies in a range of 80–220 kV, the current can be adjusted to maximally 300 mA. Possible foci are 1.3/1.2 mm or 0.7/0.9 mm using either 2.7-mm Al or a 0.2-mm Cu filter and a xenon detector. The slice thickness has to be adjusted on 1, 2, 5, 8 or 10 mm. The image matrix usually consists of 512 × 512 pixel or alternatively, 1024 × 1024 pixel.

Two different scan techniques are provided for the examination of the head and neck. In the *conventional CT*, the interesting region is recorded scan by scan. The scan time varies between 0.7 and 2 s, and the interscan time between 4 and 12 s. The *spiral CT* represents a new development of the recent years that gains great importance. In this technique, the X-ray tube is rotating while at the same time the table is moving. Scan duration lies between 12 and 40 s, table feed 1–20 mm/s. Due to the short scan time, the entire region can be examined in one single respiratory phase. Thus, respiratory-induced artifacts and gaps can be avoided. High flow contrast media application up to 4 ml/s allows dynamic examinations in combination with spiral CT. The high speed enables an optimal utilization and reduction of contrast media to one third to one half of the amount needed in conventional CT. Table feed, scan duration, start-delay after beginning the adminis-

[1] Department of Radiology, Clinic Rudolf Virchow, University of Berlin, Augustenburger Platz 1, 13353 Berlin, Germany.

tration of contrast media and injection flow are important parameters to be adjusted individually to gain optimal contrast of the interesting region.

Different postprocessing algorithms are provided to reconstruct the image matrix from the raw data. "Ultrahigh algorithms" are appropriate to visualize bony structures with high degree of accuracy, whereas "soft algorithms" are to be applied for the visualization of soft tissue. The last step of the imaging is the conversion of the X-ray densities quantified in Hounsfield Units (HU) in visible gray levels. For this, a "window" is adjusted interactively within the broad density spectrum (−1023 HU to 3072 HU) at the density range of the interesting tissue. This part of density spectrum is then projected into the maximal grey level spectrum. Thus, the display is dependent on the location and broadness of the window (soft tissue, bone and lung window).

Postprocessing algorithms allow reconstrucions of the scanned volume in further slice orientations. Three-dimensional visualization of the heads and neck is usually performed by applying two methods: The shaded surface display (SSD) for structures with high density as bones or vessels (Fig. 1), maximum intensity projection (MIP) especially for the representation of vessels similar to angiography.

Skull Base

Topography

The temporal bone, the bony basis of the middle skull base consists of four osseous parts: Tympanic cavity, mastoid, petrous and squamous segment.

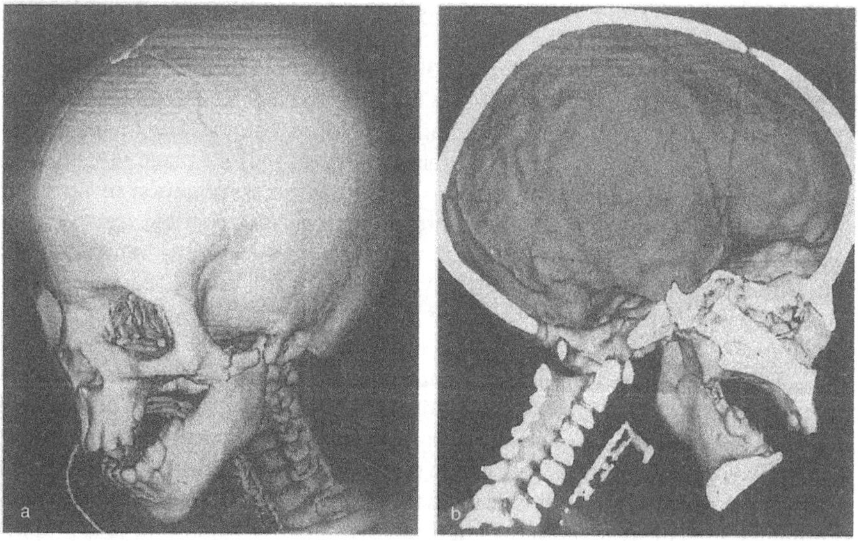

Fig. 1 **a** Three-dimensional reconstruction of the complete head and neck using a shading surface display (SSD) reconstruction algorithm and a threshold of 150 HE. **b** A postprocessing cut modus allows a view into the head

The tympanic cavity and the bony parts of the eustachian tube constitute the middle ear, which is bounded medially by the basal cochlea reduction and laterally by the tympanic membrane. Dorsally the tympanic cavity joins with the mastoid. The petrous segment contains the labyrinth, the internal carotid artery, as well al the VIIth and VIIIth cranial nerve. With the promontorium of the cochlea the petrous segment bounds laterally on the tympanic parts. The area of the temporal bone adjacent to the cerebrum constitues a part of the middle skull fossa and forms the anterolateral boundary of the posterior skull fossa. The upper parts of the posterior boundary of the temporal bone are formed by the squamous segment, which therefore, is located close to the facial canal and the mastoid.

Within the internal auditory canal and the cerebellomedullar cistern the facial nerve accompanies the superior and inferior vestibular part and the cochlear part of the vestibulocochlear nerve. In the region of the so called "Bill's bar" the facial nerve leaves the internal auditory canal toward the anterior. This course is called labyrinthian part and extends between the vestibule and the basal turn of the cochlea. At the genicular ganglion the nerve rectangularly turns off detaching the major petrous nerve. The following horizontal segment extends within the tympanic cavity to the external knee proceeding inside of the vertically positioned mastoid canal.

Pathology

The acoustic neuroma is histologically a benign neoplasm, which arises from Schwann cells of the neurilemma of the main branches of the vestibular nerve. It has its origin where the peripheral ganglionic neurilemma meets with the brainstemmneuroglia. In respect of the locus of origin acoustic neuromas are devided into lateral e.g., intrameatal growing tumors (Fig. 2), mediolateral and medial tumors.

Tumors of the glomus jugulare are second in numbers in this region and originate from chemoreceptors (glomera) which can have numerous localizations

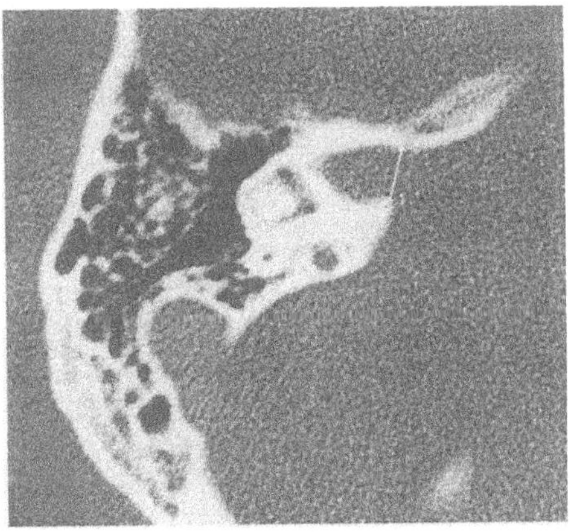

Fig. 2 A high-resolution CT of the right temporal bone shows the enlarged distance of the inner auditory canal (1), in which an acoustic neuroma is suspected. Note the regular pneumatization of the mastoid cells

throughout the human body. Histologically the tumors show precapillary arteriovenous shunts with a collection of nonchromaffin chemoreceptor cells. Most frequently the glomera in the bulbus venae jugularis are affected, as well as the tympanic plexus and the bifurcation of the carotids. The glomus tumors at the base of the skull are located in the region of the glossopharyngeal nerves extension (glomus tympanicum, jugulare and vagale).

The meningeoma of the middle skull base and the temporal bone is regarded as the third frequent tumor of this region. These clearly demarcated extraaxial tumors are located beside the convexity in the area of the sphenoid bone, the olfactory canal, the posterior skull fossa and close to cranial nerves. In difference to other tumors of the cerebellopontine angle meningeomas always show a wide contact to the pyramid and constitute a wide angle with the posterior area of the temporal bone. This fact represents the most important criterion to differentiate between meningeomas and acoustic neuromas in the majority of the patients. Acoustic neuromas show a small contact to the posterior area of the temporal bone. Based on this fact the angle between the posterior area of the temporal bone and the tumor shows wide for meningeomas and small acoustic neuromas. The majority of the meningeomas cause a demarcated exostosis of bone in the area of their origin.

The most frequent lesion of the apical pyramidal segment is the primary congenital cholesteatoma, showing a homogenous decreased density in CT. For the pretherapeutic diagnosis the exact relationship between the tumorous lesion and the facial nerve has to be documented via CT. In specific cases the pyramid apex is secondarily affected by tumors originating from surrounding structures like chordomas of the clivus, trigeminal neuromas, carcinomas of the middle ear and histiocytoses. Seldomly dermoid cysts, eosinophilic granulomas and other neoplastic structures may arise.

CT Examination

In the primary diagnostic protocol the clinical examination remains predominant as well as the performance of neuro-otological examinations (audiology, ERA, vestibular tests). Although, conventional X-ray technique (Schüller's and Stenvers's projection, konventionea tomography) provide the radiologist with low specific information, they can easily indicate processes especially in the area of the middle ear.

The examination of the temporal bone is mostly based on the use of computed tomography, in some cases combined with air cisternography for intracanalicular tumors. This technique, however, is restricted in the evaluation by a high ratio of false-positive findings ranging between 5% and 12%. The reasons for this misevaluation are soft tissue adhesions, arachnoidal cysts and abnormalities of the arachnoidal vessels like aneurysms or ectatic slings of the inferior cerebellar artery. Concerning cartilaginous and osseous structures CT is the modality of choice because of its excellent resolution. Especially the high resolution technique with slice thickness of 1 mm is important for the evalution of questions concerning the middle or inner ear (e.g., otosclerosis).

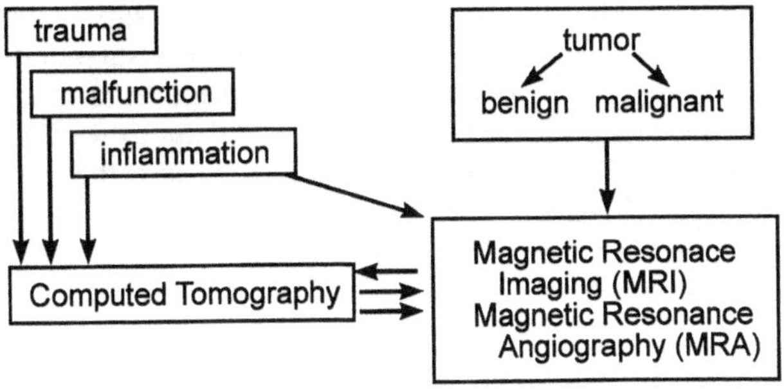

Fig. 3 Diagnostic evaluation: skull base/temporal bone

CT diagnosis was performed in order to fix the category and the expansion of glomus tumors. The high resolution technique in CT can prove the relationship to the cervical soft tissue as well as the intratympanic and intracranial expansion. In the majority of the cases glomus tumors can be differentiated from other skull base diseases by dynamic CT, that is performing several scans without table feed, and the time density profile.

For routine examinations the slice thickness should be 2 or 5 mm. The intravenous administration of iodinated contrast media (e.g., 150 ml, 1 ml/s flow, 15 s delay) improves the visualization of vessels and the detectability of tumorous and inflammatory diseases. Polytraumatic patients should be scanned in spiral technique to reduce the examination time. Limitations of CT are due to artifacts between bone and soft tissue at the skull base and to unsatisfactory differentiation of soft tissues, so that an additional MRI examination can be necessary (Fig. 3).

Orbita

Topography

The bony orbit is formed by the lacrimal, palatine, zygomatic, maxillary, ethmoid, sphenoid and frontal bone. The orbital septum (fibrous sheath lined by periosteum) forms a pre- and postseptal compartment, influencing the spread of infection.

The ophthalmic sensory nerve (N-V1) and its branches (lacrimal, frontal, nasociliary) arise from the trigeminal ganglion and pass through the superior orbital fissure into the orbit. The oculomotor nerve (N-III) also traversing the superior orbital fissure is mainly responsible for eye movements of extraocular muscles except the superior oblique and lateral rectus muscles. The trochlear nerve (N-IV) innervating the superior oblique muscle arises in the dorsal part of central nervous system and crosses the superior orbital fissure too. The abducens nerve (N-VI) supplies only the lateral rectus muscle. Intraconal attachment is reached through the superior orbital fissure accompanied by the superior ophthalmic vein. The optic nerve (N-II) as part of the white matter is surroundet by three meningeal layers containing the sclera at the posterior globe. In an sinous intraconal course medially and backward toward the orbital apex the nerve is passing the optic canal accompanied by the ophthalmic artery into the middle cranial fossa to reach the optic chiasm.

The superior ophthalmic vein, the largest and mainly visualized intraorbital vein, passes serpenginous from the trochlea to the apex and the superior orbital fissure to drain with the supraorbital and angular veins into the cavernous sinus. The ophthalmic artery arising from internal carotid artery traverses the optic canal with the optic nerve caudally located.

The motion of the eye is coordinated by six skeletal extraocular muscles. All four rectus muscles (superior, inferior, lateral, medial) arise from a tendinous ring (annulus of Zinn) forming a cone. The superior oblique muscle, the largest muscle, is supplied by the trochlear nerve, the rectus lateralis m. by the abducens nerve, all others by the oculomotor nerve. The inferior oblique muscle is the only one not to arise from the orbital apex but from orbital plate of the maxilla nearby the nasolacrimal duct.

Pathology

Pathological lesions include tumors like the retinoblastoma, the melanoma, the optic glioma (Fig. 4), intraorbital metastasis, inflammatory lesions, usually as a result of spread from adjacent structures, and traumatic lesions with fractures of the bony orbital frame. A lesion at the chiasm level classically produces a bitemporal hemianopsia or heteronymous field defects. After crossing of the fibers the information is guided over the lateral geniculate bode to the visual cortex called optic radiation (retrochiasmal part). Injuries to the visual pathway usually create homonymous hemianopsia.

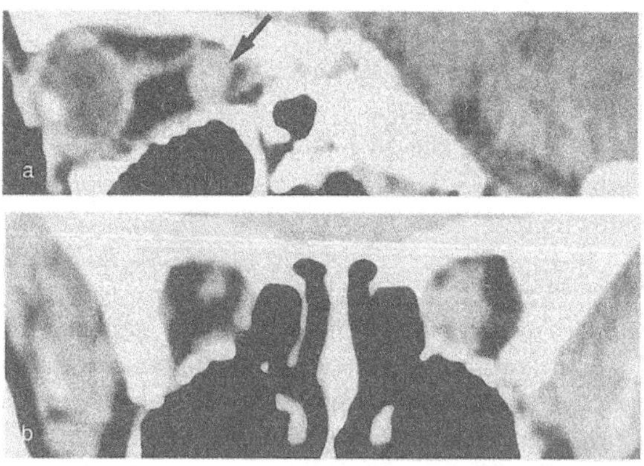

Fig. 4 **a** A sagittal reconstruction after axial CT examination visualizes a homogenous tumorous mass (*arrow*) of about 1 cm in diameter deriving from the optic nerve. **b** In a coronal orientation the tumor, which proved to be an optic glioma, cannot be differentiated from the optical nerve and the medial rectus muscle

CT Examination

CT enables an accurate visualization of the bony structures of the orbit as well as the ophthalmic muscles, the eyeball and the retroorbital fat. Slice thickness should be not more than 2 mm. The CT examination has got its indication in finding intraorbital foreign bodies and evaluation of traumatic changes. It is often necessary to gain axial and coronal sections, for example to evaluate the papyraceous lamina and the floor of the orbit, respectively. The radiation exposure of the radiosensitive eye lens can be quantified to approximately 3.2 cGy and is thus far below the threshold of radiogenous cataract of 150 cGy.

Nasopharynx and Face

Topography

The nasopharynx represents the upper part of the pharynx and is continuously connected with the nasal cavity ventrally. The roof is formed by the sphenoid bone, caudally the anatomic margin of the nasopharynx is situated at the level of the soft palate. These anatomical relationships are well demonstrated on sagittal and coronal slices. The pharyngeal recess (fossa of Rosenmueller) extends laterally in direction to the parapharyngeal space (PPR), directly neighboured to the opening of the eustachian tube. This region is often the origin of malignant neoplasms. The posterior part of the eustachian tube forms the cartilagenous torus tubarius. Laterally, the levator veli palatini muscle is to be delineated. This muscle forms, in connection with the pharyngobasilar fascia, the margin to the PPR. The PPR, which is separated from the nasopharynx by the pharyngobasilar fascia is a commen compartment of extension of nasopharyngeal neoplasms. The PPR is a fat filled, triangle space, bordered anterolaterally by the pterygoid muscles and posterolaterally by the parotid gland. Medially, the PPR is bordered by the levator and tensor veli palatini muscles. Caudally, the PPR extends to the oropharynx where it continuously leads to the digastric space. The PPR is divided into two compartments, the margin of both is formed by the styloid process. The posterior PPR (carotid space) contains the internal carotid artery, the internal jugular vein, as well as the cranial nerves IX to XII and lymphatic tissue. In this region, metastatic or inflammatory changed lymphnodes are commonly found. Laterally, the infratemporal fossa is seen, which is bordered by the maxillary sinus and the zygomatic arch and which is divided into masticator space and parotid space.

The walls and the roof of the nasopharynx are coated with lymphatic tissue. In case of hypertrophia the extension of this tissue may lead to obstruction of the tube opening and to hearing loss.

The parenchyma of the parotid gland appears to be of similar density compared to muscles. Most important anatomical structures are directly neighboured to the parotid gland and masseter muscle, the facial vein and artery as well as the retromandibular vein. The facial nerve leaves the skullbase at the stylomastoid foramen and passes through a small amount of fat before entering the parotid gland. The main trunk courses lateral to the retromandibular vein and external carotids artery or between these two structures and divides into two major branches at the posterior margin of the mandibular ramus.

The paranasal sinuses are air-filled cavities surrounded by margins of bone. The bony margins of the nose and the paranasal sinuses are cranially formed by the ethmoid bone; caudally the nose is bordered by the hard palate. The thinnest bone lies along the posteromedial boundary of the antrum. At times, this very thin area is spoken of as the membranous wall of the antrum. The infraorbital nerve, artery and vein can be found in a groove in the posterior partion of the root of the antrum. This groove becomes a canal anteriorly and later exists to the check as a foramen.

Pathology

Inflammatory changes of the nose and paranasal sinuses are commonly accidental findings in MRI examinations of the head. As a result of acute or chronical sinusitis hyperplasia of the mucosa, polyposis, retentioncysts, or mucoceles must be differentiated. The nasopharynx and the tonsil region are frequent localisation of lymphoid hyperplasia in the head and neck region. In children this disease is commonly seen, causing breath disturbances. In adults these hyperplasias are often found in patients suffering from chronic infections, such als HlV-positive patients.

A total of 5% of all malignat tumors of the head and neck region arise in the naso- and oropharynx, of which 90% histologically prove to be carcinomas. The most frequent type of malignant tumors in the pharynx are squamous cell carcinomas (Fig. 5) and lymphoepithelial neoplasms. Lymphomas however are more frequent in children. A characteristic of these tumors is the early and extensive lymphatic metastisis. Benign tumors in the pharynx are seldom, the most numerous being the juvenile angiofibroma of the nasopharynx. In spite of this fibroma being benign histologically, it clinically shows malignancy through its expansive growth. Mesenchymal tumors are mostly represented in the group of the benign tumors of the nose and the nasal sinuses. They are made up of papillomas, hemangiomas, fibromas and other seldom tumors. Histologically the gross collective can be divided into squamous cell carcinomas (60%), adenocarcinomas (20%), differentiated carcinomas (10%) and mesenchymal neoplasms.

CT Examination

The CT of the facial part of the skull base can be applied for the evaluation of traumatic and inflammatory lesions, postoperative complications as well as tumorous diseases of the nasopharynx, paranasal sinus and parotid diseases. The paranasal sinus is very well evaluable with CT because of the great density differences between air, bony structures and tumor. Compared with MRI CT allows a better evaluation of bony arrosions and destructions such as those in a chronic sinusitis. CT also gets a high sensitivity in the detection of descrete marginal and circular shadows as well as polypoid changes of the mucosa of the paranasal sinus.

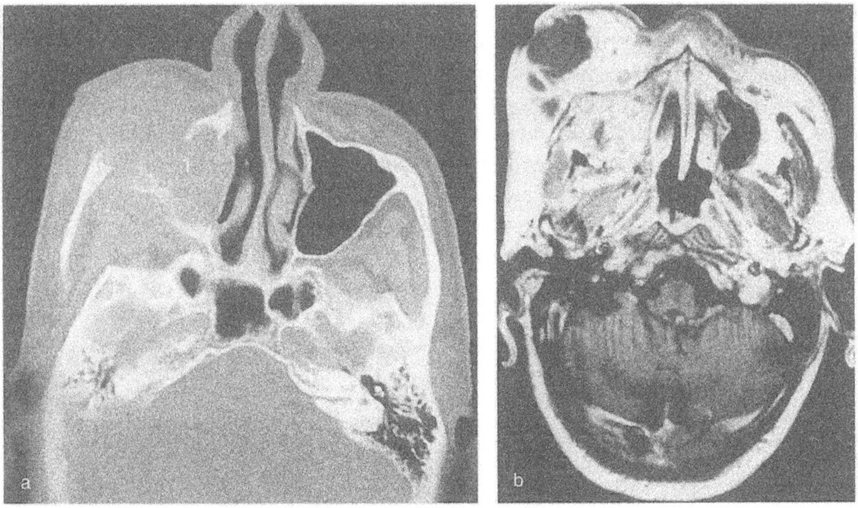

Fig. 5 **a** This transverse CT image shows a squamous cell carcinoma of the right maxillary sinus (*1*), which has already destroyed the anterior sinus wall and parts of the zygomatic bone. **b** The corresponding magnetic resonance (MR) image documents the contrast media enhancement of the tumor and a large necrotic part ulcerating the skin

The examination is usually performed with voltage of 120 kV and current of 100 mA. The slice thickness should be between 2 mm for the evaluation of thin structures like osseous lamella or 5 mm for the evaluation of bigger soft tissues. The scanned region should extend from the skull base and the roof of the orbit to the hard palate and the maxillary teeth. In contrast to most regions of the body, the facial part of the skull requires frontal sections, because in this orientation horizontally coursing osseous structures of the cranial fossa, the hard palate and the osteomeatal complex are best evaluable. Additional axial sections are required to evaluate a possible tumorous infiltration of the spheno-ethmoid recess or the papyraceous lamina. Alternatively, the CT scan is performed in one orientation followed by a reconstruction of the other orientation. This method shortens the examination time for the patient, but detailed anatomic information can be lost due to reduced resolution. Reconstructions are mostly sufficient to represent the extension of lesions in craniocaudal direction.

As a general principle, the application of iodinated contrast media is recommended for better differentiation between normal and pathologic structures. Initially, an amount of approximately 30 ml should be administered in 30 s applying a power injector. In the conventional CT a total amount up to 200 ml can be needed. Sprial CT enables a distinct reduction to one third to one half of the amount needed by conventional CT. The contrast enhancement leads to a reliable visualization of tumorous lesions and both arterial and venous vessels.

In comparison with MRI, CT requires much less examination time and is therefore less strenous for patients. Therefore CT is an ideal diagnostic tool für the documentation of interventions like punctation in order to gain histologic information (Fig. 6). Additionally, CT enables an excellent visualization of osseous and cartilaginous changes. A malignant tumor leads to an arrosion, whereas a benign process leads to a chronic elevation of the pressure thinning out osseous lamella. Besides, CT enables the analyses of a possible tumorous involvement of lymph nodes, especially jugulodigastric in the region of the angle of mandible that is frequently involved. Artifacts of metall in the region of the teeth considerably reduce the detectability of details. Another limitation of CT consists in the inability of many patients to hyperextend their head to gain frontal sections. In such cases, primary nuclear magnetic resonance (NMR) examination is recommended, as it enables acquisitions in different planes without moving the patient (Fig. 7).

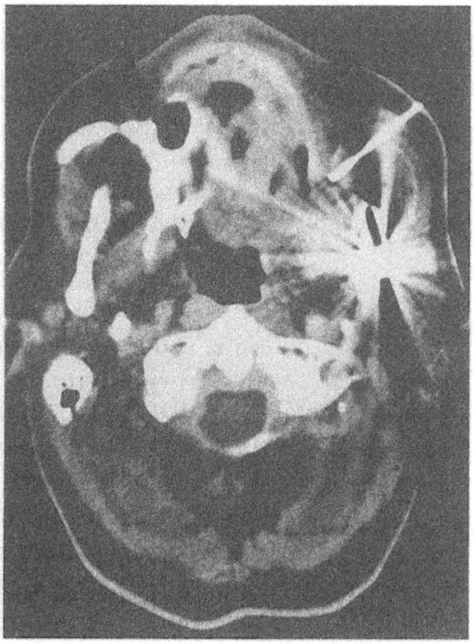

Fig. 6 Documentation of a punction needle extending from the left cheek into a recurrent tonsillar carcinoma on the left side. Artifacts from the mandible derive from a plastic reconstruction after the initial surgery

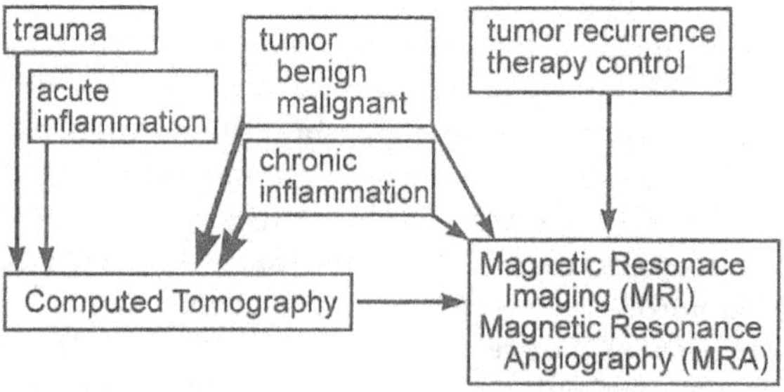

Fig. 7 Diagnostic evaluation: nose/paranasal sinuses

Oropharynx and Oral Cavity

Topography

The oral cavity and the body of the tongue are delineated by the hard and the soft palate cranial and on imagined horizontal line extending the back of the tongue caudal. The tonsils and the parapharyngeal space figure the lateral borders of the oral cavity. Although the tonsills are of low size, tumors likely spread beyond this area, because the soft tissue between the cavity and the skull base does not offer any resistance. The oropharyngeal space posterior to the tongue figures the third topographic area. It is delineated by the floor of the mouth with mylohyoid and geniohyoid muscles anterior and the glosso-epiglottic folds involving the valleculae caudal. The posterior border of the whole oropharynx is represented by the constictor pharyngeal muscle with its superior, medial and inferior part.

The paired submandibular glands are located beneath the mouth floor in the submandibular trigonum borded by the diagastric muscle and the mandible. The main portion of the submandibular gland is indented by the lingual artery along its lateral border and the common facial vein along its posterolateral border. The excretory duct originates from the anteromedial border of the gland and courses over the posterior surface of the mylohyoid muscle. It lies adjacent to the floor of the mouth, until it reaches the region of the frenulum of the tongue where it finally exits through a small papilla. The sublingual glands can be identified between mandible and tongue neighboured to the mylohyoid muscle lateral to the genohyoid/genioglossus muscle complex. The lingual and hypoglossal nerves pass close enough to the submandibular and sublingual glands to become potential pathways of perineural extension. The signal characteristics and the contrast medium dynamic are similar to that of the parotid gland.

Pathology

The oral cavity and oropharynx are parts of the aerodigestive system, whose passage is of vital importance. Inspite of the fact that benign tumors appear seldomly, all forms of neoplasms can occur in the region of the oropharynx and the oral cavity. Frequent epithelial benign neoplasms are papillomas, keratocarcinomas and adenomas. Congenital tumors are usually the hemangioma, lymphangioma and the goiter in the base of the tongue. The vast majority of malignomas in the oral cavity and the oropharynx are squamous cell carcinomas, more seldom anaplastic carcinomas. In the development of carcinomas in the oral cavity the symptomatic is strikingly minor. Inspection, palpation and endoscopy are important clinical examination techniques for the diagnosis of structures in this region. Imaging methods are indicated to grasp the exact extension in depth and the infiltration into neighboring structures.

The salivary glands may be divided into the parotid, submandibular and sublingual glands. Epithelial tumors present 90% of all salivary gland neoplasms. The remaining tumors are distributed among nonepithelial neoplasms such as hemangiomas, lymphangiomas, periglandular tumors and malignant lymphomas. A total of 85% of the benign epithelial tumors are pleomorph or monomorph adenomas. Cystic adenolymphomas (Whartin tumor) and other tumors are essentially less numerous. Malignomas of the salivary glands develop in 25%–30% of all tumors and often show a typical symptomatic with growth, pain, firm infiltration and facial paresis. Histologically acinus cell tumors are found in 15% of all cases and mucoepidermoid tumors in 30%. Carcinomas histologically show a broad variation. In a row of decreasing frequency are: adenoid cystical carcinomas (35%), adenocarcinomas (10%), squamous cell carcinoma (10%) and other seldom tumors.

CT Examination

The CT examination of the oropharynx and the oral cavity is based on the same principles as descrebed in the "nasopharynx" chapter. But as artifacts of the teeth are existent in most cases, the detectability of details is clearly reduced. Therefore, MRI gas got a greater importance in the examination of the oropharynx than CT, especially in the analysis of tumorous infiltration. Nevertheless, CT is obligatory in the evaluation of a possible infriltration of the mandible.

A special kind of examination is the so called "dental CT" as a preoperative modality before dental implants. This examination yields spiral CT using a slice thickness of 2 mm, table feed of 2 mm and an increment of 1 mm. The ultra high scan modus allows a visualization of subtle bony structures, which are reconstructed in a special sagittal postprocessing algorithm.

Larynx, Hypopharynx, and the Neck

Topography

The hypopharynx reaches from the oropharynx cranial to the supraglottic larynx caudal. Its cranial borders are the free margin of the epiglottis in the median line and the pharyngo-epiglottic folds laterally forming the valleculae epiglotticae. The preepiglottic space lies ventral the epiglottis and is filled with fatty tissue. The left and right piriform sinus form the posterior pharyngeal wall and the esophagus in their cranial/caudal growth.

The larynx is subdivided into a supraglottic, glottic and a subglottic part. The supraglottic part reaches from the false cords cranial to the true cords caudal. Ventrally it is delineated by the thyroid laminae and the thyroid notch, the aryepiglottic folds form the lateral and dorsal borders. The glottic part of the larynx contains the true cords with the vocal muscles and the laryngeal ventricle. The ventral and dorsal connection of the true cords are called anterior and posterior commisure. The cords are moved by intrinsic and extrinsic laryngeal muscles (e.g., cricoarythanoid muscle, thyreoarythaenoideus muscle) which are fixed on the arythaenoid cartilages. These small cartilages are connected with the cricoid cartilage caudal, which forms the passage to the subglottic part of the larynx. The caudal notch of the cricoid cartilage bounds the laryngeal anatomic topography and continues as trachea.

The main function of the larynx is to act as a sphincter rather than as an organ for producing sound. Keeping this function in mind simplifies an understanding of the anatomic physiology of the larynx. In addition to its role as a sphincter, the larynx is involved in respiration, deglutition and phonation.

The neck is defined as the anatomic region of the body located below a horizontal plane defined by the lower margin of the mandible and the superior nuchal line of the occipital bone. The lower margin of the neck is a horizontal plane defined by the suprasternal notch and the top of the first thoracic vertebral body. Fascial planes divide the neck into multiple compartments. For the interpretation of transverse images it is useful to define three anatomic compartments: visceral, posterior and lateral.

The visceral compartment of the neck is the most anterior and contains structures of the aerodigestive tract including the larynx, trachea and esophagus. The thyroid and parathyroid glands also lie within the visceral compartment. Sternocleidomastoid and pharyngeal constrictor muscles form the lateral and posterior boundaries, respectively, of the visceral compartment. The posterior compartment of the neck includes the cervical vertebrae, posterior extensor muscles, and anterior flexor muscles, including the scalenes, longus capiti and longus colli muscles. The lateral compartments of the neck contain the carotid sheaths.

Pathology

Malignant tumors of the hypopharynx most frequently originate in the piriform sinus, less frequently on the posterior wall of the pharynx. In over 40% of all cases the primary symptom of these tumors is a regional metastasis of laterocervical lymph nodes.

Benign as well as malignant tumors of the larynx show characteristic clinical findings, especially when they originate from the glottis level. Frequent benign neoplasms are polyps of the vocal cords, chondromas, papillomas and atypical mucosa of the voice box. The malignant carcinoma of the larynx is the most frequent among the head and neck tumors representing 45%. The result of clinical laryngoscopy lays the base for further therapeutical action such as operation, radiation therapy, or chemotherapy. In many patients imaging techniques such as CT or MRI have established themselves for the judgement of the primary tumors and the involvment of lymph nodes.

In adults, a wide variety of different causes must be considered in cervical swellings. Besides unspecific or specific lymphadenopathies, lateral and medial cervical cysts, tumors of vascular and neurogen origin, soft tissue calcification (Fig. 8) lipomas and hypertrophy of the thyroid gland have to be regarded as benign causes of neck tumors. In the diagnostic evaluation of cervical swellings, a thorough physical examination, including inspection and palpation, is absolutely mandatory. In many cases, physical examination and the patient's history will already enable the physician to establish the diagnosis.

CT Examination

Main indications for a CT examination of the hypopharynx, larynx, and the neck are tumorous and traumatic lesions as well as postoperative complications. Compared with MRI, CT enables a better detectability of osseous and cartilaginous arrosions and destructions. Moreover CT examination is shorter and therefore less strenous for patients, especially those who are not cooperative. This shorter examination time reduces the number of movement artifacts and represents a greater advantage for patients with malignant tumorous in T4 stage. Usually, the scan procedure is performed in craniocaudal direction form the skull base to the inlet of the thorax. Slice thickness should lie in the range of 2 mm and 5 mm. Coronar reconstructions of axial sections can be useful to evaluate the extent of different lesions. In special cases concerning the laryngeal skeleton, high resolution CT with slice thickness of 1 mm is often recommendable (Fig. 9).

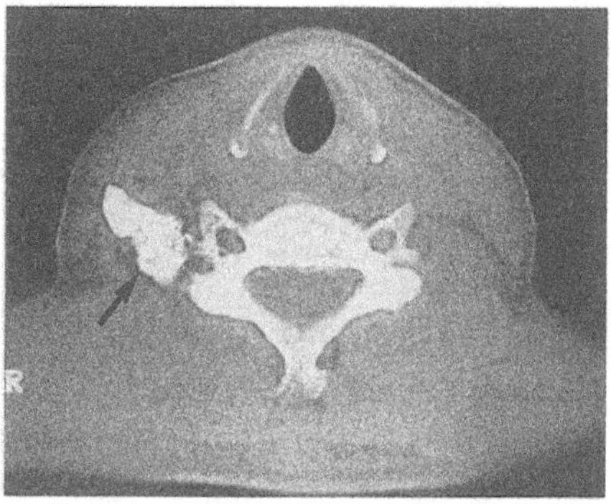

Fig. 8 Paravertebral calcification (*arrow*) in the cervical soft tissue at a subglottic level

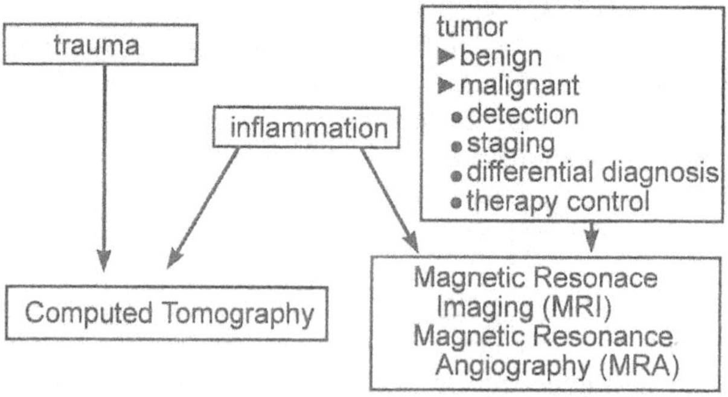

Fig. 9 Diagnostic evaluation: oropharynx, hypopharynx, larynx, and neck

CT Angiography

CT angiography is performed using a tube voltage of 120 kV and current of 165 mAs spiral CT examination. Choosing a slice thickness of 2 mm and a table feed of 4 mm a scanning volume of approximately 16 cm is enabled, extending from the skull base to the thoracic inlet along the course of the carotid arteries. After the spiral duration of 40 s, 2 mm sections have to be reconstructed with an increment of 1 mm; 120 ml iodinized contrast media should be performed with a flow of 4 ml/s and 15 s delay. CT angiography is an excellent diagnostic tool for the evaluation of the degree of stenosis and the extent of calcification. Concerning the diagnosis of calcification MIP reconstructions after CT examination showed best correlation to plain CT slices referring to lenghth and thickness (Fig. 10).

Competitive imaging methods such as color-coded duplex-sonography (ccds) can not prove mild stenosis (<30%), and in patients with sonographically suspected total occlusion vessel perfusion can be documented with CT angiography. MR angiography leeds to an overestimation in patients with high graded stenoses compared to the degree of stenosis obtained via ccds and CTA. CTA with MIP reconstructions is an excellent screening method and, in combination with ccds, CT angiography may replace digital subtraction angiography (DSA) before surgery or intervention.

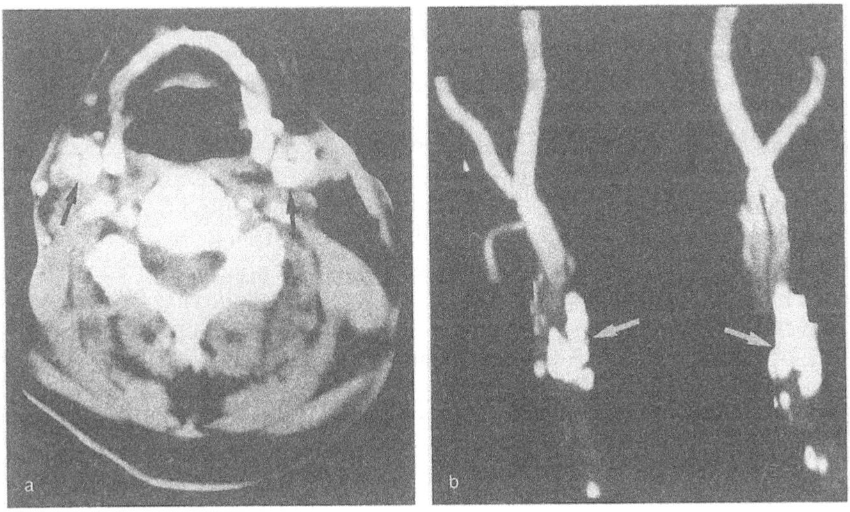

Fig. 10 **a** Circular calcification of both common carotid arteries (*arrows*) at a hypopharyngeal level. **b** CT angiography of the carotid arteries using a maximum intensity projection (MIP) reconstruction algorithm. Note the calcified plaques in the carotid bifurcation on both sides (*arrows*)

CHAPTER 9

High-Resolution Computed Tomography of Lung Diseases with Lucent Areas or Cysts

Chen Qihang, Pan Jixu and Li Guozhen[1]

High-resolution computed tomography (HRCT) is a technique that has excellent spatial resolution, and allows demonstration of the fine structure of the lung. Recently, HRCT has been very helpful in detecting and characterizing interstitial diseases or diffuse infiltrative lung diseases. We found it to be valuable in diagnosing lung disases characterized by the presence of decreased attenuation areas or cystis opacity. They include emphysema, bronchiectasis, pulmonary histiocytosis X, lymphangiomyomatosis, end-stage fibrotic disease.

Emphysema

Emphysema is defined as "a condition of the lung characterized by permanent abnormal enlargement of air spaces distal to the terminal bronchioles, accompanied by destruction of their walls, without obvious fibrosis" [1]. Emphysema is usually classified into three types: centrilobular, panlobular and paraseptal, based on the anatomic distribution of the areas of lung destruction.

Centrilobular Emphysema. This is the most common type and is often associatied with cigarrette smoking. The parenchymal destruction typically starts in the central portion of the pulmonary lobule. On HRCT, the typical findings of centrilobular emphysema are multiple small round low attenuation areas without visible walls (Fig. 1) [2, 3]. These lucent areas are usually upper lung predominant. When emphysema becomes more extensive, areas of low lucency become confluent and involve most or all of the lobule, is difficult or impossible to distinguish centrilobular emphysema from panlobular emphysema.

Panlobular Emphysema. This is less common. It may be associated with α-1-antitrypsin deficiency, and is often found in elderly people. Pathologically, there is dilatation of the entire air space distal to the terminal bronchiole. On HRCT, it appears as widespread areas of low attenuation with few vascular markings [4]. It usually predominates in the lower lobes or has diffuse distribution. The small focal lucent areas that are usually seen in centrilobular emphysema are not typically seen in this type.

---

[1] Department of Radiology, Beijing Hospital, Beijing, China.

1 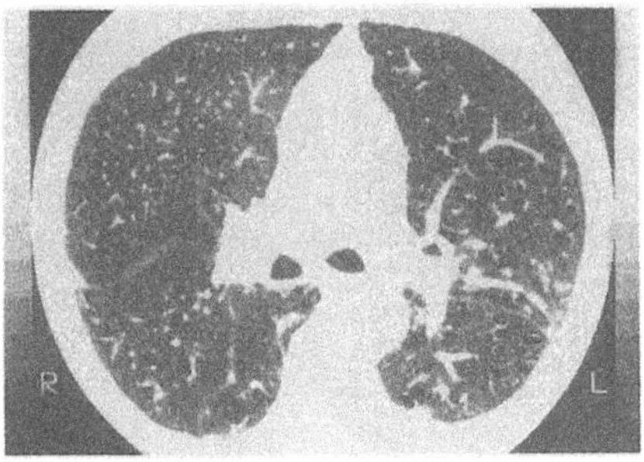

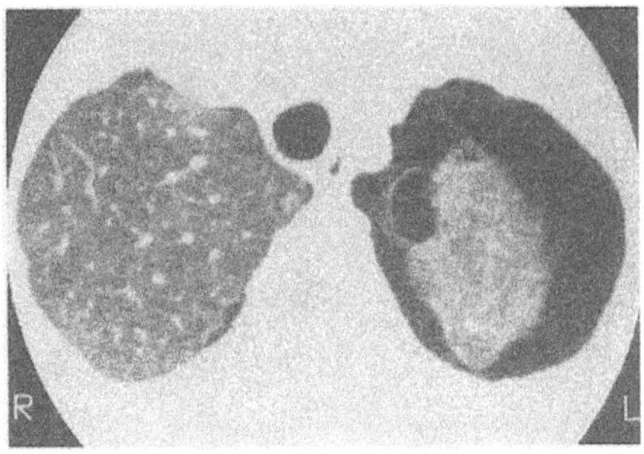 2

Fig. 1 Centrilobular emphysema. High-resolution computed tomography (HRCT) shows bilateral multifocal small lucencies that surround arteries in the lobular core, without visible walls

Fig. 2 Paraseptal emphysema in a 19-year-old man. High-resolution computed tomography (HRCT) shows left pneumothorax, multiple small subpleural cysts and bullae through lung apices

Paraseptal Emphysema. This is more common. It is often the cause of spontaneous pneumothorax in young adults and often occurs in association with centrilobular emphysema. It involves the distal part of the pulmonary lobule and demonstrates overexpansion of air spaces adjacent to the pleural. HRCT shows the bullae or air cysts of the subpleural region with very thin walls. HRCT is useful in the early detection of apical subpleural bullae in young adults with idiopathic spontaneous pneumothorax (Fig. 2) [5].

HRCT is the most sensitive imaging modality and has a high specificity for diagnosing emphysema. Correlation between HRCT findings and pathologic findings in patients with emphysema is excellent. On HRCT, emphysema can easily be distinguished from cystic air spaces and honeycombing by the absence of any visible walls.

Bronchiectasis. Bronchiectasis is characterized by a permanent abnormal dilatation of the medium-sized cartilaginous bronchi. Reid divided bronchiectasis into three types based on pathologic and bronchographic findings: cylindrical, varicose and cystic [6]. Bronchiectasis usually results from infection. The other possible initiating factors include inhaled chemical toxins or immunoactive substances, bronchial obstruction and parenchymal traction on bronchi [7].

Bronchiectasis may be focal or diffuse. The lower lobes are the commonest sites of bronchiectasis, especially the left lower lobe. Each type of bronchiectasis has a characteristic appearance on HRCT. Cylindrical bronchiectasis shows smooth bronchial dilatation which is recognized as "tram tracks" when oriented horizontally to the scan plane. When oriented vertically or obliquely to the section, it gives the appearance of a "signet ring" (Fig. 3) with a large, round, thickwalled, air-containing structure (dilated bronchi) accompanied by a smaller round density (normal size accompanying pulmonary artery) [8, 9]. Varicose bronchiectasis results in a similar appearance, except that the dilated bronchi have an irregular, beaded contour (Fig. 4). Cystic bronchiectasis results in more grossly enlarged

3 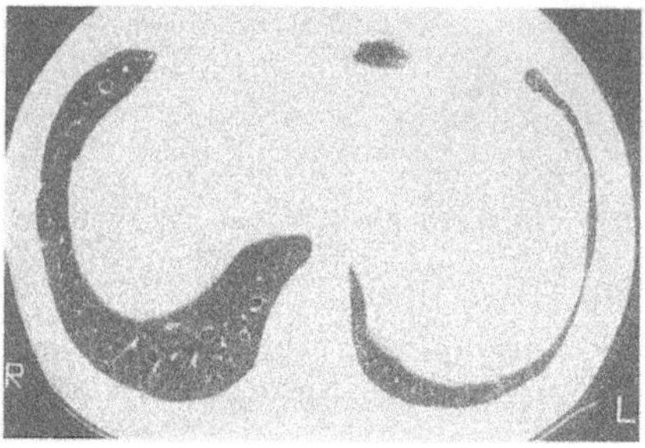

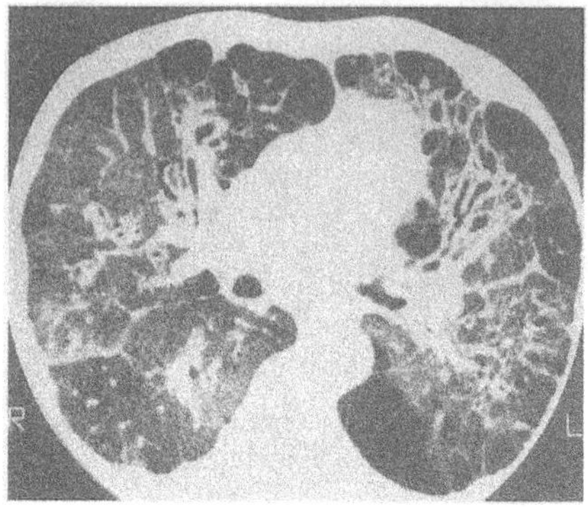 4

Fig. 3 Cylindrical bronchiectasis. High-resolution computed tomography (HRCT) shows typical "signet ring" sign in right lung base

Fig. 4 Varicose bronchiectasis. Dilated bronchi show irregular or beaded contour on High-resolution computed tomography (HRCT)

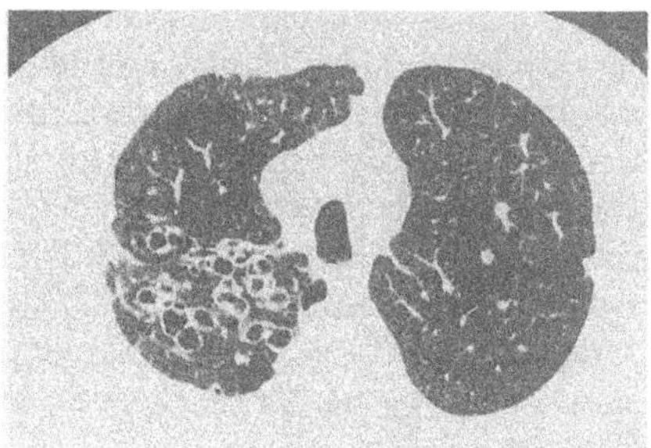

Fig. 5 Cystic bronchiectasis. High-resolution computed tomography (HRCT) image through the upper lung level shows appearance of a cluster of cysts with thicker walls

cystic spaces. They may show a string or cluster of cysts (Fig. 5). Airfluid levels within the dilated bronchi are specific sign of cystic bronchiectasis.

Routine chest radiography has a low sensitivity for diagnosing bronchiectasis. The sensitivity of conventional CT is 60%–80%. However, Grenier et al. confirmed a sensitivity of 97% and a specificity of 93% using HRCT [10]. HRCT is the procedure of choice for diagnosing bronchiectasis. Bronchography is no longer routinely performed in the evaluation of patients with possible bronchiectasis, unless surgery is being considered.

Pulmonary Histiocytosis X

Pulmonary histiocytosis X (also known as pulmonary eosinophilic granuloma) is an uncommon disease. It occurs most commonly in young or middle-aged adults, up to 97% of patients are smokers [11]. In early stage, pulmonary histiocytosis X is characterized pathologically by granulomatous nodules containing Langerhans histiocytes and eosinophils. In its later stage, the cellular granulomas are replaced by fibrosis and cysts.

On HRCT, almost all patients show lung cysts. Pulmonary cysts are found in patients in all stages of histiocytosis X. The cysts may vary markedly in size but are usually lees than 10 mm in diameter, although they may be larger than 10 mm in some patients. Cysts may be round or bizarre in shape. These cysts have walls that range from being barely perceptible to being several millimeters in thickness. The presence of nodules is a frequent manifestation of pulmonary histiocytosis X. In the majority of cases, the nodules are small (less than 10 mm in diameter). The combination of thin-walled cysts and small nodules on HRCT is virtually diagnostic of pulmonary histiocytosis X [11, 12]. It is predominant in the upper or mid-lung zones and the costophrenic sulci are relatively spared. The cysts of histiocytosis X are easily distingushed from emphysematous areas, because they have visible thin walls.

Lymphangiomyomatosis

Lymphangiomyomatosis (LAM) is a rare disease that occurs exclusively in female patients. The majority of patients are of child-bearing age. LAM is characterized by progressive proliferation of spindle cells in pulmonary lymphatics, along the bronchioles and vessels. Proliferation of spindle cells can obstruct bronchioles by air trapping and the formation of cysts, and obstruct lymphatic vessels leading to chylothorax [13, 14].

On HRCT, patients with LAM characteristically show numerous well-defined, air-filled round areas surrounded by a thin, regular wall (Fig. 6). Most cysts are round and vary from 2 to 60 mm in diameter [14]. Their size tends to increase with progression of the disease. In the majority of patients the cysts are distributed diffusely throughout the lung: no lung zone is spared. Lung parenchyma between cysts appears normal in most patients. LAM has a characteristic appearance on HRCT. It should be noted, however, that normal findings at HRCT examination do not rule out early disease in patients with LAM.

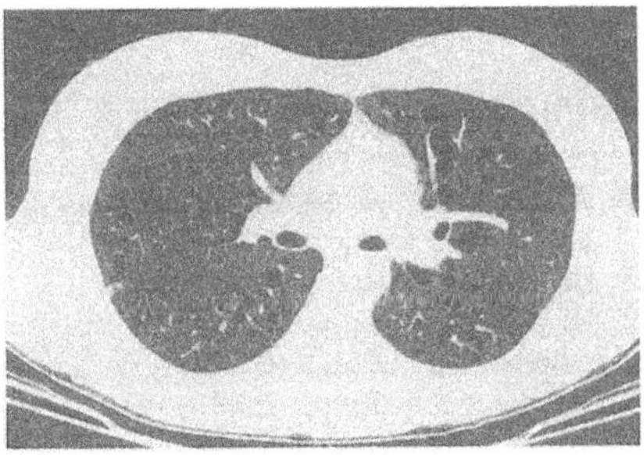

Fig. 6 Lymphangiomyomatosis in a 24-year-old woman. High-resolution computed tomography (HRCT) shows diffuse, small cysts with thin walls. The lung parenchyma between the cysts appears normal

End-Stage Fibrotic Disease

End-stage fibrotic diseases include idiopathic pulmonary fibrosis, collagen vascular disease, and asbestosis [15]. They are characterizid by a honeycomb appearance. Although they have different pathogenesis and clinical features, the pathologic and radiographic characteristics are similar. On HRCT, the patients with end-stage fibrotic disease show cystic spaces that are characterized by thick, clearly, fibrous walls (Fig. 7). In the majority of patients, these cysts are less than 10 mm in diameter, having a peripheral or subpleural predominance. These diseases are predominantly basal. There is gross distortion of lung architecture, and the secondary lobules are no longer discernible.

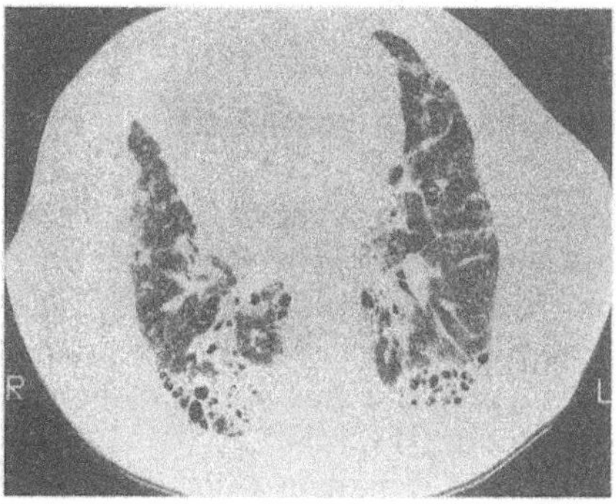

Fig. 7 End-stage idiopathic pulmonary fibrosis. Typical honeycomb cysts are present in the subpleural regions

Conclusion

HRCT has significantly improved our ability to image morphologic abnormalities associated with decreased attenuation area or cysts. It is more sensitive and more specific than conventional CT or chest radiography. In most cases, correct diagnosis can be suggested on the basis of HRCT findings.

References

1. Snider GL, Kleinerman J, Thurbeck WM et al. (1985) The definition of emphysema. Report of a National heart, Lung, and Blood Institute, Division of Lung Diseases Workshop. Am Rev Respir Dis 1985:132:182
2. Hruban RH, Meziane MA, Zerhoum EA et al. (1987) High resolution computed tomography of inflation fixed lungs. Pathologic-radiologic correlation of centrilobular emphysema. Am Rev Respir Dis 136:935
3. Webb WR, Stein MG, Finkbeiner WE et al. Normal and diseased isolated lungs: high-resolution CT. Radiology 1988; 166:81
4. Murata K, Khan A, Herman PG (1989) Pulmonary parenchymal disease: evaluation with high-resolution CT. Radiology 170:629

5. Lesur O, Delorme N, Fromaget JM et al. (1990) Computed tomography in the etiologic assessment of idiopathic spontaneous pneumothorax. Chest 98:341
6. Reid LM (1950) Reduction in bronchial subdivision in bronchiectasis. Thorax 5:233
7. Cherniack NS (1991) Chronic obstructive pulmonary disease. W. B. Saunders P319
8. McGuinness G, Naidich DP, Leitman BS et al. (1993) Bronchiectasis: CT evaluation. AJR 160:253
9. Hartman TE, Primack SL, Lee KS et al. (1994) CT of bronchial and bronchiolar disease. RadioGraphics 14:991
10. Grenier P, Maurice F, Musset D et al. (1986) Bronchiectasis: Assessment by thin-section CT. Radiology 161:95
11. Kulwiec EL, Lynch DA, Aguayo SM et al. (1992) Imaging of pulmonary histiocytosis X. RadioGraphics 12:515
12. Moore ADA, Godwin JD, Muller NL et al. (1989) Pulmonary histiocytosis X: comparison of radiographic and CT findings. Radiology 172:249
13. Aberle DR, Hansell DM, Brown K et al. (1990) Lymphangiomyomatosis: CT, chest radiographic, and functional correlations. Radiology 176:381
14. Lenoir S, Grenier P, Brauner MW et al. (1990) Pulmonary lymphangiomyomatosis and tuberous sclerosis: comparison of radiographic and thin-section CT findings. Radiology 175:329
15. Gamsu G (1992) Computed tomography of the body with magnetic resonance imagmg. second edition, Volume one. WB Saunders, P171

CHAPTER 10

Computed Tomography of Tracheal Tumors

Jung-Gi Im[1]

Introduction

The diagnosis of a tracheal mass is commonly delayed, frequently under the impression of bronchial asthma, because the detection of the mass on chest radiography is difficult and clinical symptoms and signs mimic bronchial asthma [1]. Computed tomography (CT) scans are usually performed after the detection of the mass on bronchoscopy. CT scan is the mainstay of radiological examination in the detection, evaluation of the disease extent, and in characterization of tracheal tumors.

A variety of diseases can cause tracheal masses [2]. Primary malignant neoplasms, such as squamous cell carcinoma and tracheobronchial gland tumors, are the most common. Others include malignant tumors of adjacent organs, benign neoplasms of the trachea, and granulomas.

Because surgical resection and anastomosis is the ultimate goal in most tracheal neoplasms, the evaluation of the disease extent is particularly important in planning the treatment. The application of two- and three-dimensional images in the evaluation of the tracheobronchial disease is especially useful for these purposes [3].

Primary Malignant Neoplasms

Carcinoma

Tracheal carcinoma accounts for less than 1% of carcinomas of the respiratory tract [4–6]. Average age of the patients is about 55 years, and there is male preponderance. The clinical presentation is variable. Initial symptoms are nonspecific, including dyspnea, wheezing, stridor, hemoptysis, or dysphasia. As with other causes of tracheal narrowing, the patient may initially be treated for bronchial asthma. Most of the lesions are typically visible on chest radiographs but are rarely identified prospectively.

Bronchoscopy continues to be the mainstay of diagnosis and is highly successful in identifying and in evaluating the intraluminal portion of the tumor [2].

[1] Department of Radiology, Seoul National University College of Medicine, Seoul, Korea.

However, it is impossible to assess the extraluminal extension of the tumor with this modality. Sometimes bronchoscopic biopsy is not warranted when the mass occupies a major portion of the tracheal lumen and especially when the mass is hypervascular.

CT enables the comprehensive evaluation of the extraluminal portion of the tumor, as well as the status of the bronchi distal to the tight stenosis. Routine axial CT scans tend to underestimate the longitudinal extent of the tumor. Two- and three-dimensional reformatted images from volumetric scan data with spiral or helical CT scanners are helpful, especially in the evaluation of the longitudinal extent, which is critical for planning surgery [3, 7].

The most common primary tracheal malignant tumors are squamous cell carcinoma, constituting 50% or more of cases in various series and being four times as common in men as in women [8]. Adenoid cystic carcinoma (Fig. 1) is slightly less common than squamous cell carcinoma and shows no sex predilection. Mucoepidermoid carcinoma (Fig. 2), carcinoid tumor and glomus tumor are less common tumors.

Squamous cell carcinoma commonly appear as an infiltrating and polypoid tumor. Adenoid cystic carcinoma is the most common subtype of tracheobronchial gland tumor comprising about 80%. Approximately 80% of these tumors arise in the trachea and mainstem bronchi. This tumor accounts for 31–35% of primary malignant tumor of the trachea [9]. The tumor characteristi-

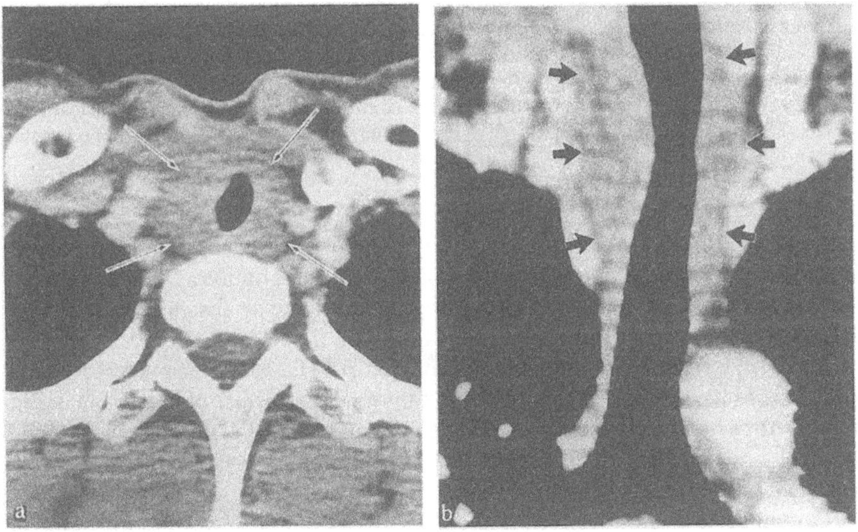

Fig. 1 a, b A 65-year-old woman with adenoid cystic carcinoma of the trachea. **a** Routine axial CT scan obtained after intravenous contrast medium injection at the level of thoracic inlet shows circumferential thickening of the tracheal wall and narrowing of the tracheal lumen (*arrows*). Transtracheal extension of the tumor and the relationship with the adjacent great vessels are best demonstrated in this axial image. Note laterally displaced great vessels. **b** Coronal reformatted image (3 mm collimation, 4 mm table feed, 1 mm reconstruction interval) clearly shows longitudinal extent of the tumor (*arrows*)

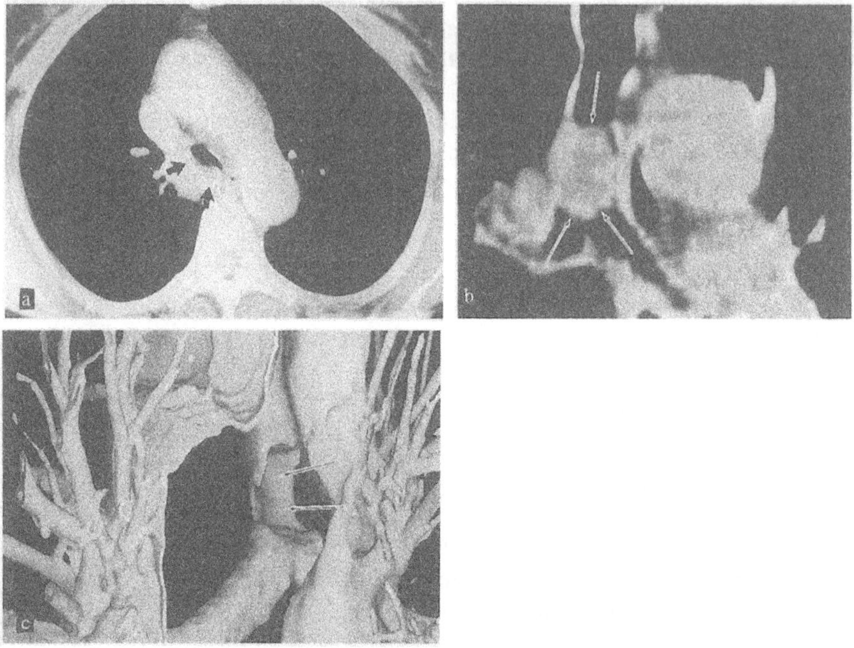

Fig. 2 a–c A 67-year-old woman with mucoepidermoid carcinoma of the trachea. **a** Routine contrast enhanced axial CT scan at the level of the aortic arch shows endotracheal mass posteriorly (*arrows*). The mass is confined to the lumen of the trachea. **b** Coronal two-dimensional reformatted image (3 mm collimation, 4 mm table feed, 1 mm reconstruction interval) clearly shows longitudinal extent of the endotracheal mass (*arrows*). **c** Posterior view of the shaded surface display three-dimensional image comprehensively shows endotracheal mass (*arrows*). The longitudinal extent as well as the character of the mass are clearly demonstrated

cally grows into the airway lumen forming a smooth-surfaced, somewhat polypoid tumor; occasionally growth is circumferential and annular. CT is definitely a useful technique, particularly in assessing the presence or absence of the mediastinal extension.

Mucoepidermoid carcinoma accounts for 0.2–0.5% of primary bronchial neoplasms [10, 11]. The majority of the tumors are typically of low grade malignancy with a benign clinical course. The tumor arises most commonly in proximal bronchi and tracheal involvement is less common. The tumors are typically confined to the tracheobronchial wall.

Carcinoid and glomus tumor typically show dense contrast enhancement because of hypervascularity of the tumor [5].

Invasion by Adjacent Malignant Tumors

Invasion from adjacent tumors such as esophageal carcinoma, thyroid carcinoma, or malignant mediastinal mass can cause tracheal mass. On CT scan, the recognition of the primary site is possible in most of the patients. However, sometimes it is impossible, especially when the tumors show infiltrative growth.

Primary Benign Neoplasms

Papillomas

Multiple tracheobronchial papillomas are typically found 10–34 years after the initial diagnosis of laryngeal papillomatosis in childhood. About 2% of patients with laryngeal papillomas develop lower respiratory tract lesion. Implantation of fragments of inhaled papillomas from the larynx and multifocal viral infection are the possible pathogenesis of papilloma formation in the lower respiratory tract. Pathologically, the tumors consist of sessile or broadly stalked papillary growths lined by a squamous epithelium. Typical radiographic findings are atelectasis and obstructive pneumonia due to airway obstruction. Involvement of distal airways results in multiple nodular opacities frequently associated with cavitation [12]. CT scans demonstrate endotracheal mass, distal bronchiectasis, nodules and cavitary lesions more clearly. Shaded surface display of three-dimensional images is especially informative in the evaluation of the multiple endotracheal masses. The wall of the cavitary lung lesions typically shows a smooth surface and uniform thickness [12].

Hamartoma

Hamartomas arising in the tracheobronchial tree are very rare. Typical endotracheal or endobronchial hamartomas appear as fleshy, polypoid tumors attached to the tracheobronchial wall by a narrow stalk. The central portion of the tumor is usually composed of a core of adipose tissue.

Typical radiographic findings are post-obstructive atelectasis or recurrent pneumonic consolidation. CT scan can demonstrate fatty endotracheal or endobronchial mass which is pathognomonic for hamartoma [13]. Most of the lipomas arising from the tracheobronchial wall are considered to be hamartomas.

Mesenchymal-Origin Tumors

Leiomyoma, neurilemmoma, fibroma, fibrous histiocytoma, and chondroma are rare benign tumors of mesenchymal origin. Radiological findings are those of a well-circumscribed endotracheal mass.

Granulomas

Tuberculosis of the trachea is caused by repeated implantation of the organism from a cavitary pulmonary lesion which contains abundant *Mycobacterium tuberculosis*. Another mechanism is local extension from adjacent mediastinal tuberculous lymphadenitis. Higher prevalence of both tracheobronchial tuberculosis and mediastinal tuberculous lymphadenitis in young adult women supports this causal relationship [14]. CT findings of tracheobronchial tuberculosis depend on the stage of the disease. In patients with active caseation process, irregular thickening of the tracheobronchial wall is seen with some degree of enhancement on post-contrast scan. Sometimes, nodular endotracheal granuloma can mimic tracheal tumor. In patients with healed fibrotic lesion, smooth and diffuse narrowing of the tracheal lumen without thickening or contrast enhancement is typically seen [15]. Differentiation from bronchogenic carcinoma can usually be made by their smooth and diffuse narrowing of the lumen without intraluminal mass and by the patient's younger age.

Other causes of granulomatous tracheal mass include fungal infection, rhinoscleroma, and Wegener's granulomatosis.

Amyloidosis

Amyloidosis can cause infiltration of fibrillar protein in the lung and tracheobronchial tree or other organs. When the disease involves the trachea, the pattern is either diffuse submucosal infiltration or multiple submucosal nodules. Rarely, a single submucosal nodule can occur. The tracheal mucosa is usually normal and sometimes submucosal nodules contain calcification or ossification [2, 16].

CT findings are thickening of the tracheal wall with or without narrowing of the lumen, and sometimes calcification in the thickened wall. Thickening of the entire circumference of the tracheal wall is typical for amyloidosis, in contrast to typical sparing of the membranous portion in patients with tracheopathia osteochondroplastica [6, 16].

Tracheopathia Osteochondroplastica

Tracheopathia osteochondroplastica is characterized by multiple submucosal osteocartilagenous growths along the inner anterolateral surface of the trachea sparing the membranous portion. Men are more frequently affected than women (3:1). The etiology is unknown. Theories have been advanced linking this disorder to chronic inflammation, degenerative processes, amyloidosis, and frank neoplasia [16].

Typically the radiograph reveals multiple sessile nodular tumors, with or without calcification, extending over a long segment of the trachea. CT scan typically shows irregular nodular protrusion of the nodules into the tracheal lumen commonly with calcifications [17]. Sparing of the membranous portion is important in differentiation from amyloidosis.

References

1. Felson B (1983) Letter from the editor. Semin Roentgenol 18:1-3
2. Kwong JS, Müller NL, Miller RR (1992) Diseases of the trachea and main-stem bronchi: correlation of CT with pathologic findings. RadioGraphics 12:645-657
3. Im J-G, Song JG, Chung MJ, Yeon KM, Han MC (1994) Clinical utility of 2-D and 3D spiral CT in the evaluation of tracheobronchial diseases. RSNA Scientific Program : 261
4. Gamsu G, Webb WR (1983) Computed tomography of the trachea and mainstem bronchi. Semin Roentgenol 18:51-59
5 Naidich DP (1990) CT/MR correlation in the evaluation of tracheobronchial neoplasia. Radiol Clin North Am 28:555-571
6. Felson B (1983) Neoplasms of the trachea and mainstem bronchi. Semin Roentgenol 18:23-37
7. Remy-Jardin M, Remy J, Petyt L, Wannebroucq J (1994) Spiral CT tracheobronchography with multiplanar and 3D reformations. RSNA Scientific Progam : 261
8. Fraser RG, Pare JAP (1988; 1989) Diagnosis of the diseases of the chest. Philadilphia; Saunders, 3rd ed
9. Cleveland RH, Nice CM, Ziskind J (1977) Primary adenoid cystic carcinoma (cylindroma) of the trachea. Radiology 122:597-600
10. Turnbull AD, Huvos AG, Coodner JT, Foote AW (1971) Mucoepidermoid tumors of the bronchial glands. Cancer 28:539-544
11. Axelsson C, Burcharth F, Johansen A (1973) Mucoepidermoid lung tumors. J Thorac Cardiovasc Surg 65:902-908
12. Kramer SS, Wehunt WD, Stocker JT, Kashima H (1985) Pulmonary manifestations of jubenile laryngotracheal papillomatosis. AJR 144:687-694
13. Ahn JM, Im J-G, Seo JW, et al. (1994) Endobronchial hamartoma: CT findings in three patients. AJR 163:49-50
14. Im J-G, Song KS, Kang HS, et al. (1987) Mediastinal tuberculous lymphadenitis: CT manifestations. Radiology 164:115-119
15. Im J-G, Itoh H, Yeon KM, Han MC (1994) Computed tomography in pulmonary tuberculosis. Seoul J Medicine 35:51-71
16. Choplin RH, Wehunt WD, Theros EG (1983) Diffuse lesions of the trachea. Semin Roentgenol 18:38-50
17. Onitsuka H, Hirose N, Watanabe K, et al. (1983) Computed tomography of tracheopathia osteoplastica. AJR 140:268-270

CHAPTER 11

High-Resolution Computed Tomography Technology for the Chest

Philippe Grenier[1]

Introduction

High-resolution computed tomography (HRCT) has revolutionized the radiological approach to diagnosing lung diseases. The key to the interpretation of HRCT is an understanding of the anatomy of the secondary pulmonary lobule [4, 73]. HRCT can show many features of the secondary pulmonary lobule in both normal and abnormal lungs. For an adequate assessment of lung disease, volumetric scanning involves continuous data acquisition while the patient is advanced at a constant rate through the CT gantry, eliminating any interscan delay. HRCT and volumetric helical CT can be used in combination to give adequate assessment of focal lung diseases and airway diseases [15].

CT Technique

High-resolution scanning should be performed with thin slices (1 to 2 mm), a high spatial frequency algorithm for reconstruction, and a fast scan time (1 s or less) to reduce artifacts from respiratory motion and cardiac pulsation. Patients are routinely scanned in a supine position, but scans with the patients prone can be helpful for better definition of the lung basis [71]. Oblique scans using a 20°–25° cranial angulation of the gantry improves the CT analysis of segmental and subsegmental bronchi (64). For assessing diffuse lung disease, scans should be obtained from the apex of the lungs to the diaphragm with 10-mm intersection spacing. For areas of particular interest, scans should be performed at suspended end inspiration, but additional examination may occasionally be required in expiration to demonstrate air trapping. A 512×512 matrix should be used; a 15- to 25-cm field of view is recommended for retrospectively targeting images. Window settings of –600/1600 H are recommended for viewing pulmonary disease.

Spiral volumetrical scanning represents a considerable improvement compared to conventional CT due to the ability to utilize thin sections to detect subtle structures as well as the elimination of misregistration that results from slight variations in respiration [52]. Because of its ability to survey the entire volume of the lung continuously, spiral scanning enhances detection of nodules [13]. This

[1] Service de Radiologie générale, Hôpitaux de Paris, Paris France.

has proved especially important in those portions of the lung difficult to evaluate because of respiratory motion, for example in the lung basis adjacent to the diaphragm where the potential for misregistration is greatest [65]. In addition to nodule detection, spiral CT is especially valuable for evaluating nodular structure and vascularity. Intravenous injection of iodinated contrast medium is required. Usually 65–90 ml non ionic contrast medium (300–370 mg/l) is injected at a rate of 2–3 ml/s after a 25–35-s delay. Spiral CT can be valuable in assessing the relationship between nodules and adjacent airways [52]. Similarly spiral CT has proved valuable in assessing patients who have suspected pulmonary arterio-venous malformation [61].

It may be helpful to use HRCT and spiral CT in combination, particularly in assessing focal lung lesion or bronchiectasis [15]. In patients suspected of having bronchiectasis or suffering from hemoptysis, we recommend the following CT protocol:

1. HRCT scanning, 20–25° cranial inclination of the gantry
2. From the apex of the lungs to the carina:
   - With 1- to 1.5-mm collimation and 10-mm interspacing
3. Spiral CT scanning from the carina during a 20-s breath hold:
   - 3-mm collimation
   - Pitch, 1.6
   - Reconstruction of images every 2 mm
   - High spatial frequency reconstruction algorithm
4. From the bottom line of spiral CT acquisition volume to the lower part of the diaphragm:
   - HRCT scans with 1- to 1.5-mm collimation and 10-mm interspacing
5. Complementary scans at expiration:
   - HRCT scans with 30-mm slice interspacing from the apex of the lungs to the diaphragm or
   - Spiral HRCT during a 10-s forced expiratory vital capacity maneuver

Spiral HRCT may also be used to search for air trapping during active expiration. The technique consists of a 15-mm-thick lung volume selected in the region of interest with 1.5-mm collimation, a pitch of 1, and caudocranial increment of the table. Ten slices are obtained during the 10-s period as the patient performs forced expiration. The series of ten images can be viewed in a cine view in which the ten individual images can be rapidly displayed in a sequential fashion.

Clinical Application

Focal Lung Disease

Focal lung disease is often encountered in the interpretation of chest radiographs. In most cases, comparison with findings from a previously performed chest radiograph, can definitively aid in the diagnosis. In other cases, a definitive diagnosis of a benign process can be made with CT, thus obviating surgery. Indeed many focal nodular and nodular lung lesions, including aspergilloma, pulmonary infarct, hamartoma, lipoid pneumonia, round atelectasis and arteriovenous malformation, have characteristic findings at CT [54].

Nodules measuring 2.5 cm or less with smooth edges and demonstrating focal collection of fat (or fat alternating with areas of calcifications) permits a firm diagnosis of hamartoma and should be conservatively managed. The detection of oily substances with a CT number in the range of fatty tissues in a pulmonary infiltrate is a pathognomonic sign of lipoid pneumonia. Pulmonary arteriovenous malformation can be recognized by the demonstration of large feeding and draining vessels connected to the malformation. These lesions can be recognized with or without contrast injection because of their typical morphology [61]. Pulmonary infarcts typically present as wedge shaped, peripheral, pleural based densities on CT [68]. Often these wedge densities demonstrate a lucent center. Another important finding is the presence of rim-enhancement of the infarct after contrast injection probably reflecting the inflammatory response of the lung at the periphery of the infarct. More specific diagnosis is made if a vessel is demonstrated at the apex of the wedge density. Rounded atelectasis is a condition observed in patients with asbestos exposure or after pleural fluid collection. The most indicative CT features of rounded atelectasis are (a) contiguity to areas of focal or diffuse pleural thickening, (b) a lentiform or wedge shaped outline, (c) evidence of volume loss in the adjacent lung, and (d) the characteristic comet tail of vessels and bronchi sweeping into the margins of the mass [41,67].

Regarding the diagnosis of solitary pulmonary nodule, it was demonstrated that HRCT is more sensitive than other techniques in depicting benign pattern calcification. Diffuse, target or laminated calcification is indicative of a calcified granuloma. Popcorn classification is indicative of pulmonary hamartoma.

In undeterminate cases, CT can help select the most appropriate route for biopsy of the focal lung lesion. If CT shows that a bronchus leads up to a lung nodule, bronchoscopic evaluation should yield a substantially higher likelihood of a positive biopsy. In other cases, percutaneous needle biopsy can be performed under CT control. The value of needle biopsy of nodules in patients unsuitable for surgery is well established. But, on the other hand, it proved to be of limited value in the management of solitary nodule which has a high clinical suspicion of malignancy and the patient is a candidate for surgery.

Chronic Infiltrative Lung Disease

Over the last 10 years, several studies have shown that CT can play a major role in the assessment of patients with chronic infiltrative lung disease (CILD).

Although chest radiography is the first imaging technique used to demonstrate the presence of pulmonary infiltration in patients suspected of CILD, the radiograph may be normal in about 10%–16% of patients with proven disease. The sensitivity of radiography in depicting infiltrative lung disease was 80% compared with 94% for CT [57]

Confronted with a patient having abnormalities consistent with a CILD, a physician must consider a formidable list of entities. Many of these entities have a characteristic pattern on CT scans [46, 47]. Three studies have concluded that CT is superior to chest radiography for correctly diagnosing CILD [19, 23, 39].

As most CILD have a patchy distribution in the lung parenchyma, HRCT is helpful in determining the area and the type of biopsy that is most likely to provide the correct diagnosis. The two entities that can be consistently and reliably diagnosed on the basis of the findings of bronchial or transbronchial biopsy are lymphangitic carcinomatosis and sarcoidosis [39]. Most other diseases require open lung biopsy for a definitive diagnosis. When open lung biopsy is indicated, CT is helpful in guiding the surgeon to the optimal biopsy site, the specimen including tissue from a representative area of lung and avoiding areas of extensive honeycombing.

CT can be helpful in distinguishing potentially reversible active inflammation from irreversible fibrosis [48]. Reticular lines, small cystic spaces or traction bronchiectasis within areas of ground glass are suggestive of fibrosis [8, 51]. In a CT pathologic correlation study of 33 patients with pulmonary infiltration, air-space opacification was pathologically associated with potentially treatable or reversible disease in 88% of cases [37]. Ground glass may represent reversible disease only when it is seen without any findings of fibrosis visible in the same area [63].

CT is helpful in demonstrating the presence of super imposed complications and in deciding what is the most appropriate method to reach a definitive diagnosis. In patients with asbestos exposure and focal abnormality on the radiograph, HRCT has a role to differentiate typical rounded atelectasis from undeterminate lung opacity [38]. In patients with silicosis or coalworker pneumoconiosis, when malignancy is suspected or the chest radiographic findings are not typical for progressive massive fibrosis, HRCT should be performed to more accurately assess pulmonary abnormalities before further investigations and biopsy. CT was demonstrated as useful in assessment of patients with pulmonary complications related to sarcoidosis, including bronchiectasis and cavitary lesions.

Chronic Obstructive Lung Disease

This group of diseases is defined by the presence of abnormal pulmonary function rather than specific morphologic findings. Imaging studies have a limited role in the diagnosis and evaluation of patients with chronic obstructive lung disease. HRCT, however, has significantly improved the ability to image morphologic abnormalities associated with chronic airflow obstruction [72].

Emphysema

CT allows direct demonstration of lung destruction by showing areas of abnormally low attenuation, surrounded by normal lung zone but without any visible wall, which allows emphysema to be distinguished from cystic airspaces and honeycombing. Centrilobular emphysema is characterized on HRCT scans by the presence of small round areas of low density, several millimeters in diameter, grouped near the center of the secondary pulmonary lobule [17]. Panlobular emphysema is characterized by uniform destruction of the pulmonary lobule, leading to widespread areas of abnormally low density. In severe panlobular emphysema, extensive lung destruction, and paucity of vascular markings are easily distinguished from normal lung parenchyma, but on the other hand, mild and moderately severe panlobular emphysema can be very difficult to detect. Paraseptal emphysema is detected in a subpleural location and adjacent to peripheral interlobular septa. Irregular emphysema is easily detected when the associated fibrosis is identified [17].

Correlation between HRCT findings and pathologic findings in patients with centrilobular emphysema is excellent. However, as emphysema may be missed on CT, this investigation can not be used to definitely rule out the diagnosis.

In clinical practice, HRCT is rarely used in an attempt to diagnose emphysema. One exception, however, is its use for patients having shortness of breath and low diffusing capacity without evidence of airway obstruction on pulmonary function tests and chest radiograph. If significant emphysema is found on HRCT, no further evaluation is necessary, especially lung biopsy is not needed [32]. Also, HRCT can be used in the preoperative assessment of patients with bullous emphysema, who are being considered for bullectomy. CT allows for an assessment of the extent of bullous disease, the degree of compression of underlying lung, and the severity of emphysema in the remaining lung parenchyma [10, 16, 43].

Cystic Lung Disease

The term lung cyst is used to describe a thin-walled (usually less than 3 mm) air-containing lesion. Two lung diseases, histiocytosis X and lymphangiomyomatosis are commonly associated with the presence of lung cysts. In histiocytosis X, the lung cysts have walls that range from being barely perceptible to being several millimeters in thickness [44]. They appear round, but they also can have bizarre shapes due to fusion of several cysts. An upper lobe predominance is common and the intervening lung parenchyma appears normal without evidence of fibrosis. Small nodules may be also present [7]. In lymphangiomyomatosis, HRCT scans show numerous thin-walled lung cysts surrounded by relatively normal lung parenchyma. The cysts are distributed diffusely throughout the lungs and no lung zone is spared [1, 36, 45].

Bronchiectasis

HRCT is now the imaging technique of choice for the diagnosis of bronchiectasis (Fig. 1). It is comparable in accuracy to bronchography [22]. The CT diagnosis of varicose and cystic bronchiectasis is easy [20, 21]. A group or cluster of multiple air-filled cysts is a common finding, in cystic bronchiectasis. Air fluid levels in the dependent portions of the dilated bronchi are a specific sign of this entity. Varicose bronchiectasis is seen as dilated bronchi with a beaded appearance or as a string of pearls. The only limitation of CT in the assessment of bronchiectasis

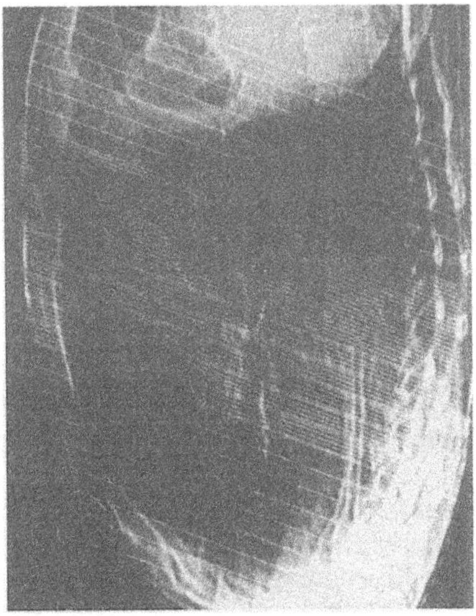

Fig. 1 Lateral scout view illustrating the position of high-resolution and spiral CT scans for assessing bronchiectasis

concerns cylindrical pattern. Cylindrical bronchiectasis is characterized on HRCT by the presence of thick-walled bronchi, which extend to the lung periphery and fail to show normal tapering. Depending on their orientation relative to the scan plane they can simulate tram tracks or can show the signet-ring sign in which the dilated thick-walled bronchus and its accompanying pulmonary artery are seen adjacent to each other. Dilated bronchi can be filled with fluid, mucus or pus. Surgery is still performed on some patients when the bronchiectasis is localized. In such cases, accurate assessment is required on segmental basis. Traditionally, surgery has been an indication for bronchography. However, this view is being challenged and more surgeons are now prepared to operate on the basis of high quality HRCT examination [11].

Abnormalities of Small Airways

Morphologic abnormalities of the small airways in patients with chronic obstructive lung disease include wall thickening, narrowing or obliteration of the bronchiolar lumen, bronchiolar dilatation and mucous plugging. On HRCT abnormal bronchioles filled with fluid, mucus or pus can appear as small centrilobular tubular, branching, linear or nodular structures. These can be associated with peribronchiolar or centrilobular ill-defined nodular opacities if inflammation of the adjacent lung is present. If air-filled bronchi or bronchioles are visible in the peripheral lung, it usually indicates bronchial or bronchiolar wall thickening and/or dilatation [24]. Diseases associated with bronchiolar abnormalities visible on HRCT include panbronchiolitis [55], cystic fibrosis, diseases associated with chronic bronchial sepsis, bronchopneumonia, bronchiolitis obliterans [24, 72], respiratory bronchiolitis [62] and hypersensitivity bronchiolitis [66]. In many patients with small airways abnormalities visible on HRCT, large airways abnormalities such as bronchiectasis or bronchial wall thickening are also visible [2].

Patchy areas of varying lung attenuation are often visible on HRCT in patients with small airways abnormalities [20, 72]. These often indicate the presence of perfusion abnormalities occuring as a result of abnormal regional lung ventilation (mosaic perfusion). The denser lung regions visible in these patients are better ventilated and better perfused [72]. Air trapping contributes to this phenomenon of mosaic perfusion. This is particularly well demonstrated on HRCT scans performed at expiration.

Acute Diffuse Lung Disease in Immunocompromised Patients

It has been demonstrated that HRCT can be helpfully indicated in the immunocompromised patient who has acute pulmonary complications: (a) to assess those patients who have normal or questionable radiographic findings; (b) to narrow the differential diagnosis in patients who have non specific findings on the radiograph; and (c) to guide the optimal type and site of lung biopsy [30, 53, 60].

The presence of areas of ground glass attenuation in a perihilar angiographic distribution in hypoxemic immunocompromised patient is very suggestive of *Pneumocystis carinii* pneumonia (PCP) [5, 35]. Ground glass opacities can be also observed in drug toxicity, pulmonary hemorrhage, viral infection and bronchiolitis obliterans with organizing pneumonia (BOOP) [3, 9, 56].

CT may allow early recognition of invasive pulmonary aspergillosis by the characteristic appearance of nodules with a surrounding halo of ground-glass attenuation (CT halo sign representing hemorrhagic necrosis) [33]. This sign, however, has also been described in patients with candidiasis, cytomegalovirus (CMV) and herpes simplex virus pneumonia [59]. Air crescent formation is another relatively common finding in invasive pulmonary aspergillosis, but this finding is a late manifestation representing air between retracted, infarcted lung and the adjacent lung parenchyma. Another characteristic manifestation is the presence of segmental or subsegmental consolidation due to pulmonary infarction.

CT has also been shown to be more accurate in the detection of septic pulmonary emboli [34]. The most characteristic findings of septic emboli on CT are multiple well-defined pulmonary nodules in various stages of cavitation and subpleural wedge-shaped infiltrates. The pulmonary nodules often have definable feeding vessels associated with them [27]. In a patient with AIDS, the presence of ill defined nodules or areas of consolidation in peribronchovascular distribution is suggestive of Kaposi sarcoma [53, 74] and the presence of one or more well-defined pulmonary nodules is strongly suggestive of lymphoma [69]. In patients who have undergone transplant and are receiving cyclosporine, multiple well-defined nodules are suggestive of post transplantation lymphoproliferative disorders, and reduction of immunosuppression is essential to obtain regression or complete resolution of pulmonary lesions [14].

Small centrilobular opacities including nodular or branching linear, 2–4 mm in diameter is suggestive of tuberculosis or atypical mycobacteria [28]. Diffuse nodules of 1 to 3 mm in diameter associated with nodular thickening of the vessels, interlobular septa, interlobar fissures, are suggestive of hematogeneously disseminated tuberculosis or histoplasmosis [40].

Conclusion

HRCT has gained wide acceptance as the imaging modality of choice after chest radiography in the evaluation of focal and diffuse lung diseases. HRCT is used: (a) to detect lung disease, (b) to characterize lung disease morphologically, (c) to guide lung biopsy procedures, (d) to determine the presence and extent of reversible and irreversible lung disease and (e) to follow patients who are being treated in order to monitor the success or failure of the treatment being employed.

Spiral scanning is highly recommended to detect pulmonary nodules, particularly when pulmonary metastases are suspected. Spiral HRCT can be used over focal lung lesions (nodular or non nodular) after bolus injection of contrast medium to improve its characterization and its anatomic relationships with pleura and airways. Spiral HRCT can also be recommended in the assessment of bronchiectasis and to search for air trapping.

References

1. Aberle DR, Hansell DM, Brown SK, Tashkin DP (1990) Lymphangiomyomatosis: CT, chest radiographic, and functional correlations. Radiology 176:380–388
2. Akira M, Kitatani F, Lee Y-S et al. (1988) Diffuse panbronchiolitis: evaluation with high-resolution CT. Radiology 168:433–438
3. Bellamy EA, Husband JE, Blaquiere RM, Law MR (1985) Bleomycin-related lung damage: CT evidence. Radiology 156:155–158
4. Bergin C, Roggli V, Coblentz C, Chiles C (1988) The secondary pulmonary lobule: normal and abnormal CT appearances. AJR 151:21–25
5. Bergin CJ, Wirth RL, Berry GJ, Castellino RA (1990) Pneumocystis carinii pneumonia: CT and HRCT observations. J Comput Assist Tomogr 14:756–759
6. Bhalla M, Turcios N, Aponte V et al. (1991) Cystic fibrosis: scoring system with thin-section CT. Radiology 179:783–788
7. Brauner MW, Grenier P, Mouelhi MM, Mompoint D, Lenoir S (1989) Pulmonary histiocytosis X: evaluation with high resolution CT. Radiology 172:255–258
8. Brauner MW, Lenoir S, Grenier P, Cluzel P, Battesti JP, Valeyre D (1992) Pulmonary sarcoidosis: CT assessment of lesion reversibility. Radiology 182:349–354
9. Brown MJ, Miller RR, Müller NL (1994) Acute lung disease in the immunocompromised host: CT and pathologic examination findings. Radiology 190:247–254
10. Carr DH, Pride NB (1984) Computed tomography in pre-operative assessment of bullous emphysema. Clin Radiol 35:43–45
11. Cole P, Flower CDR, Lavender JP (1993) Clinical and imaging aspects of bronchiectasis. In: Pulmonary Radiology. The Fleischner Society. Potchen EJ, Grainger RG, Greene R, WB Saunders Company ed, Philadelphia
12. Corcoran HL, Renner WR, Milstein MJ (1992) Review of high-resolution CT of the lung. Radiographics 12:917–939
13. Costello P, Anderson W, Blume D (1991) Pulmonary nodule: evaluation with spiral volumetric CT. Radiology 179:875–876

14. Dodd GD III, Ledesma-Medina J, Baron RL, Fuhrman CR (1992) Post transplant lymphoproliferative disorder: intrathoracic manifestations. Radiology 184:65
15. Engeler CE, Tashjian JH, Engeler CM, Geise RA, Holm JC, Ritenour ER (1994) Volumetric high-resolution CT in the diagnosis of interstitial lung disease and bronchiectasis: diagnostic accuracy and radiation dose. AJR 163:31–35
16. Fiore DW, Biondetti PR, Sartori F et al. (1982) The role of computer tomography in the evaluation of bullous lung disease. J Comput Assist Tomogr 6:105–108
17. Foster WL Jr, Gimenez EI, Roubidoux MA, Sherrier RH, Shannon RH, Roggli VL, Pratt PC (1993) The emphysemas: radiologic-pathologic correlations. Radiographics 13:311–328
18. Foster WL, Pratt PC, Roggli VL, Godwin JD, Halvorsen RA, Putman CE (1986) Centrilobular emphysema: CT-pathologic correlation. Radiology 159:27–32
19. Grenier P, Chevret S, Beigelman C, Brauner MW, Chastang C, Valeyre D (1994) Chronic diffuse infiltrative lung disease: determination of the diagnostic value of clinical data, chest radiography, and CT with bayesian analysis. Radiology 191:383–390
20. Grenier P, Cordeau MP, Beigelman C (1993) High-resolution computed tomography of the airways. J Thorac Imag 8:213–229
21. Grenier P, Lenoir S, Brauner M (1990) Computed tomographic assessment of bronchiectasis. Semin US, CT, MR 11:430–441
22. Grenier P, Maurice F, Musset D, Menu Y, Nahum H (1986) Bronchiectasis: assessment by thin-section CT. Radiology 161:95–99
23. Grenier P, Valeyre D, Cluzel P, Brauner MW, Lenoir S, Chastang C (1991) Chronic diffuse interstitial lung disease: diagnostic value of chest radiography and high-resolution CT. Radiology 179:123–132
24. Gruden JF, Webb WR, Warnock M (1994) Centrilobular opacities in the lung on high-resolution CT: diagnostic considerations and pathologic correlation. AJR 162:569–574
25. Hansell DM, Wells AU, Rubens MB, Cole PJ (1994) Bronchiectasis: functional significance of areas of decreased attenuation at expiratory CT. Radiology 193:369–374
26. Hruban RH, Meziane MA, Zerhouni EA et al. (1987) High resolution computed tomography of inflation fixed lungs: Pathologic-radiologic correlation of centrilobular emphysema. Am Rev Respir Dis 136:935–940
27. Huang RM, Naidich DP, Lubat E, Shcinella R, Garay SM, McCauley DI (1989) Septic pulmonary emboli: CT radiographic correlation. AJR 153:41–45
28. Im JG, Itoh H, Shim YS, Lee JH, Ahn J, Han MC, Noma S (1993) Pulmonary tuberculosis: CT findings-early active disease and sequential change with antituberculous therapy. Radiology 186:653–660
29. Itoh H, Murata K, Konishi J, Nishimura K, Kitaichi M, Izumi T (1993) Diffuse lung disease: pathologic basic for the high-resolution computed tomography findings. J Thorac Imag 8:176–188
30. Janzen DL, Adler BD, Padley SPG, Müller NL (1993) Diagnostic success of bronchoscopic biopsy in immunocompromised patients with acute pulmonary disease: predictive value of disease distribution as shown on CT. AJR 160:21–24
31. Kalender WA, Seissler W, Klotz E et al. (1990) Spiral volumetric CT with single-breath-hold technique, continuous transport, and continuous scanner rotation. Radiology 176–181–183
32. Klein JS, Gamsu G, Webb WR, Golden JA, Müller NL (1992) High-resolution CT diagnosis of emphysema in symptomatic patients with normal chest radiographs and isolated low diffusing capacity. Radiology 182:817–821
33. Kuhlman JE, Fishman EK, Siegelman SS (1985) Invasive pulmonary aspergillosis in acute leukemia: characteristic findings on CT, the CT halo sign and the role of CT in early diagnosis. Radiology 157:611–614
34. Kuhlman JE, Fishman EK, Teigen C (1990) Pulmonary septic emboli: diagnosis with CT. Radiology 174:211–213
35. Kuhlman JE, Kavuru M, Fishman EK, Siegelman SS (1990) Pneumocystis carinii pneumonia: spectrum of parenchymal CT findings. Radiology 175:711–714

36. Lenoir S, Grenier P, Brauner MW et al. (1990) Pulmonary lymphangiomyomatosis and tuberous sclerosis: comparison of radiographic and thin-section CT findings. Radiology 175:329–334
37. Leung AN, Miller RR, Müller NL (1993) Parenchymal opacification in chronic infiltrative lung diseases: CT-pathologic correlation. Radiology 188:209–214
38. Lynch DA, Gamsu G, Ray CS, Aberle DR (1988) Asbestos-related focal lung masses: manifestations on conventional and high-resolution CT scans. Radiology 169:603–607
39. Mathieson JR, Mayo JR, Staples CA, Müller NL (1989) Chronic diffuse infiltrative lung disease: comparison of diagnostic accuracy of CT and chest radiography. Radiology 171:111–116
40. McGuinness G, Naidich DP, Jagirdar J, Leitman B, McCauley DI (1992) High-resolution CT findings in miliary lung disease. J Comput Assist Tomogr 16:384–390
41. McHugh K, Blaquiere RM (1989) CT features of rounded atelectasis. AJR 153:257–260
42. Miller RR, Müller NL, Vedal S, Morrisson NJ, Staples CA (1989) Limitations of computed tomography in the assessment of emphysema. Am Rev Respir Dis 139:980–983
43. Morgan MDL, Strickland B (1984) Computed tomography in the assessment of bullous lung disease. Br J Dis Chest 78:10–25
44. Moore AD, Godwin JD, Müller NL, et al. (1989) Pulmonary histiocytosis X: comparison of radiographic and CT findings. Radiology 172:249–254
45. Müller NL, Chiles C, Kullnig P (1990) Pulmonary lymphangioleiomyomatosis: correlation of CT with radiographic and functional findings. Radiology 175:335–339
46. Müller NL, Miller RR (1990) Computed tomography of chronic diffuse infiltrative lung disease. Part 1 Am Rev Respir Dis 142:1206–1215
47. Müller NL, Miller RR (1990) Computed tomography of chronic diffuse infiltrative lung disease. Part 2 Am.Rev Respir Dis 142:1440–1448
48. Müller NL, Staples CA, Miller RR, Vedal S, Thurlbeck WM, Ostrow DN (1987) Disease activity in idiopathic pulmonary fibrosis: CT and pathologic correlation. Radiology 165:731–734
49. Murata K, Itoh H, Todo G, et al. (1986) Centrilobular lesions of the lung: demonstration by high-resolution CT and pathologic correlation. Radiology 161:641–645
50. Murata K, Khan A, Herman PG (1989) Pulmonary parenchymal disease: evaluation with high-resolution CT. Radiology 170:629–635
51. Murdoch J, Müller NL (1992) Pulmonary sarcoidosis: changes on follow-up CT examination. AJR 159:473–477
52. Naidich DP (1994) Helical computed tomography of the thorax. Clinical applications. In: The radiologic Clinics of North America. Advances in chest radiology. Godwin JD, WB Saunders Company, Philadelphia, 759–774
53. Naidich DP, McGuinness G (1991) Pulmonary manifestations of AIDS: CT and radiographic correlations. Radiol Clin North Am 29: 999–1017
54. Naidich DP, Zerhouni EA, Siegelman S (1991) Computed tomography and magnetic resonance of the thorax. 2nd ed New York: Raven Press
55. Nishimura K, Kitaichi M, Izumi T, Itoh H (1992) Diffuse panbronchiolitis: correlation of high-resolution CT and pathologic findings. Radiology 184:779–785
56. Padley SPG, Adler BD, Hansell DM, Müller NL (1992) High-resolution computed tomography of drug-induced lung disease. Clin Radiol 46:232–236
57. Padley SPG, Adler BD, Müller NL (1993) High resolution computed tomography of the chest: current indications. J Thorac Imaging 8:189–199
58. Paranjpe DV, Bergin CJ (1994) Spiral CT of the lungs: optimal technique and resolution compared with conventional CT. AJR 162:561–567
59. Primack SL, Hartman TE, Lee KS, Müller NL (1994) Pulmonary nodules and CT halo sign. Radiology 190:513–515
60. Primack SL, Müller NL (1994) High-resolution computed tomography in acute diffuse lung disease in the immunocompromised patient. Radiol Clin North Am 32:731–744

61. Remy J, Remy-Jardin M, Giraud F, Wattinne L (1994) Angioarchitecture of pulmonary arteriovenous malformations: clinical utility of three-dimensional helical CT. Radiology 191:657–664
62. Remy-Jardin M, Boulenguez C, Edme JL, Sobazek A, Wallaert B, Rémy J (1993) Morphologic effects of cigarette smoking on airways and pulmonary parenchyma in healthy adult volunteers: CT evaluation and correlations with pulmonary function tests. Radiology 186:107–115
63. Remy-Jardin M, Giraud F, Remy J, Copin MC, Gosselin B, Duhamel A (1993) Importance of ground-glass attenuation in chronic diffuse infiltrative lung disease: pathologic-CT correlation. Radiology 189:693–698
64. Remy-Jardin M, Remy J (1988) Comparison of vertical and oblique CT in evaluation of bronchial tree. J Comput Assist Tomogr 12:956–962
65. Remy-Jardin M, Remy J, Giraud F et al. (1993) Pulmonary nodules: detection with thick-section spiral CT versus conventional CT. Radiology 187:513–520
66. Remy-Jardin M, Remy J, Wallaert B, Müller NL (1993) Subacute and chronic bird breeder hypersensitivity pneumonitis: sequential evaluation with CT and correlation with lung function tests and bronchoalveolar lavage. Radiology 189:111–118
67. Ren H, Hruban RH, Kuhlman JE, Fishman EK, Wheeler PS, Zerhouni EA, Hutchins GM (1988) Computed tomography of rounded atelectasis. J Comput Assist Tomogr 12:1031–1034
68. Ren H, Kuhlman JE, Hruban RH, Fishman EK, Wheeler PS, Hurchins GM (1990) CT of inflation-fixed lungs: wedge-shaped density and vascular sign in the diagnosis of infarction. J Comput Assist Tomogr 14:82–86
69. Sider L, Gabriel H, Curry DR, Pham MS (1993) Pattern recognition of the pulmonary manifestations of AIDS on CT scans. Radiographics 13:771–784
70. Stern EJ, Franck MS (1994) Small-airway diseases of the lungs: findings at expiratory CT. AJR 163:37–41
71. Webb WR (1989) High resolution CT of the lung parenchyma. Radiol Clin North Am 27:1085–1097
72. Webb VR (1994) High-resolution computed tomography of obstructive lung disease. Radiol Clin North Am 32:745–757
73. Webb WR, Stein MG, Finkbeiner WE, Im JG, Lynch D, Gamsu G (1988) Normal and diseased isolated lungs: high-resolution CT. Radiology 166:81–87
74. Wolff SD, Kuhlman JE, Fishman EK (1993) Thoracic Kaposi sarcoma in AIDS: CT findings. J Comput Assist Tomogr 17:60–62

CHAPTER 12

Computed Tomography in the Diagnosis of Cystic Lesions of the Liver

Huay-Ben Pan, Jer-Shyung Huang and Chien-Fang Yang[1]

The cystic lesions of liver in computed tomography may present in a variety of pathologic entities. As has been well documented, a pure cyst has a well-demarcated thin wall, ovoid shape, homogenous near water content, and lack of contrast enhancement. Thick-walled lesions represent infected cysts or liver abscess. Increased density of the content of a liver cyst is seen in hemorrhage or infection. The cystic lesion containing solid parts represents cystic tumor, either benign or malignant. Irregular shape of the cystic lesion can be noted in liquefied hematoma, liver infarct, or dilated intrahepatic ducts. In this paper, we categorized all the cystic lesions of the liver into six groups in addition to the pure liver cysts.

Cysts with Increased Density

A pure cyst has computed tomography (CT) numbers between 8 and 20 HU. Higher values of the cyst usually a result of hemorrhage, infection, high protein content of the cystic fluid or just an effect of partial volume artifacts. An infected cyst is easily recognized if the nearby cysts are available for comparison. Precontrast CT is more reliable in this situation. Blood clots in the dependent portion suggest the possibility of hemorrhage (Fig. 1), while gas bubbles in the independent portion indicate an infectious nature. The clinical information of traumatic history or fever are important for diagnosis. However, the traumatic history may be too subtle to be traced, especially in cases of polycystic liver disease. Besides, blood clots within the cyst may simulate soft tissue components in cystic tumor. Additional image modalities such as doppler ultrasonography or magnetic resonance imaging may provide useful information in this situation. Sometimes a tumor with complete necrosis will give the same picture as a mature abscess or liquefied hematoma. However, the border of the cyst will be more irregular in the former. On the other hand, an edematous zone surrounding a cystic lesion of the liver indicates a rapid development of the lesion with resultant compression of the surrounding parenchyma. It is more often seen in abscess, especially pyogenic, rather than in a tumor with complete necrosis. However, aspiration or drainage is necessary to confirm the diagnosis and to treat the lesions. Even with total resection of a completely necrotic tumor, it may be difficult to get adequate tissue to make the diagnosis of neoplasm not to mention a more specific diagnosis.

---

[1] Department of Radiology, Veterans General Hospital-Kaohsiung, Kaohsiung, Taiwan.

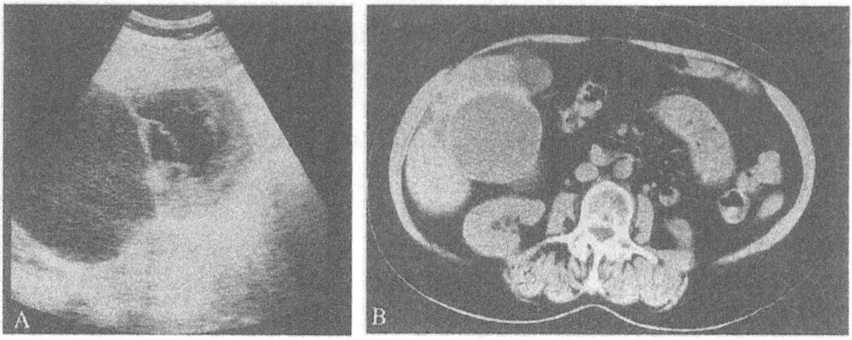

Fig. 1 A, B A simple cyst complicated with hemorrhage simulating cystic neoplasm under sonography. A hyperdense component is seen in dependent parts of the cystic lesion. Aspiration and biopsy showed bloody fluid with old blood. No definite tumor cell identified

Cysts with Mural Nodules

Cysts with mural nodules may be seen in cases of metastasis, mucinous cystadenoma or cystadenocarcinoma of liver, and other necrotic solid primary tumors. The cystic metastasis has been classified into four types of presentation [1], i.e., septations, fluid-fluid level in the cystic lesion, thick wall, and mural nodules of the cystic wall. The former two can be more precisely demonstrated by sonography than CT scan. The latter two are well demonstrated in postcontrast CT scans especially with spiral CT technique. The spiral CT and contrast-enhanced magnetic resonance imaging (MRI) can provide information about dynamic enhancement of the mural nodules. Color doppler ultrasound may detect the doppler shift at the solid part of the cystic tumor but is more time-consuming. The pitfalls of color doppler in diagnosing the mural nodules of cystic lesion may occur in a pure cyst with vessels passing the cystic wall or in a pure cyst with previous hemorrhage causing local thickening of the cystic wall. However, in this situation, the cystic wall should not appear enhanced in CT scan and MRI. Once the viable mural nodules have been demonstrated, tumor growth has to be considered. Cystic metastases are most commonly seen in epidermoid carcinoma in our experience (Fig. 2). However, leiomyosarcoma and carcinoma of the ovary and colon have also been found. A primary malignant history with multiple lesions in the liver parenchyma should lead to the consideration of cystic metastasis. The presence of dilated bile duct without definite stones or tumor compression may suggest the diagnosis of mucin-producing cystadenoma or cystadenocarcinoma. Distinguishing these two lesions microscopically is not quite reliable. However, the more solid part is found, the greater the possibility of malignancy. The biliary cystadenoma or cystadenocarcinoma usually present with a solitary tumor rather than multiple lesions. Their hypersecretion of mucin account for the non-obstructive dilatation of bile ducts. In cystic liver lesions with irregular border and the associated findings of liver cirrhosis and portal vein thrombosis,

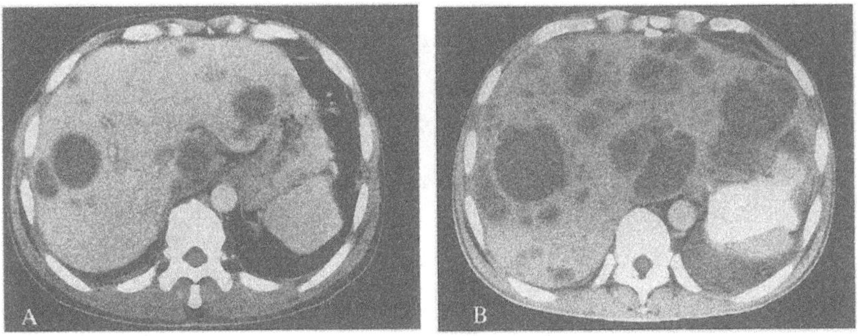

Fig. 2 A,B Cystic metastasis from nasopharyngeal carcinoma. **A** Multiple cystic lesions were noted in both lobes of liver with small mural nodules identified. **B** Follow-up CT scan showed progressive enlargement of these cystic lesions and mural nodules.

hepatocellular carcinoma with necrosis is strongly suggested. The internal architecture of cystic lesions is more clearly depicted by sonography than CT scan although sometimes the internal echogenicities from pus formation, mucous, or necrotic tissue may mimic a solid tumor in sonogram.

Tumors with Cystic Part

Necrosis and hemorrhage of the liver tumor may result in a cystic appearance. They are usually caused by a hypervascular tumor with insufficient blood supply or rupture of the vessels. Cavernous hemangioma is the most common benign tumor with hypervascularity in the general population. The image diagnosis of cavernous hemangioma is well-established and characterized by dense and thick peripheral enhancement with slowly, centripetal fill-in towards isodensity over several minutes up to an hour. On magnetic resonance imaging, in addition to a very bright signal in T2-weighted image, the characteristic enhancement pattern in CT scans can also be demonstrated in dynamic study. Cystic degeneration of cavernous hemangioma is rare. The non-enhanced portion of cavernous hemangioma is mostly due to fibrosis or thrombosis. The other common hypervascular tumor is hepatocellular carcinoma. Once a necrotic liver tumor is associated with a thrombosed portal vein, hepatoma is highly suggestive. Considering the 80% percent of hepatocellular carcinoma occuring in liver with preexisting cirrhosis, we should keep in mind the possibility of hepatocellular carcinoma in liver cirrhosis with cystic liver lesions (Fig. 3). It is characteristically accompanied by central cleft necrosis. The hypervascular metastases of liver mainly form from leiomyosarcoma, renal cell carcinoma, islet cell carcinoma, thyroid cancer, pheochromocytoma, melanoma, choriocarcinoma, and carcinoid tumor. In the cases of known primary malignancy especially from the above mentioned organs, metastasis is suggestive. Biopsy is needed to confirm the diagnosis.

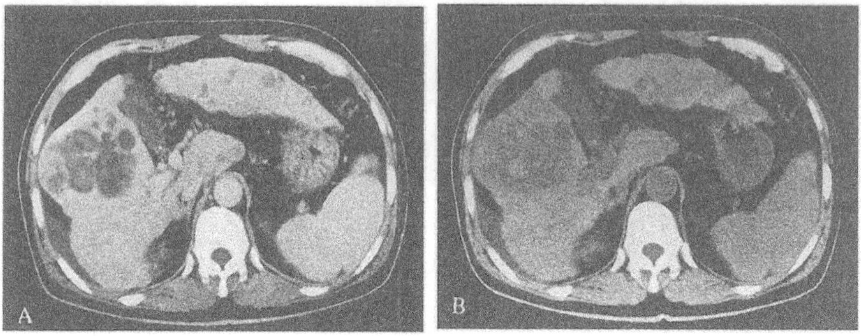

Fig. 3 A, B Hepatocellular carcinoma with hemorrhage and cystic components. **A** The pre-contrast CT scan showed liver cirrhosis and a bulging mass lesion at the anterior segment. Hemorrhage was noted. **B** Cystic components were evident at the post-contrast CT scan

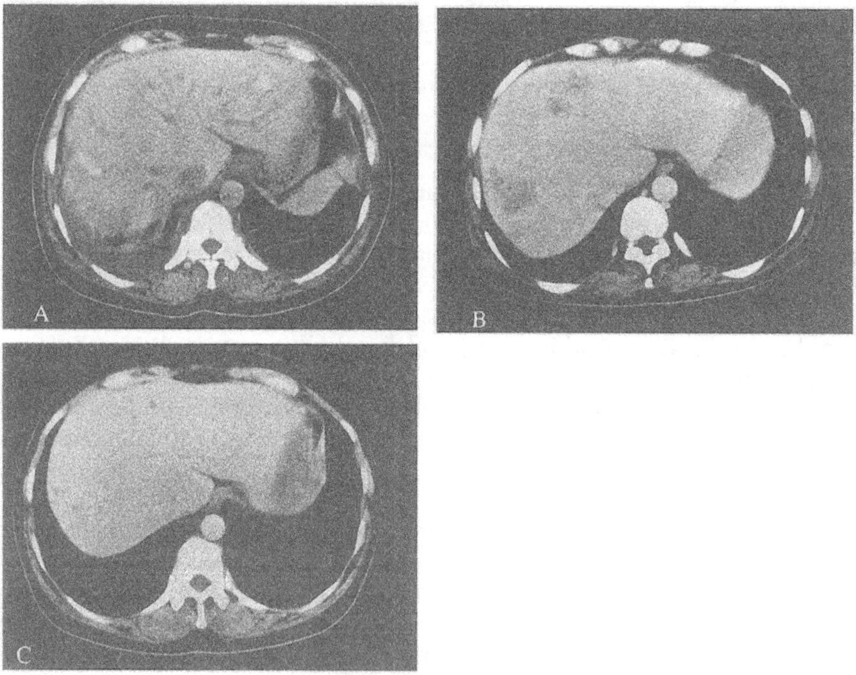

Fig. 4 A A 56-year-old male patient presented with persistent fever and multiple tiny hypodense lesions in both lobes of liver parenchyma. The aspiration failed to prove the etiology. **B** Progression of the lesions was noted, 3 weeks later despite administration of antibiotics. Tuberculosis (TB) was found in aspiration at this time. **C** After 3 months of anti-TB medication, calcification of the lesions was noted

Cysts developing or Disappeared in a Short Period

In the situation that a cystic lesion developed in a short period, the clinical history is important to approach the diagnoses. In the presence of fever or immunosuppression, microabscess is the most likely diagnosis (Fig. 4). In post-traumatic cases, liquefied hematoma or biloma should be included in the differential diagnosis. If the patient has received TAE in the previous few days, biloma or tumor necrosis should be first considered. If the tumor transforms from a solid to a cystic one, cystic necrosis should be considered. Although lipiodol-filled component of hepatoma in patients after transarterial embolization is generally accepted as a non-viable component of the tumor, complete necrosis presents as a simple cystic lesion is not a reliable sign of complete eradication of the tumor cells in this nodule. In our experience, close follow-up is necessary because the relapsed lesion of the hepatoma has been noted. Disappearance of the cystic lesions in a short period of time is most likely due to an absorbed microabscess or small hematoma.

Persistent Tiny Cystic Lesions

Persistent tiny cystic lesions in the liver are mostly due to simple cyst, hemangioma, peliosis hepatitis or biliary hamartoma. It is hard to make a definite diagnosis. Blind biopsies of the liver parenchyma may be necessary. Among them, early diagnosis of peliosis hepatitis is important to avoid complications including hepatocellular dysfunction, portal hypertension, and potential rupture of the liver. Peliosis hepatitis is most strongly associated with the use of anabolic steroids and may be solved if the steroid use is discontinued. Because peliosis hepatitis is caused by multiple blood-filled cavities in the liver, it may appear isodense on the post-contrast CT scan as hemangioma does, or present as cystic lesions due to blood clots or thrombosis. Follow-up is recommended in this group of cystic lesions.

Tubular Structure

The transaxial image of dilated tubular structures may present as cystic lesions. On the contrary, the transaxial images of thrombosed portal veins may present as a solid nodule and be misinterpreted as solid tumors. Usually, the bile duct dilation is seen in the cases of bile duct obstruction, such as tumor compression, stone or mucous impaction. If the intrahepatic bile duct dilation is not proportionally dilated to the common bile duct (CBD) and is present as cylindrical or cystic dilation, Caroli disease or sclerosing cholangitis should be distinguished. The dilatation of the bile duct may be more extensive in Caroli disease than in sclerosing cholangitis. These two diseases are more common in oriental countries. Segmental Caroli disease is hard to distinguish from simple biliary inflammation and dilatation by stone obstruction.

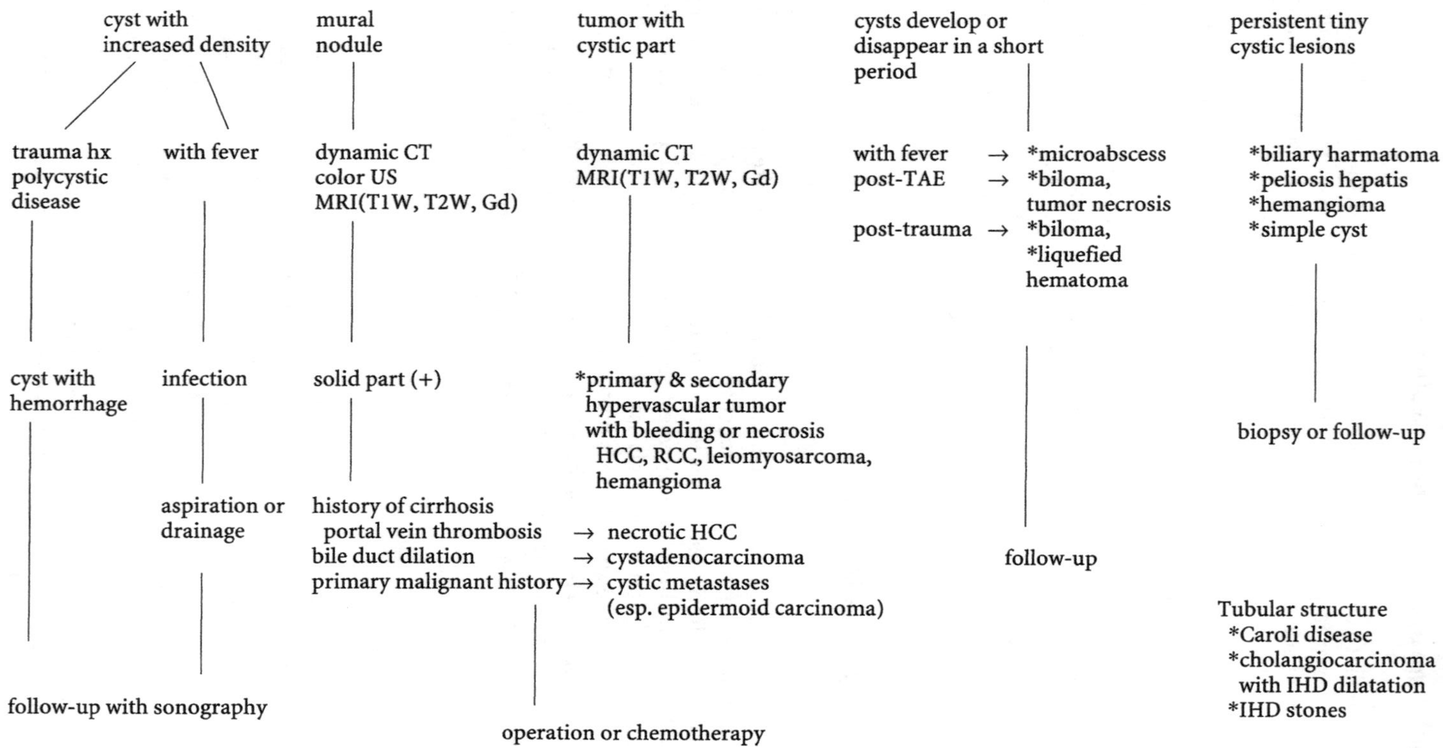

Fig. 5 Computed tomography (CT) scans for cystic lesions of the liver. *MRI*, magnetic resonance image; *W*, weighted; *Gd*, gadolinium; *HCC*, hepatocellular carcinoma; *RCC*, renal cell carcinoma; *US*, ultrasonography

Conclusion

Most cystic lesions of the liver can be specifically diagnosed with CT scans, as discussed above (Fig. 5). However, in some small nodules, pitfalls do exist such as mass with partial volume effect, change of the background of liver parenchyma in fatty metamorphosis or hemochromatosis, solid tumor with poor enhancement, double lesions (figure 5), and extrahepatic cystic lesions mimicking intrahepatic ones. Measurement the CT number of the cystic content, further evaluation by ultrasound or MRI, the application of dynamic CT scan, needle aspiration or follow-up in a short period of time are the methods to solve the problem of pitfalls in diagnosis.

References

1. Murphy BJ, Casillas JC, Ros PR, Morillo G, Rolfes DB (1989) The CT appearance of cystic masses of the liver. Radiographics 9 (2): 307–321
2. Chiang JH et al. (1985) Correlation of the images of computed tomography and angiography in hepatic tumors. Chinese J Radiology 10: 183–191
3. Friedman AC et al. (1987) Focal disease. In: Friedman AC (ed) Radiology of theliver, biliary tract, and spleen. W & W, Baltimore, p 214
4. Stephens DH, Johnson CD (1990) Benign masses of the liver. In: Silverman PM, Zeman RK (eds) CT & MRI of the liver & biliary system. Churchill Livingstone, New York, pp 98–112
5. Nagasue N (1984) Successful treatment of Caroli's disease by hepatic resection: report of six patients. Ann Surg 200: 718
6. Berland L, Lee JKT, Stanley RJ (1989) Liver & biliary tree. In: Lee JKT, Sagel SS, Stanley RJ (eds) Computed body tomography with MRI correlation. Raven, New York, p 620

Solid Liver Tumor: Spiral Computed Tomography During Angiography in Hepatocellular Carcinoma

Yun Hwan Kim[1]

Indications

The indication for combined spiral computed tomography (CT) during hepatic arteriography (CTHA) and CT during arterial portography (CTAP) was mainly to detect nodular lesions, which are associated with liver cirrhosis on pre-existing imagings, such as conventional CT scans (non-contrast CT, contrast enhanced CT or hepatic arterial phase of IV bolus spiral CT), MR, ultrasonography (US) and US-guided percutaneous biopsy, etc. Most of the patients at high risk of hepatocellular carcinoma (HCC) had at least one or two nodules suspected on previous images. Our interests were to evaluate how many more nodules were detected on combined CTHA and CTAP or either one or the other and which would be better to depict the entire nodules in the liver.

Routinely, follow-up combined CTHA and CTAP were recommended usually with 2- to 6-month interval, to evaluate previous lesions and newly developed lesions after transarterial chemoembolization (TACE).

CT Technique and Required Contrast Media Application

Arterial vascular access was obtained by bilateral punctures of the common femoral artery utilizing the Seldinger technique. Angiographic catheters (5 F) were then selectively placed in the proximal celiac artery and superior mesenteric artery (SMA). Celiac and SMA angiographies were performed initially in all patients. Intraarterial digital subtraction arteriography (DSA) was performed to reduce the total volume of contrast material used during arteriography and subsequent spiral CTHA and CTAP. The primary goal of arteriography was to depict the vascular anatomy for the surgeon and interventional radiologist to perform either surgery or TACE. The total amount of contrast material used during angiography varied, but was less than 40ml in all cases. The catheters were secured in place, and the patients were then transferred to the CT scanner.

Initially, Spiral CTHA was performed with 10 mm collimation and a table speed of 10 mm/s during a transcatheter infusion of 20–35 ml (0.5 ml/kg) nonionic contrast medium (Ultravist, 300 mg I/ml, Schering, Germany). Contrast material

[1] Department of Diagnostic Radiology, Korea University Hospital, Korea University, College of Medicine, 126-1, 5-Ka, Anam-Dong, Sungbuk-Ku, Seoul, 136–705, Korea.

was injected through the catheter in the common or proper hepatic artery at a rate of 1 to 1.5 ml/s through a power injector (Medrad, Pittsburgh, Pa). CTAP followed the same CT parameters, injecting contrast medium via the catheter into the superior mesenteric or splenic artery at a rate of 2.0–2.5 ml/s. A total of 60–80 ml (1.5 ml/kg) of contrast medium was used. Spiral scanning usually began 5 s (for CTHA) and 25 or 40 s (for CTAP) from the start of the injection. In the case of CTAP, we usually wait 40 s after the start of infusion, because the majority of our patients have cirrhotic liver with portal hypertension. All of the spiral CT angiographic studies were performed on a Somatom Plus S(Siemens, Erlangen, Germany). The patients were instructed to hold their breath during spiral scanning to eliminate motion artifacts. Spiral CT scans were obtained at 210 mAs and 120 kVp. Scan duration was 15–25 s, with craniocaudal table incrementation.

The Value of Spiral CTHA and CTAP in Comparison to Other Imaging Procedures

The numerous imaging techniques available for detecting small HCC and regional differences have resulted in various diagnostic standards and comparative studies. The relative efficacies of various techniques for detecting HCCs less than 3 cm in diameter have been evaluated. Reviewing previous reports reveals a wide variation in accuracy for US, CT, and angiography, as a variety of techniques, scanners, and protocols were used for each procedure. The sensitivity for detecting HCCs less than 3 cm in diameter is 55%–84% with US, 46%–84% with CT, 61%–81% with angiography, 82% with CTHA, 72%–94% with CTAP, 71%–96% with lipidiol CT, 86% with US angiography, and 94%–96% with intraoperative US. In most comparative analyses, the senstivities of intraoperative US, CTAP, and lipidiol CT are significantly higher than those of US, conventional CT, CTHA, or angiography.

According to recent reports, the hepatic arterial phase of spiral CT, after intravenous bolus injection, greatly improved the detection of HCC as compared with the delayed phase, which is comparable with conventional CT. This report indicates that it is advantageous to perform hepatic arterial phase of CT in the detection of hypervascular tumor, such as HCC. Based on our experience, the more pure hepatic arterial phase of CT, such as CTHA, can surely provide a high contrast resolution in spite of minimal arterial flow in HCC. However, the report for the sensitivity of combined CTHA and CTAP in benign and malignant nodules with liver cirrhosis are rare. To our knowledge, no report has been published on combined CTHA and CTAP with use of spiral CT.

Combined spiral CTHA and CTAP consist of obtaining rapid CT scans during a bolus injection of contrast material administered through a transfemoral catheter, the tip of which is located in the hepatic artery (arteriography) or the superior mesenteric artery (arterial portography). The evidence of CTHA or CTAP in the detection of HCC lies in the differences in perfusion between normal liver(blood supply from the hepatic artery and portal vein) and HCC (blood supply from the hepatic artery only). Most of HCC are seen as hyperattenuating nodules on CTHA and as perfusion defects on CTAP, because most of these tumors have no portal supply.

Matsui et al. found that intranodular portal blood flow tends to decrease as the grade of malignancy increases. Unlike adenomatous hyperplasia, almost all HCC of Edmondson grade 2 or greater had a definite decrease in the intranodular portal supply on CTAP. In intermediate lesions, such as early HCC and well-differentiated (Grade 1) HCC, the intranodular portal blood supply tended to decrease progressively as the grade of malignancy increased, whereas the intranodular hepatic arterial supply increased. Unlike early HCCs, adenomatous hyperplasias are not visualized on CTAP because of portal blood flow in these lesions. The relationship between the portal and arterial blood supplies in the hepatocytic lesions found in cirrhotic liver was considered to be reciprocal on imaging. Therefore, the combination of CT arteriography and CT arterial portography is more accurate than either alone in determining the nature of the nodular lesions associated with liver cirrhosis.

The precise diagnosis of small HCC is not always easy, not only by imaging but also by percutaneous needle biopsy, because of the existence of various types of hepatocytic nodular lesions with inner heterogeneity in the cirrhotic liver. When difficulty exists in determining the grade of malignancy of these lesions, evaluation of the intranodular blood supply by imaging is very useful. From this point of view, the combination of CTHA and CTAP may provide the precise diagnosis of hepatocytic lesions associated with cirrhotic liver.

In our institute, 180 cases of combined CTHA and CTAP were performed on 105 patients with nodular HCC during a period of 18 months from March 1993 to September 1994. According to our unpublished data, 30 patients (28.6%) showed the same nodules on either initial spiral CTHA or CTAP, as compared with pre-existing imagings. In 75 patients (71.4%), combined CTHA and CTAP revealed more HCC lesions, except for confirmed and suspected pseudolesions. It was easy to detect small exophytic and subcapsular lesions on CTHA in seven patients, as compared with CTAP (Fig. 1). These tumors ranged from a few millimeters (Fig. 2) to less than 15 mm in diameter.

Adenomatous hyperplasias associated with regenerative nodules were well delineated with hypoattenuating nodules on CTHA in 31 patients (29.5%), because of isoattenuation on CTAP. Therefore, CTHA is definitely superior to CTAP in the detection of regenerative nodules and adenomatous hyperplasias.

Intermediate lesions, such as atypical adenomatous hyperplasia, early HCC and well differentiated HCC, had partly different dual blood supply. In these lesions, the combination of CTHA and CTAP is important to detect more accurately hepatic arterial and portal flows respectively.

On follow-up spiral CTHA and CTAP, who had more than one TACE, residual or new lesions were well noted, including a stepwise development of HCC from adenomatous hyperplasia or intermediate lesions, suggestive of increased hepatic arterial and decreased portal flow (Fig. 3).

Evaluating the blood supply is also useful for selecting treatment methods, because transarterial chemoembolization (TACE) is not effective in the treatment of well differentiated HCC, atypical adenomatous hyperplasia (AH), or AH with malignant foci with an intranodular portal blood supply.

The advantage of combined CTHA and CTAP was the easy detection of adenomatous hyperplasia, early HCC and small definite HCC with vascular flow

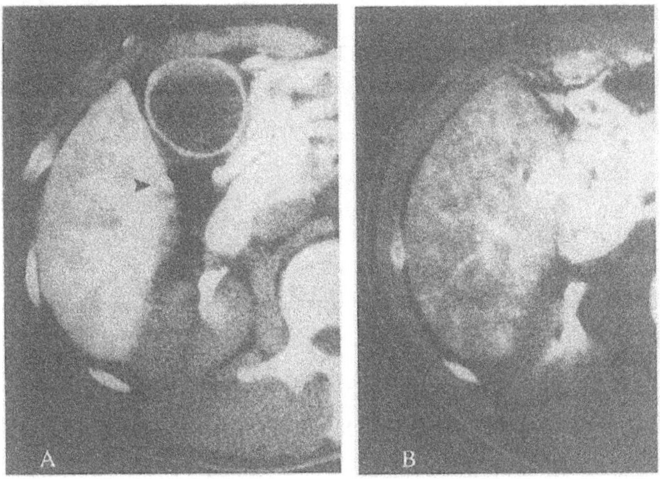

Fig. 1 A–B This patient had left lobectomy, due to a small hepatocellular carcinoma (HCC; 3.0 cm in diameter) on segment 3, after initial computed tomography during hepatic arteriography (CTHA) and arterial portography (CTAP). A small hyperattenuating daughter nodule, (arrowhead) 5 mm in diameter, is seen on subcapsular portion along medial aspect of segment 6. CTAP does not reveal this lesion. **B** Follow-up CTHA, 7 months after initial CTHA and lobectomy, shows marked enlargement (17 mm in diameter) of the previously tiny nodule on segment 6. The gallbladder is not seen, due to previous cholecystectomy

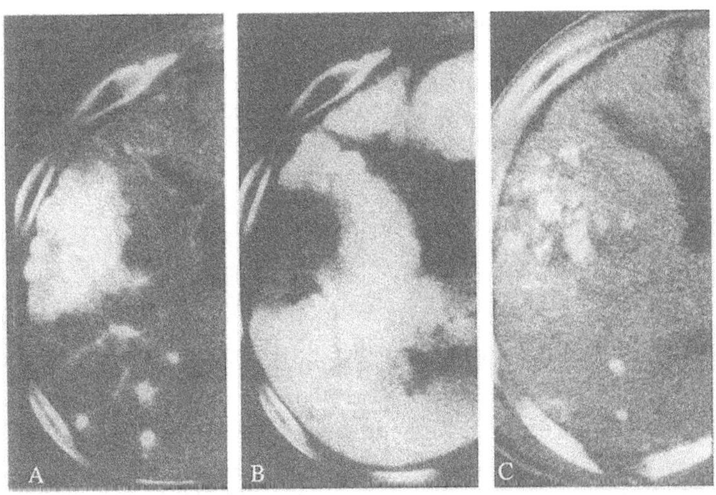

Fig. 2 A Computed tomography during hepatic arteriography (CTHA) shows confluent hyperattenuating nodules on segment 5 and tiny small hyperattenuating nodules on segment 6, which are less than 5 mm in diameter. **B** CT during arterial portography (CTAP) shows less sensitivity on segment 5 and 6 lesions in contrast to CTHA, showing as only one perfusion defect in confluent nodules, probably due to tumor thrombus of small portal venous branch. **C** Lipiodol CT shows similar lesions with CTHA, 1 week after transarterial chemoembolization (TACE)

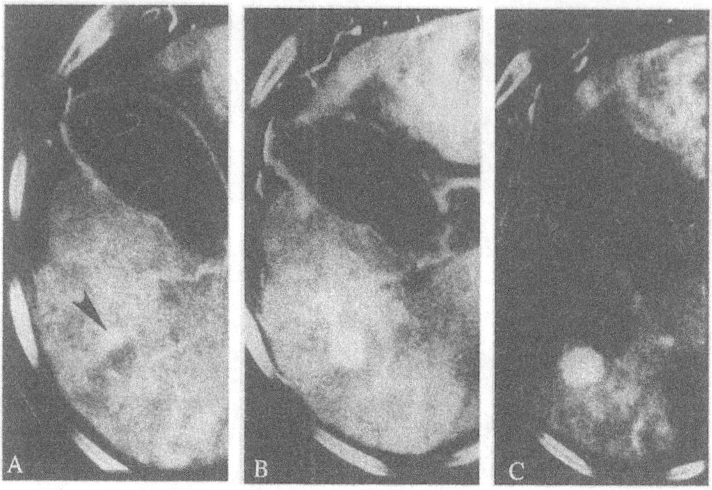

Fig. 3 A–C This patient has been treated seven times, with transarterial chemoembolization (TACE) for 4 years. **A** Spiral computed tomography during hepatic arteriography (CTHA) shows a hyperattenuating focus on the eccentric site of a round hypoattenuating mass, suggestive of malignant focus (arrowhead) with adenomatous hyperplasia (AH; early hepatocellular carcinoma, HCC). **B** Follow-up CTHA, 6 months later, shows total replacement of hyperattenuating area, suggestive of small HCC. **C** Follow-up CTHA, another 3 months after TACE, shows a slightly more enlarged hyperattenuating nodule, 1.2 cm in diameter. These serial CTHA shows a stepwise development of HCC from AH in cirrhotic liver, with angiogenesis

mapping of hepatocytic nodules. The other advantages were easy understanding of the hemodynamics, and complementary compensation of false negative lesions due to lamina flow, spasm, or technical error in performing either CTHA or CTAP. The disadvantages of combined CTHA and CTAP were the difficulty in interpretation due to pseudolesions, and the difficulty of the technique.

In our experience, the sensitivity of Lip-CT depends on the scanning date after lipiodol injection, the amount of lipiodol used, and variation in the lipiodol injection technique, including size and position of catheters. Due to above mentioned causes, CTHA seems to be the standard imaging to evaluate Lip-CT after TACE.

Position Within the Cascade of Imaging Procedures

Early detection of HCC is important as a complete surgical resection of these tumors is the most effective treatment. Therefore, screening and regular follow-up with imaging techniques have been introduced in patients at high risk of HCC.

If the nodules are small and appear benign (such as regenerating nodules or AH) on CTHA and magnetic resonance (MR) images, interval serial scanning is currently the only practical method of follow-up. In such cases, the final diagnosis based on histologic findings alone, after percutaneous biopsy, is difficult because entire pathologic specimens are needed for histologic diagnosis.

If imaging findings suggest that nodules are malignant, staging of the nodules by using spiral CTHA, CTAP, and Lip-CT is necessary. The selection of techniques for staging might be difficult, because the decision as to which imaging techniques are state-of-the art and the levels of familiarity with certain techniques will vary among institutions.

Conclusions

Recent advances in various imaging techniques have led to an increase in the detection of other hepatic nodular lesions such as regenerating nodules, adenomatous hyperplasia, atypical AH, and early HCC in the cirrhotic liver. Although the definitions of AH and early HCC are still controversial, the concept of these borderline lesions is expected to prevail gradually. Some of lesions are maligant nodules; therefore, the distinction between benign and malignant nodules is clinically important.

Though difficulties in technique and interpretation of combined CTHA and CTAP exist, it is our opinion that the combination of CTHA and CTAP in patients at high risk for HCC will be helpful for the early detection and treatment planning of HCC as the precise diagnosis of benign, intermediate and malignant lesions.

References

1. Soyer P, Levesque M, Elias D, Zeitoun G, Roche A (1992) Preoperative assessment of resectability of hepatic metastases from colonic carcinoma: CT portography vs sonography and dynamic CT. AJR 159:741–744
2. Karl RC, Morse SS, Halpert RD, Clark RA (1993) Preoperative evaluation of patients for liver resection: appropriate CT imaging. Ann Surg 217:226–232
3. Soyer P, Levesque M, Caudron C, Elias D, Zeitoun G, Roche A (1993) MRI of liver metastases from colorectal cancer vs CT during arterial portography. J Comput Assist Tomogr 17:67–74
4. Matsui O, Takashima T, Kadoya M, et al. (1985) Dynamic computed tomography during arterial portography: the most sensitive examination for small hepatocellular carcinomas. J Comput Assist Tomogr 9:19–24
5. Heiken JP, Weyman PJ, Lee JKT, et al. (1990) Detection of focal hepatic masses: prospective evaluation with CT, delayed CT, CT during arterial portography, and MR imaging. Radiology 175:47–51.
6. Merine D, Takayasu K, Wakao F (1990) Detection of hepatocellular carcinoma: comparison of CT during arterial portography with CT after intraarterial injection of iodized oil. Radiology 175:707–710
7. Utsunomiya T, Matsumata T, Adachi E, Honda H, Sugimachi K (1992) Limitations of current preoperative liver imaging techniques for intrahepatic metastatic nodules of the hepatocellular carcinoma. Hepatology 16:694–701
8. Soyer P, Bluemke DA, Hruban RH, Sitzmann JV, Fishman EK (1994) Primary malignant neoplasms of the liver: detection with helical CT during arterial portography. Radiology 192:389–392
9. Choi BI, Takayasu K, Han MC (1993) Small hepatocellular carcinoma and associcated nodular lesions of the liver: pathology, pathogenesis, and imaging findings AJR 160:1177–1187

10. Takayasu K, Moriyama N, Muramatsu Y et al. (1990) The diagnosis of small hepatocellular carcinomas: efficacy of various imaging procedures in 100 patients. AJR 155:49–54
11. Heiken JP, Brink JA, Vannuer MW (1993) Spiral (helical) CT. Radiology 189:647–656
12 Zeman RK, Fox SH, Silverman PM et al. Helical(spiral) CT of the abdomen. AJR 1993; 160:719–725
13 Urban BA, Fishman EK, Kuhlma JE, Kawachima A, Hennessey JG, Siegelman SS (1993) Detection of focal hepatic lesions with spiral CT: comparison of 4- and 8-mm interscan spacing. AJR 160:783–785
14. Okuda K, Kojiro M (1987) Small hepatocellular carcioma. In: Okuda K, Ishak KG, eds. Neoplasms of the liver. Tokyo: Springer-Verlag, 215–216.
15. Ohta G, Nakanuma Y (1987) Comparative study of three nodular lesions in cirrhosis: adenomatoid hyperplasia, adenomatoid hyperplasia with intermediate lesions and small hepatocellular carcinoma. In: Okuda K, Ishak KG, eds Neoplasms of the liver. Tokyo: Springer-Verlag, 177–188.
16. Matsui O, Kadoya M, Kameyama T, et al. (1989) Adenomatous hyperplastic nodules in the cirrhotic liver: differentiation from hepatocellular carcinoma with MR imaging. Radiology 173:123–126
17. Matsui O, Kadoya M, Kameyama T et al. (1991) Benign and malignant nodules in cirrhotic livers: distinction based on blood supply. Radiology 178:493–497
18. Matsui O, Takahashi S, Kadoya M, Yoshikawa J, et al. (1994) Pseudolesion in Segment IV of the liver at CT during arterial portography: correlation with aberrant gastric venous drainage. Radiology 193:31–35
19. Matsui O, Takashima T, Kadoya M et al. (1987) Staining in the liver surrounding gallbladder fossa on hepatic arteriography caused by increased cystic venous drainage. Gastrointestinal Radiol 12:307–312
20. Paulson EK, Baker ME, Spritzer CE, Leder RA, Gulliver DJ, Meyers WC (1993) Focal fatty infiltration: a cause of nontumorous defects in the left hepatic lobe during CT arterial portography. J Comput Assist Tomogr 17:590–595
21 Fernandez MP, Bernardino ME (1991) Hepatic pseudolesions: appearance of focal low attenuation in the medial segment of the left lobe at CT-arterial portography. Radiology 181:809–812
22. Freeny PC, Marks WM (1986) Hepatic perfusion abnormalities during CT angiography: detection and interpretation. Radiology 159:685–691
23. Kudo M, Hirasa M, Takakuwa H et al. (1986) Angiography of small hepatocellular carcinioma: analysis of 105 resected tumors. AJR 147:525–529
24. Choi BI, Park JH, Kim BH et al. (1989) Small hepatocellular carcinoma: detection with sonography, computed tomography (CT), angiography and lipiodol-CT. Br J Radiol 62:897–901
25. Kudo M, Tomita S, Tochio H et al. (1992) Small hepatocellular carcinoma: diagnosis with US angiography with intraarterial CO2 microbubbles. Radiology 182:155–160
26. Choi BI, Han JK, Song IS et al. (1991) Intraoperative sonography of hepatocellular carcinoma: detection of lesions and validity in surgical resection. Gastrointest Radiol 16:329–333
27. Takayasu K, Moriyama N, Muramatsu Y et al. (1990) The diagnosis of small hepatocellular carcinomas: efficacy of various imaging procedures in 100 patients. AJR 155:49–54
28. Matsui O, Kameyama T, Yoshikawa J et al. (1988) Angiographic diagnosis of hepatocellular carcinoma including CT arteriography and CT arterial portography (in Japanese) J Med Imaging 8:1289–1300
29. Hayashi N, Yamamoto K, Tamaki N et al. (1987) Metastatic nodules of hepatocellular carcinoma: detection with angiography, CT and US. Radiology 165:61–63
30. Choi BI, Cho JM, Han JK, Kim SH, Han M (1994) Spiral CT for the detection of hepatocellular carcinoma: relative value of two-phase scanning. presented (1383) at the meeting of RSNA

31. Chezmar JL, Bernardino ME, Kaufman SH, Nelson RC (1993) Combined CT arterial portography and CT hepatic angiography for evaluation of the hepatic resection candidate. Work in progress. Radiology 189:407–410
32. Freeny PC, Marks WM (1983) Computed tomographic arteriography of the liver. Radiology 148:193–197
33. Takayasu K, Makuuchi M, Hirohashi S et al. (1989) Imaging of adenomatous hyperplastic lesions containing and not containing hepatocellular carcinoma in the liver(in Japanase). Nippon Shokakibyo Gakkai Zasshi 86:2404–2412

CHAPTER 14

Fatty Infiltration of Liver

Jae Mun Lee[1]

Hepatic fatty infiltration (metamorphosis or steatosis) is a metabolic complication where excessive neutral fat (triglycerides) accumulates within the cytoplasm of the hepatocytes. It is associated with a variety of clinical disorders, including obesity, diabetes mellitus, alcoholic liver disease, malnutrition, total parenteral nutrition, chemotherapy, glucocorticoid therapy and hepatotoxin [1–3]. The fatty infiltration is clinically silent in most cases and the liver function test is usually normal. However, mild to moderate hepatomegaly, with vague right upper quadrant abdominal pain and tenderness may be present and is often associated with abnormal liver chemistry [1, 3, 4].

Computed Tomographic Diagnosis of Fatty Liver

Computed tomography (CT) is the best noninvasive technique for the detection of fatty liver because there is an excellent correlation between the hepatic parenchymal CT attenuation value and the amount of hepatic triglycerides [5, 6]. On noncontrast scans, the attenuation of the normal liver is 50–75 HU, which is at least as much as, but usually 8–10 HU greater than, the attenuation of the spleen [7, 8].

Diffuse Fatty Liver

Hepatic parenchymal fatty infiltration decreases the mean hepatic CT attenuation value. There is a homogeneous, diffuse decrease in the hepatic density with diffuse fatty infiltration of various grades [9].

In a mild case (grade 1), the diagnosis can be made by comparing the CT attenuation value of the nonenhanced liver and the spleen, with the liver attenuation being slightly less than that of spleen. In a moderate case (grade 2), the liver becomes less dense with more pronounced contrast between the lower-attenuation liver and spleen. Intrahepatic vessels are not seen or are of a slightly higher attenuation than the liver. In a severe case (grade 3), the hepatic attenuation is markedly reduced with a sharp contrast between the liver and intrahepatic

[1] Department of Radiology, St. Mary's Hospital, Catholic University Medical College, Seoul, Korea.

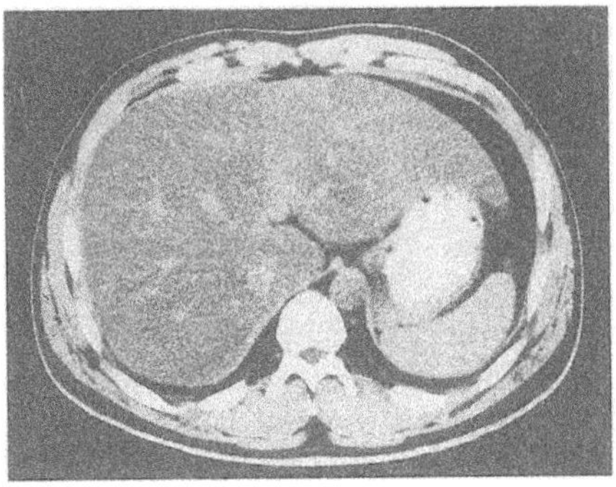

Fig. 1 Diffuse fatty infiltration of the liver. Nonenhanced computed tomography (CT) scan shows diffuse decrease of hepatic attenuation. The intrahepatic vessels appear as relatively high attenuation structures

vessels. The portal and hepatic veins appear as high-attenuation structures surrounded by a background of lower attenuation hepatic parenchyma (Fig. 1). Dilated biliary trees or low attenuation lesion within the liver may be obscured due to little contrast between them and the decreased attenuation hepatic parenchyma [10].

Focal Fatty Liver

The pattern of focal fatty infiltration is variable; lobar, segmental, wedge-shaped, nodular or patchy with discrete or vague margin, bizarre geographic, heterogeneous irregular, or diffuse small nodular [10–19]. When fatty infiltration is lobar, segmental or wedge-shaped, it is not difficult to differentiate it from other focal hepatic lesions, but when the fatty metamorphosis is nodular, patchy, bizarre geographic or heterogeneous irregular, differentiation from primary or metastatic tumor is problematic (Fig. 2a). There are several helpful differentiating features: portal and hepatic venous branches normally run through the fatty area without displacement. The focal fatty infiltration does not usually cause local contour abnormality and does not show significant mass effect for the size of the lesion [4]. It may also have a linear margin [3]. The pattern of fatty infiltration can be transient, rapidly appearing and disappearing (Fig. 2b) [20, 21]. Occasionally, discrete focal areas of fatty replacement have a central core of normal appearing tissue, which is the reverse of the typical tumor necrosis pattern [14, 17]. The medial segment of the liver adjacent to the falcifarum ligament is particularly susceptible to focal fatty infiltration [22]. It may result from nutritional ischemia because it is as watershed of the arterial blood supply.

Earthquake patterns of focal fatty infiltration have been reported; scattered irregular low density lines zigzagging through an otherwise normally dense liver parenchyma, which is similar to liver laceration by trauma [9]. Diffuse heterogeneous, irregular or small nodular fatty infiltration may be very similar to an infiltnating primary or metastatic tumor, requiring further imaging studies or biopsy (Fig. 2a).

Occasionally small islands of normal hepatic parenchyma ("skip" areas of spared parenchyma) within otherwise fatty infiltration may mimic primary or metastatic tumors, or regenerating nodules [23, 24]. Frequent sites of focal spared parenchyma in fatty liver are the inferomedial portion of the liver, along the gallbladder fossa adjacent to the interlobar fissure, subcapsular portion of the liver, around the porta hepatis and caudate lobe (Fig. 3). Direct vascular communications between the portal system and the capsular or accessory cystic vein are found in the spared regions, and it is postulated that these areas are perfused by systemic blood from the capsule and gallbladder rather than by splanchnic venous blood from the portal veins ("a third blood" supply) [24]. A glove pattern of focal sparing, high density finger-like interdigitations of spared liver parenchyma on a background of low-density fatty infiltration, has been reported [9].

Occasionally focal hepatic lesions in a diffuse fatty liver can be mistaken for focal areas of spared liver parenchyma or it can be difficult to make a differential diagnosis because there is altered contrast between the lesion and lowered hepatic parenchymal attenuation (Fig. 2) [25]. Needle biopsy, Xenon scan, radionuclide liver scan, or magnetic resonance imaging may be necessary to diagnose and differentiate the lesion.

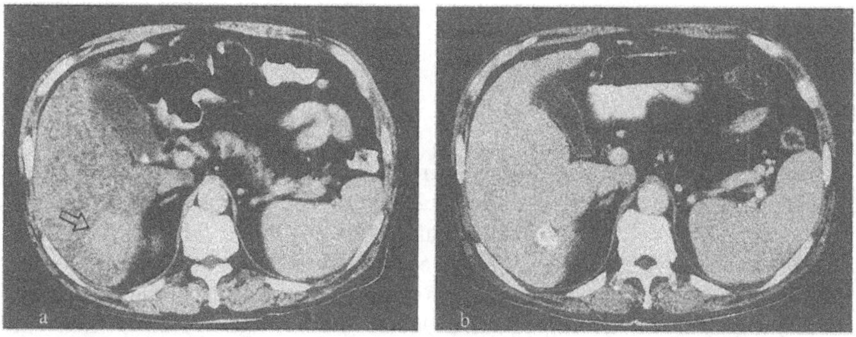

Fig. 2a, b Focal fatty infiltration of the liver with hepatocellular carcinoma. **a** Contrast CT scan shows diffuse nodular hypodensities in the liver. There is a poorly defined hyperattenuation area posteromedially (*arrow*). **b** On follow-up CT scan with TAE (3 weeks later), the nodular hypodensities are not apparent, representing the rapid change of fatty infiltration. The tumor is significantly regressed with TAE

Fig. 3 Focal sparing of normal hepatic parenchyma around the porta hepatis

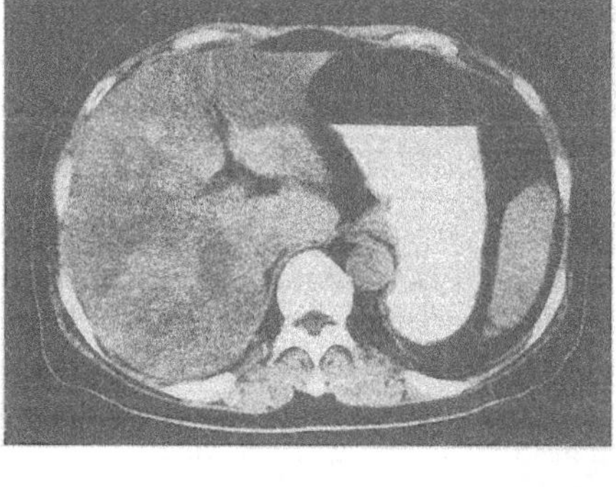

References

1. Isselbacher KJ, Podolsky DK (1994) Infiltrative and metabolic diseases affecting the liver. In: Isselbacher KJ, Braunwald E, Wilson JD, Martin JB, Fauci AS, Kasper DL. Harrison's principle of internal medicine. 13th ed Vol 2, MaGraw-Hill, Inc. 1498–1499
2. Berland L, Lee JKT, Stanley RJ (1989) Liver and biliary tract. In: Lee JKT, Sagel SS, Stanley RJ. Computed body tomography with MRI correlation. 2nd ed New York: Raven Press, 627–630
3. Baron RL, Freeny PC, Moss AA (1992) The liver. In: Moss AA, Gamsu GG, Genant HK. Computed tomography of the body with magnetic resonance imaging. 2nd ed Vol 3, Philadelphia: WB Saunders Co 751–755
4. Gore RM (1994) Diffuse liver disease. In: Gore RM, Levine MS, Lanfer I. Textbook of gastrointestinal radiology. Vol 2 Philadelphia: WB Sauders Co 1968–1972
5. Ducommun J-C, Goldberg HI, Korobkin M, Moss AA, Kressel HY (1979) The relation of liver fat to computed tomography numbers: A preliminary experimental study in rabbits. Radiology 130:511–513
6. Kawata R, Sakata K, Kunieda T, Saji S, Doi H, Nozawa Y (1984) Quantitative evaluation of fatty liver by computed tomography in rabbits. AJR 142:741–746
7. Piekarski J, Goldberg HI, Royal SA, Axel L, Moss AA (1980) Difference between liver and spleen CT numbers in the normal adult: its usefulness in predicting the presence of diffuse liver disease. Radiology 137:727–729
8. Bydder GM, Chapman RWG, Harry D et al. (1981) Computed tomography attenuation values in fatty liver. Comput Tomogr 5:33–38
9. Jain KA, McGahan JP (1993) Spectrum of CT and sonographic appearance of fatty infiltration of the liver. Clinical Imaging 17:162–168
10. Kawashima A, Suehiro S, Murayama S, Russel WJ (1986) Focal fatty infiltration of the liver mimicking a tumor: sonographic and CT features. J Comput Assist Tomogr 10:329–331
11. Brawer MK, Austin GE, Lewin KJ (1980) Focal fatty change of the liver, a hitherto poorly recognized entity. Gastroenterology 78:247–259
12. Scott WW, Sanders RC, Siegelman SS (1980) Irregular fatty infiltration of the liver: diagnostic dilemmas. AJR 135:67–71
13. Halvorsen RA, Korobkin M, Ram PC, Thompson WH (1982) CT appearance of focal fatty infiltration of the liver. AJR 139:277–281
14. Flournoy JG, Potter JL, Sullivan BM, Gerza CB, Ramzy I (1984) CT appearance of multifocal hepatic steatosis. J Comput Assist Tomogr 8:1192–1194
15. Baker ME, Silverman PM (1985) Nodular focal fatty infiltration of the liver: CT appearance. AJR 145:79–80
16. Tang-Barton P, Vas W, Weissman J, Salimi Z, Patel R, Morris L (1985) Focal fatty liver lesion in alcoholic liver disease: A broad spectrum of CT appearances. Gastroint Radiol 10:133–137
17. Yates CK, Streight RA (1986) Focal fatty infiltration of the liver simulating metastatic disease. Radiology 159:82–84
18. Adkins MC, Halvorsen RA, duCret RP (1990) CT evaluation of atypical fatty metamorphosis. J comput Assist Tomogr 14:1013–1015
19. Flueckiger F, Steiner H. Leitinger G, Hoedl S, Deu E (1991) Nodular focal fatty infiltration of the liver in acquired porphyria cutanea tarda. Gastroint Radiol 16:237–239
20. Bashist B, Hecht HL, Harley WD (1982) Computed tomographic demonstration of rapid changes in fatty infiltration of the liver. Radiology 142:691–692
21. Clain JE, Stephens DH, Charboneau JW (1984) Ultrasonography and computed tomography in focal fatty liver. Gastroint Radiol 87:948–952
22. Yoshikawa J, Matsui O, Takashima T et al. (1987) Focal fatty changes of the liver adjacent to the falcifarum ligament: CT and sonographic finding in five surgically confirmed cases. AJR 149:491–494
23. Arai K, Matsui O, Takashima T, Ida M, Nishida Y (1988) Focal spared areas in fatty liver caused by regional decreased portal flow. AJR 151:300–302

24. Silverman PM, Baker ME (1985) Nodular focal fatty infiltration of the liver: CT appearance. AJR 145:79–80
25. Lewis E, Bernardino ME, Barnes PA et al. (1983) The fatty liver: Pitfalls in the CT and angiographic evaluation of metastatic disease. J Comput Assist Tomogr 7:235–241

Detection and Diagnosis of Small Hepatocellular Carcinoma: Techniques of Computed Tomography and Imaging Modalities

Kang-Rong Zhou, Meng-Su Zeng, Bing Wang, and Bei Zhang[1]

Hepatocellular carcinoma (HCC) is the predominant type of primary cancer accounting for over 90% of cancers in China [1]. The incidence of HCC varies greatly from country to country and is particularly prevalent in coastal regions of China. It is the third cause of death in males and the fourth cause of death in females from malignant tumors. It is recognized that early detection is of great clinical importance since HCC has a high possibility of surgical resection, which is considered the best method of treatment with a 5-year survival rate (50%–70%) according to our statistics. In contrast, advanced cases of HCC have low resectability and a poor prognosis. Currently, detection of HCC has been improved significantly with many imaging modalities available and in common use, but for small HCC, (SHCC), and in particular for less than 1 cm lesions, there are problems in early detection and differential diagnosis. Our aim as radiologists is to carry out research work to detect HCC lesions as early as possible and as small as possible, i.e., less than 4.5 cm (Okuda), less than 2.0 cm, and even less than 1.0 cm in diameter.

Detection of SHCC

Numerous imaging techniques are available for the detection of SHCC and various diagnostic standards and comparitive studies have been made. In most comparative analyses and according to our statistics based on 118 patients with 180 lesions of HCC (< = 3.0 cm in diameter), the sensitivities of computed tomography (CT) angiography (CTA) and CT arterial portography (CTAP) are significantly higher than those of other conventional CT or angiography modalities [2]. Intraoperative ultrasonography (US) and iodized-oil CT are also relatively high in sensitivity [3]. Bolus dynamic incremental CT (BDICT) is more sensitive than conventional contrast enhancement CT, but much less sensitive than CTA or CTAP [4]. Noncontrast enhancement CT and US are even less effective in detecting lesions smaller than 1.0 cm and PMT is almost valueless. Results of magnetic resonance imaging (MRI) for 1.0-cm SHCC are controversial and considered supplementary to CT [5]. Spiral (or helical) CT permits scanning of the whole liver in a single breath hold and so respiratory misregistration between adjacent scan

[1] Department of Radiology, Zhongshan Hospital, Shanghai Medical University 200032.

slices can be eliminated. In addition, because imaging with spiral CT is extremely rapid, the scans can be completed during the interval of peak hepatic contrast enhancement. Thus, small hepatic lesions would be missed much less frequently than with conventional dynamic CT. If a combination of a spiral scan of the arterial, portal and parenchymal phase is done after rapid IV injection of contrast medium by power injector, the detection of SHCC would be significantly increased [6]. The advantages of CTA and CTAP performed with spiral CT would be more evident than those with conventional CT in this regard [7].

As lipiodol tends to accumulate within the hepatic tumor when it is combined with lipophilic anticancerous agents and introduced through catheterization and approach of HA for treatment, CT, after lipiodol infusion (oil CT), is one of the most useful and sensitive methods for detecting SHCC. It can enhance a greater number of small nodules which may not be displayed on conventional CT (Fig. 1).

The high sensitivity of CTA for SHCC detection has been well established by us and other authors. It derives from the fact that HCC are fed by the hepatic artery and not by the portal vein, so that HCC have a very high attenuation compared with the surrounding normal liver in CTA. They have very low attenuation and appear to have a negative defect within the high-attenuation hepatic tissue in CTAP. A small lesion is very conspicuous compared with the surrounding liver because of the marked difference in density between the lesion and the liver in both CTA and CTAP images. With SHCC confirmed surgiopathologically, we performed CTA and CTAP in 35 and 30 patients, respectively. CTA demonstrated a sensitivity of 80% and CTAP a sensitivity of 85% for lesions less than 1 cm (Figs. 2, 3).

On the basis of the various advantages and disadvantages or pitfalls of different imaging modalities, we suggest the following techniques for improving detectability of SHCC:

1. BDICT should be perfomed routinely and followed by US and precontrast CT. Spiral CT would be preferable (if available).
2. CT can be delayed in selected cases, namely repeated scanning 4–5 h after BDICT if there is any clinical suspicion or doubt about images.

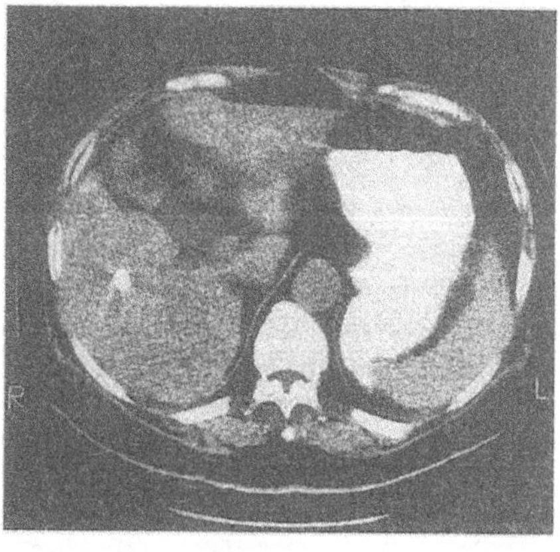

Fig. 1 Oil CT after TAE treatment shows accumulation of lipiodol within the recurrent small heptacellular carcinoma (HCC) nodule which cannot be demonstrated with conventional CT scans

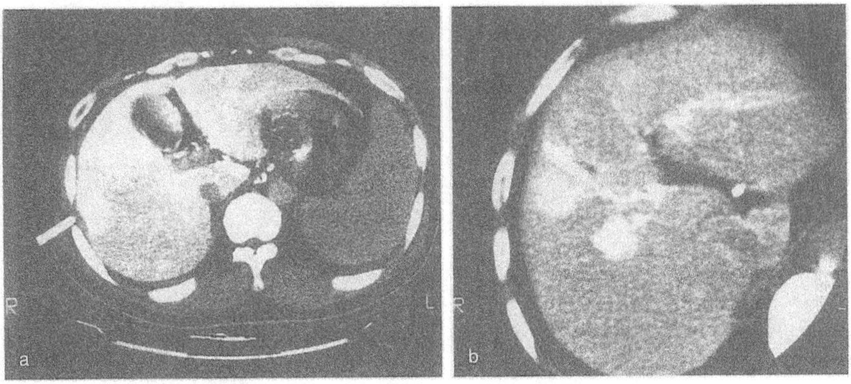

Fig. 2 a, b. CT angiography (CTA) performed in two patients with highly suspicious recurrent clinical lesions not indicated by US or conventional CT. **a** An oval-shaped high-density lesion adjacent to a wedge resection site of the right lobe. **b** Two highly opacified nodules and their feeding vessels are seen on CTA

3. Because of their invasive nature, CTA and CTAP should only be performed after all other procedures have been performed and only in carefully selected patients.
4. Oil CT can be performed 10–15 days after infusion of lipiodol for displaying small satellite nodules and daughter lesions and for examining the distribution of oil in the tumor in the treatment of proven cases.
5. Intraoperative US is useful for confirming the presence or absence of suspicious lesions found before the operation, since a small tumor may not be seen or palpated from the surface of the liver during the operating procedure. An additional advantage of this technique is its ability to show liver lesions and adjacent structure tissue simultaneously and so is helpful for the surgeon's determination of operativity and the best operative method to use.
6. Organ-specific contrast media such as EOE-13 (CT), an early development, and supermagnetic iron oxide (ferrite) particles (MR), which has been developed recently, can be used soon. These are both very specific and highly sensitive in detecting SHCC but are still in clinical development due to certain drawbacks, technical limitations and side effects.

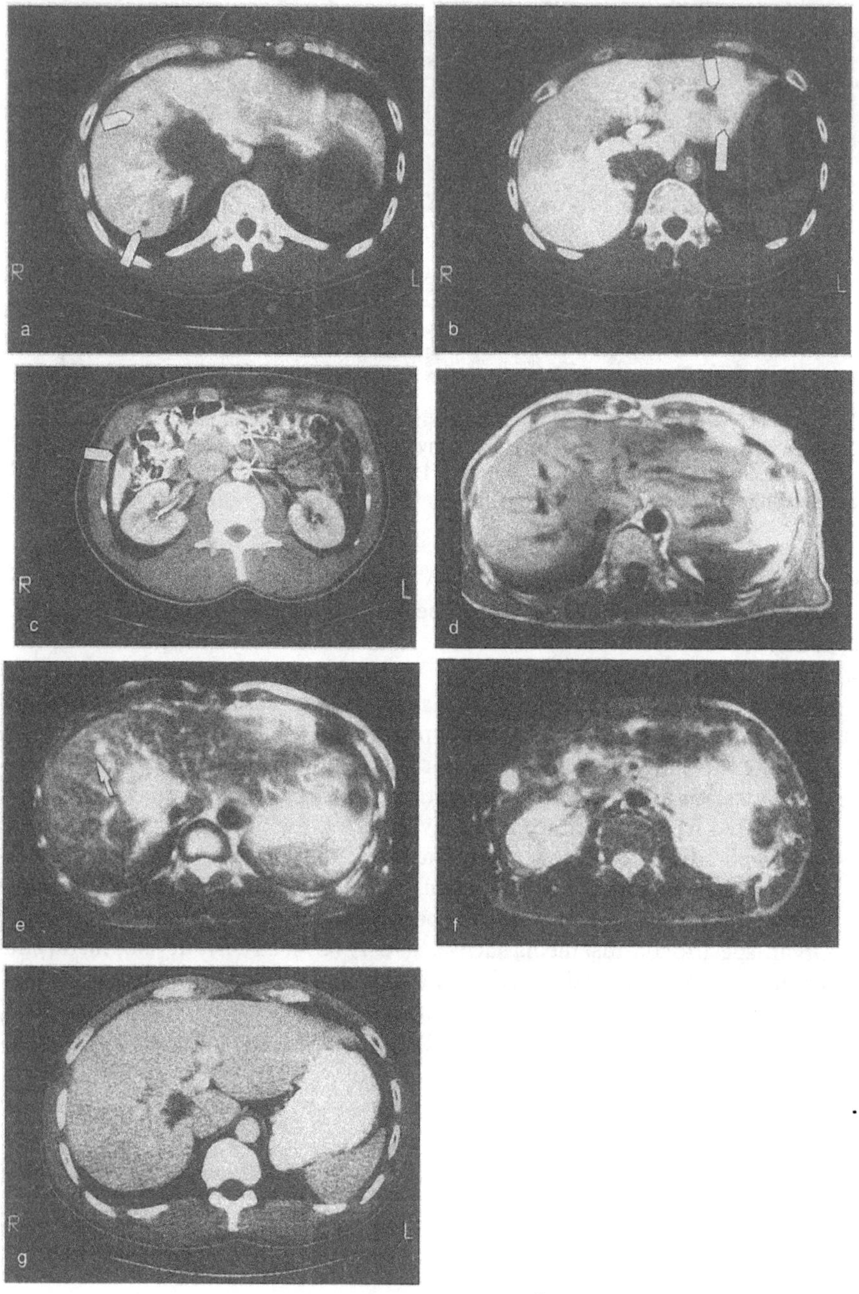

Fig. 3 a–g CT arterial portography (CTAP) performed in a patient with hepatocellular carcinoma (HCC) and compared with magnetic resonance imaging (MRI) and CT. **a–e** CTAP images in three levels show a large lesion in the right lobe near porta hepatis and small nodules in different segments of right and left lobes. **d–f** Corresponding level T1- and T2-weighted MRI images in which one lesion in the posterior part of the right lobe and three lesions in the left lobe cannot be shown. **g** Contrast enhancement CT shows large lesions but does not show all small lesions

Diagnosis and Differentiation of SHCC

The precise diagnosis and differentiation from other lesions is another major problem in SHCC. Understanding their pathological features is a fundamental factor in establishing the correct diagnosis and the differentiation of SHCC from other liver lesions such as hemangioma, liver cirrhotic nodule, granuloma and fatty infiltration etc.:

1. Hypervascularity with full or predominant blood supply from the hepatic artery and an A-V shunt within the tumor in the majority of SHCC.
2. Fatty component or fatty metamorphosis (Fig. 4).
3. An expansive growing type of HCC, associated with liver cirrhosis caused by hepatitis B as the underlying disease, is much more common in oriental patients than in western patients. A fibrous capsule (or pseudocapsule) is a very important feature, represented by a smooth margin or halo sign in CT, US and MRI imaging.
4. Infiltrative growing type associated with high incidence of hepatic venous invasion or thrombosis (Fig. 5).

The following are key points for correct diagnosis and differentiation:

1. A halo sign encapsulated in a SHCC is one of the characteristic images seen in CT, US and MRI. A thin peripheral fibrous band, called a halo, may be represented as hypointense attenuation in CT, hypoechoic in CT and a hypointense signal in MRI (Figs. 6, 7).
   It must be noted that in individual cases, a halo sign may be displayed in all three modality images or in only one or two of them.
2. Early high and transient enhancement after a bolus injection of contrast medium and rapid rising and falling of the curved enhancement line, well established in BDCT (single level). This is similar to dynamic MRI using gadolininum diethylene triamine penta-acetate (Gd-DTPA) or other contrastmedia and fast magnetic nuclear resonance (MNR) techniques, as well as in dynamic US using CO_2 microbubbles [8].

For differential diagnosis, the following examination techniques can be used:

1. Single-level (or modified) BDICT is the most useful and common way of making a definitive diagnosis [3] (Fig. 8).
2. Dynamic enhancement MRI and US are new technique procedures and need to be studied further (Fig. 7).
3. CTA is sensitive and also specific for detecting and diagnosing SHCC. Differentiation between SHCC and regenerating nodules is sometimes diffucult using conventional CT and US, but simple using CTA. The hepatic artery provides the main blood supply for a SHCC whereas the regenerating nodule derives its supply from the portal vein.
4. SHCC usually retain iodized oil (oil CT) whereas the regenerating nodule does not.
5. Doppler US or color Doppler US can provide information about blood flow and its patterns that is useful in differential diagnosis.
6. MRI using SE T1 weighted scans and multiple T2 weighted scans can help to differentiate SHCC from hemangioma.

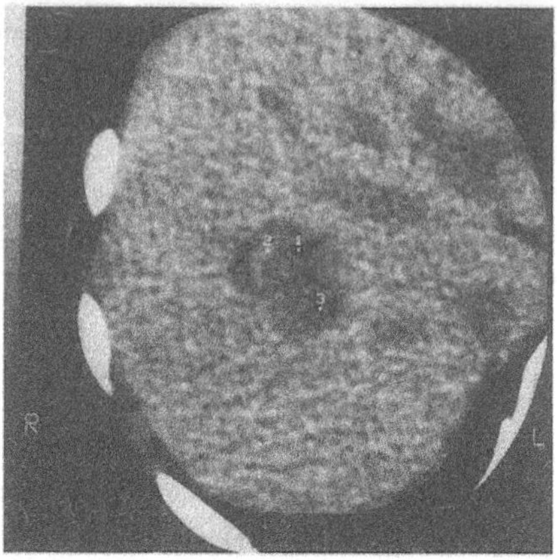

Fig. 4 Inhomogenous density of small hepatocellular carcinoma (SHCC) with low attenuation (-35 Hu) representing the fatty component shown on a precontrast CT scan

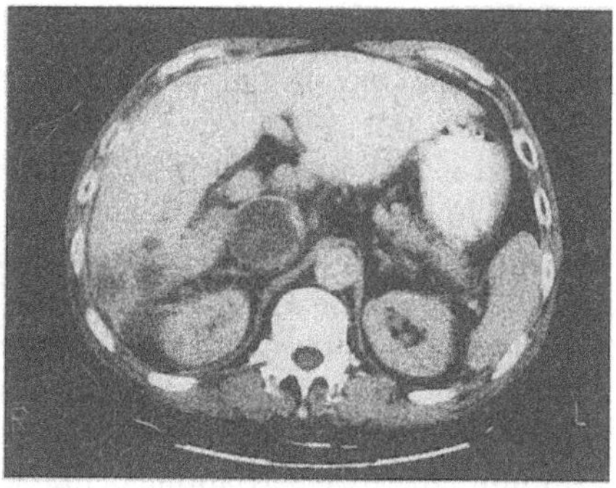

Fig. 5 Contrast enhancement CT scan shows infiltrative type of small hepatocellular carcinoma (SHCC) in the posterior segment of the right lobe of the liver, associated with cancercous thrombosis in the inferior vena cava (IVC)

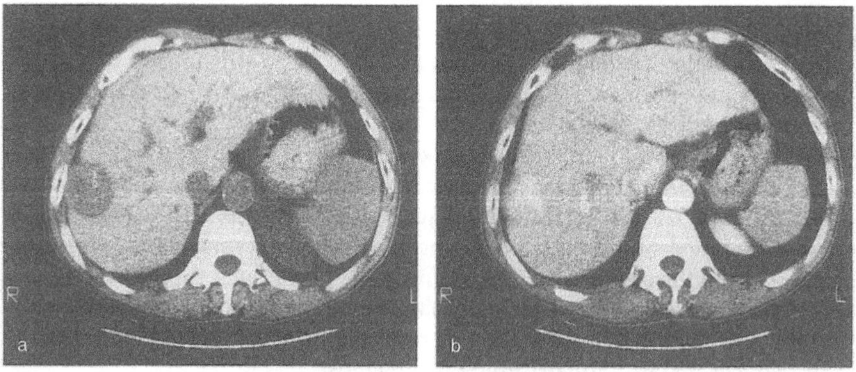

Fig. 6 a, b Precontrast **a** and postcontrast **b** CT scans show halo sign indicating the presence of pseudocapsule of small hepatocellular carcinoma (SHCC)

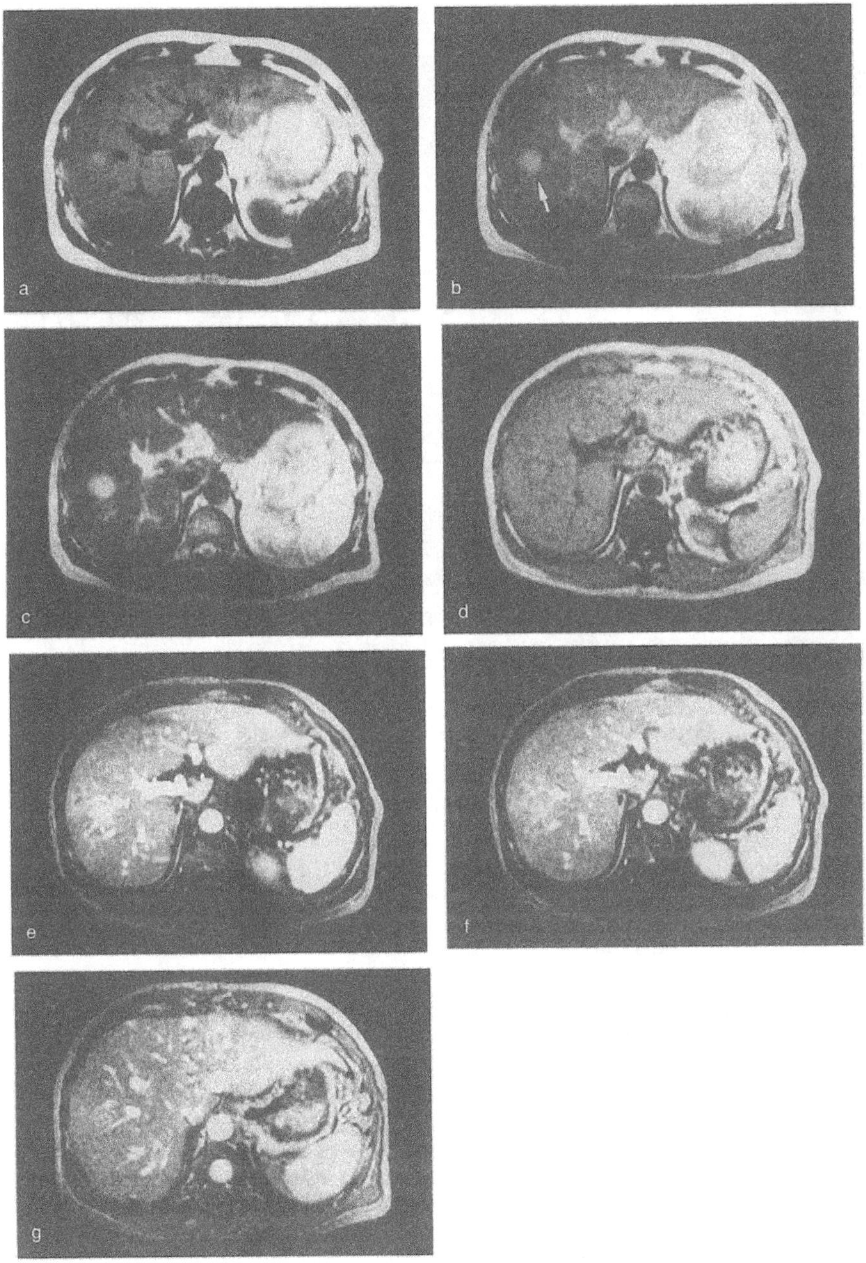

Fig. 7 a–g Typical features of small hepatocellular carcinoma (SHCC) on magnetic resonance imaging (MRI) and dynamic enhancement MRI. **a** T1W image (TR 540, TE 16) shows small nodule with slightly high signal in the right lobe of the liver. **b** Proton image (TR 2000, TE 30) and T2W image (TR 2000, TE 80) show some degree of increase of signal **d–g** SPGR images (**d** precontrast and **e–f** postcontrast Gd-DTPA) show dynamic changes of enhancement of SHCC similar to BDICT. In **a**, **d**, **e** and **f** the halo sign can be seen

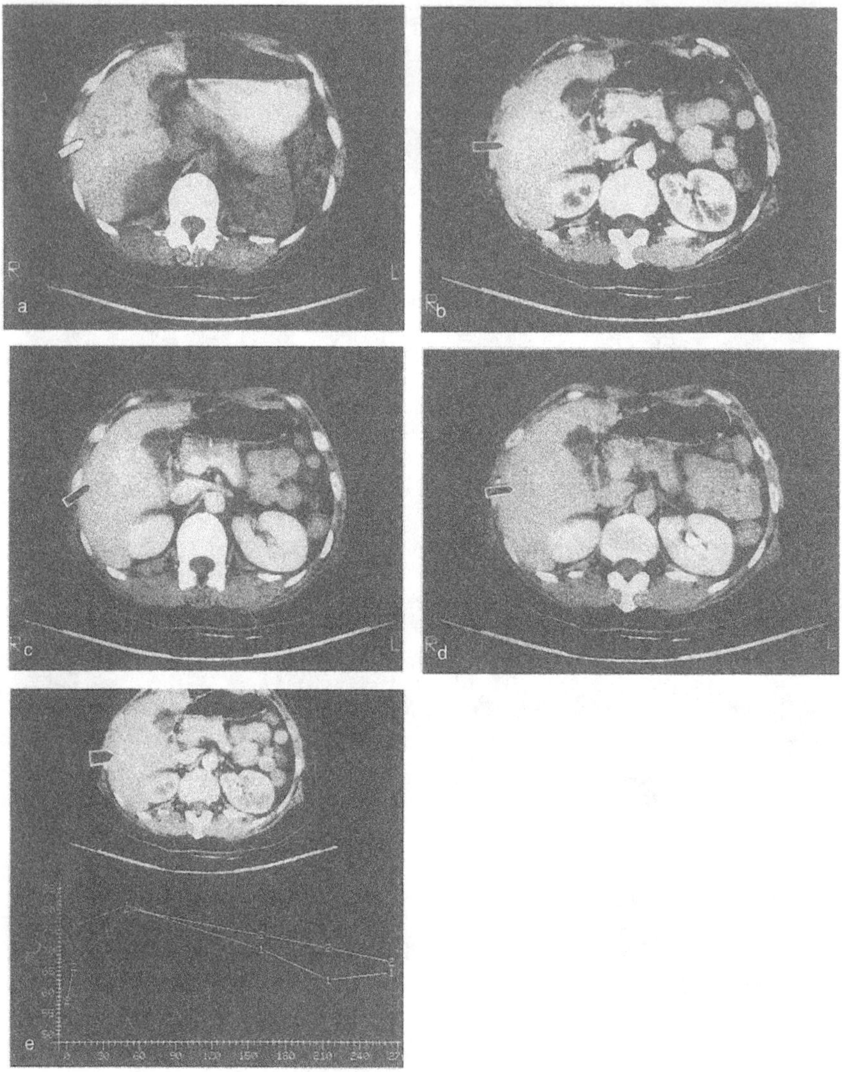

Fig. 8 a–e Bolus dynamic CT in the center of the lesion shows characteristic findings of enhancement and time-density curve line of small hepatocellular carcinoma (SHCC). **a** Pre-contrast CT demonstrated low attenuation small lesion in the right lobe of the liver. **b–d** Nonincremental postcontrast CT shows dynamic changes of enhancement from high density in arterial phase (**b**), isodensity in portal phase (**c**) to low density in parenchymal phase (**d**). **e** Typical time-density curve line, line 1 and line 2 representing HCC and liver parenchyma, respectively

Conclusion

The early detection rate of SHCC increased significantly with the improvement of imaging instruments and techniques. The sensitivity of SHCC detection has increased in the past few years but is still low for lesions of less than 1.0 cm. We believe that early detection and precise diagnosis will improve further on with the application of properly selected CT techniques and protocol, combined with the advantages of other modalities and with the development of new methods in the future.

References

1. Zhou KR (1993) CT of the Abdomen, Shanghai, Shanghai Medical University Publishing House 7
2. Takayasu K, Moriyama N, Muramatsu U et al. (1990) The diagnosis of SHCC: Efficacy of various imaging procedures in 100 patients. AJR 155:49–54
3. Foley WD (1989) Dynamic hepatic CT. Radiology 170:617–622
4. Choi BI, Han JK, Song IS et al. (1991) Intraoperative sonography of HCC: detection of and validity in surgical resection. Gastrointest Radiol 16:329–333
5. Heiken JP, Wergman PE, Lee JKT et al. (1989) Detection of focal hepatic masses: prospective evaluation with CT, delayed CT, CTAP, and MR imaging. Radiology 1989: 174:47–51
6. Zeman RK, Fox SH, Silverman PM et al. (1993) Helical CT of the abdomen. AJR 160:719–725
7. Bluemke DA, Fishman EK (1993) Spiral CT arterial portography of the liver. Radiology 186:576–579
8. Kodo M, Tomity S, Tochio H et al. (1992) SHCC diagnosis with US angiography with intra-arterial CO_2 microbubbles. Radiology 182:155–160

CHAPTER 16

Computed Tomography of Pancreatic Tumors

Heoung Keun Kang[1]

Introduction

Computed tomography (CT) has been a useful modality for the assessment of pancreatic lesions, because it can display excellent pancreatic anatomy and complex relationships between neighboring structures. CT imaging of the pancreas developed initially from outlining of the organ contour to visualize even subtle parenchymal detail [1, 2]. The later improvements came about largely because of advanced scanning technology and the administration of an intravenous bolus injection of contrast material. Good bolus technique, rapid scanning, and conventional dynamic CT scanning, have made it possible to demonstrate pancreatic parenchymal changes, pancreatic and bile duct abnormalities, vascular changes, and metastases to lymph node and liver. Recent development of helical (spiral) scanning offers many advantages over conventional dynamic CT scanning: (a) scanning during the phase of maximum vascular enhancement, with improved visualization of the splanchnic vasculature; (b) multiple thin sections through the enhancement; (c) lack of misregistration of data since a volume data set is rapidly acquired during a single breath hold (with less patient motion); and (d) capability to view these data both as axial slices and as a multiplanar (coronal and sagittal) display [3, 4].

This paper describes the important technical considerations and clinical applications of CT, especially of helical CT, in the diagnosis and staging of pancreatic tumors.

CT Technique Including Contrast Material Application

Patients should receive adequate oral contrast material (e.g., 500 ml 2% Gastrografin) to define more clearly the boundaries of the pancreas, to increase the accuracy of the detection of adenopathy, and also to avoid confusion of nonopacified bowel loops with intraperitoneal fluid collections. After a topogram, an unenhanced scan is obtained to center the image field. Intravenous contrast material offers three distinct advantages: (a) it enhances normal parenchyma, allowing visualization of small lesions and pancreatic duct; (b) it fills peripan-

[1] Department of Radiology, Chonnam University Medical School, Kwangju, Korea.

creatic arteries and veins, allowing for an assessment of vascular invasion versus patency; and (c) it enhances normal hepatic parenchyma, maximizing conspicuity, and ultimately detectability of hepatic metastases [5]. The methods of intravenous contrast enhancement and scanning parameters are varied according to commercially available CT scanners.

Conventional CT

A total of 150 ml intravenous contrast material (300 mgI/ml) should be delivered as a biphasic bolus (2.5 ml/s for 20 s and 1 ml/s for 100 s) using a power injector. Scanning is performed during the latter phase of the injection. However, newer CT technology ("cluster" scan) allowing 1-s scan time, combined with more rapid table incrementation, can obtain six contiguous scans during the single breath hold, so a total 150 ml of contrast material could be delivered as a uniphasic bolus at a rate of 2.5 ml/s with scanning starting 40 s after the start of intravenous injection.

Scanning parameters are variable; commonly with a tube voltage of 120–130 kVp, a tube current of 150–200 mAs, and a section thickness of 5–10 mm. Most routine body CT uses 10-mm collimation. Scanning with 5-mm sections provides improved contrast between neoplasm and adjacent structures because of decreased volume averaging. Newer scanners allow collimation at 1.5 or 3 mm. In using 1.5- or 3-mm sections, however, there will be some noise, which is inversely related to the square of the section thickness. To compensate, one must increase mAs and hence the exposure [5].

Helical CT

A total of 100–120 ml intravenous contrast material should be delivered as a bolus at a rate of 2–3 ml/s using a power injector. The contrast between parenchyma and pancreatic tumor is maximal during the arterial phase of the bolus injection. Therefore, data acquisition begins 40 s after the injection of contrast material (Fig. 1). Completion of the injection occurs 10 s before the completion of scanning. The helical scans of the pancreas are obtained from the bottom of the pancreas (level of the third portion of the duodenum), and scans are extended cranially ("bottom-up").

Scanning parameters are a tube voltage of 120–140 kVp and tube current of 210–280 mAs. The helical protocol of the pancreatic region is 5-mm collimation and table incrementation of 5 mm/s (1:1 pitch), and reconstruction at 2-mm intervals. Evaluation of the pancreas requires about 7–9 cm scanning area, therefore, the patient is instructed to hold his breath for 20 s while helical CT scanning is performed. Total scanning length is 10 cm. After the scanning of the pancreas, the liver and the rest of the abdomen are scanned at 7-mm slice thickness and 1:1 pitch.

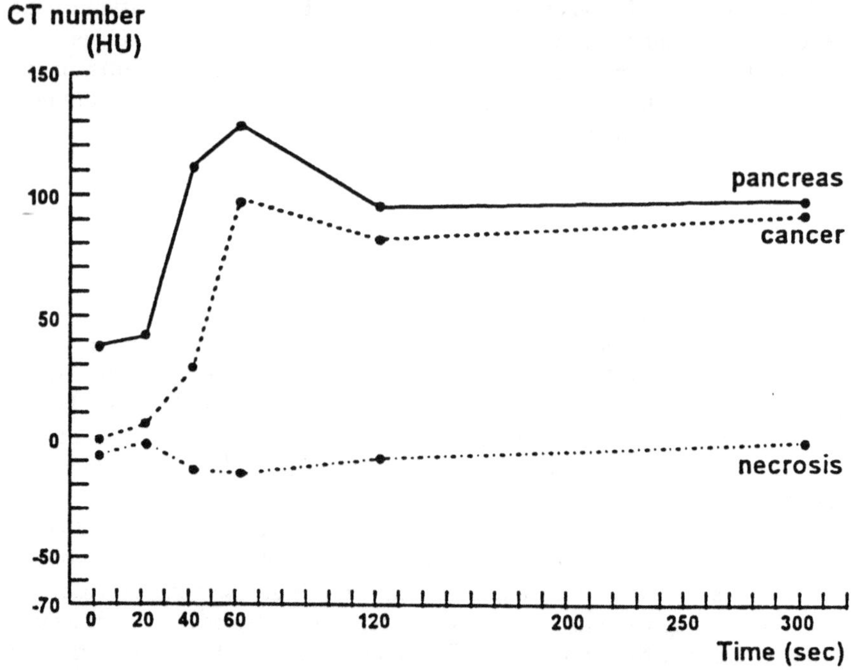

Fig. 1 Time-density curve of pancreas and pancreatic cancer (contrast material, 2 ml/s, total, 100 ml)

Value of CT in Pancreatic Adenocarcinoma

CT is extremely accurate both in confirming or excluding the presence of a suspected pancreatic mass and in staging tumor. In both instances, helical CT improves diagnostic confidence.

Diagnosis

The diagnosis of pancreatic tumor is performed on the basis of the focal mass(contour, texture, CT attenuation) with associated pancreatic or bile duct dilatation, and ancillary findings such as local tumor extension, invasion of neighboring organs and vessels, and metastatic lesion [6–8].

The focal mass enlarges a region of the pancreas and produces either an abrupt or a gradual change in contour. Very small peripheral masses may be detected by virtue of disruption of the normal surface lobularity caused by peripancreatic areolar tissue dipping in between parenchymal lobules [9]. In the elderly or the obese, the pancreatic parenchyma is often marbled because of fatty infiltration. These focal losses of peripheral lobularity and marbling are often subtle and can

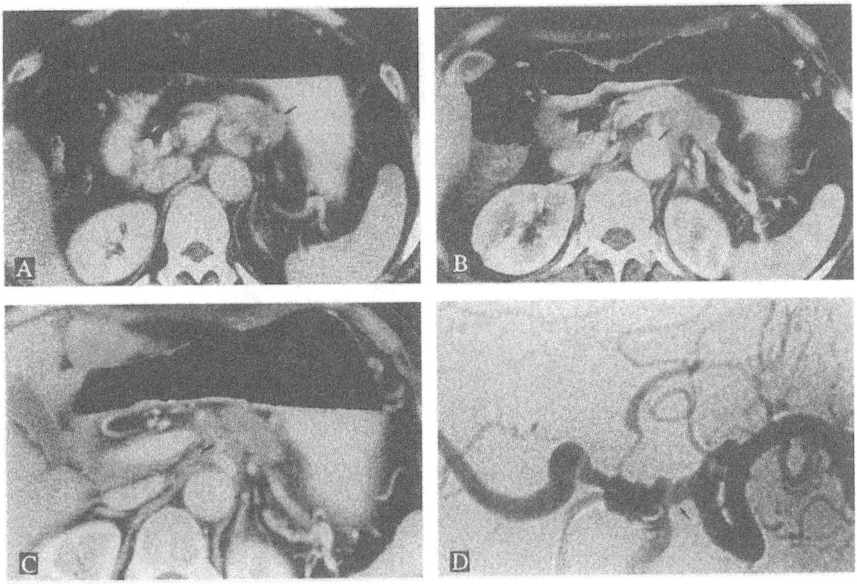

Fig. 2 Pancreatic carcinoma. **A** Conventional CT scan demonstrates a subtle mass (*arrow*) in the distal body and proximal tail of the pancreas and retropancreatic region. **B, C** Helical CT scans show a low-attenuation mass (*arrow* in **B**), which encases the celiac artery and its branches (*arrow* in **C**) and the splenic vein. Rich collateral vessels are also noted. **D** Celiac arteriogram shows irregular encasement of celiac artery and its branches (*arrow*) and rich collateral vessels, similar to helical CT scans

be difficult to recognize, but these abnormalities can be recognized by evaluating the texture of the suspected lesion and compared with the surrounding pancreatic parenchyma. Changes in the size, contour or shape are the most frequent features of pancreatic adenocarcinoma, occurring in 95% of patients [10].

Pancreatic adenocarcinoma demonstrates a hypoattenuating central zone, compared with the surrounding parenchyma. The pathophysiologic characteristics of this finding reflect the hypovascular, scirrhous and fibrous nature of this tumor [4, 11]. This change is well demonstrated in 78% on the bolus phase of dynamic, thin section CT, as opposed to 24% on conventional CT (Fig. 2) [5, 11].

In addition to focal mass, secondary signs such as pancreatic duct and/or bile duct dilatation may lead to the detection of the pancreatic mass. Dilatation of the main pancreatic duct proximal to the obstructing tumor is well delineated in 88% of pancreatic head adenocarcinoma with 5-mm slice thickness and good contrast enhancement [10]. Furthermore, 2-mm interval reconstruction by using helical CT improves the detectability of pancreatic duct dilatation [3, 12]. Adenocarcinoma of the head of the pancreas causes obstructive jaundice and biliary dilatation on CT scans in 86% [10]. CT typically shows abrupt obstruction of the common bile duct, usually at the level of the pancreatic head. An associated mass is usually detected in addition to an abrupt obstruction of bile ducts from pancreatic carcinoma. Some-

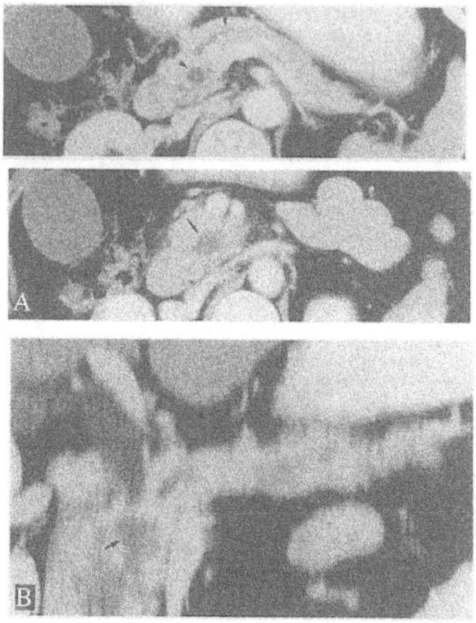

Fig. 3 A, B Pancreatic carcinoma. **A** Axial helical CT scans show dilated ducts (*arrowheads*) and a low-attenuation mass (*arrow*) in the pancreatic head. **B** Coronal view of multiplanar imaging defines the relationship of pancreatic mass (*arrow*) to dilated ducts

times the most caudally visible portion of the obstructed duct will be an irregular ring with contrast enhanced, uneven thickness on CT [13]. Since helical CT improves the visualization of small mass and biliary duct and can represent the CT cholangiographic image by using multiplanar reformation, the determination level and cause of biliary obstruction is improved (Fig. 3).

Differential Diagnosis of Pancreatic Adenocarcinoma

Focal pancreatic masses with or without pancreatic or bile duct dilatation are nonspecific for adenocarcinoma and can be caused by chronic pancreatitis, islet cell carcinoma, lymphoma, and metastasis.

Chronic pancreatitis presenting with a focal mass is difficult to distinguish from adenocarcinoma [15]. The helpful findings for focal pancreatitis are the presence of foci of calcification within the mass and almost complete isodensity to the normal parenchyma in bolus enhanced CT. Although the pattern of pancreatic duct dilatation (beaded, irregular, or smooth) is not helpful, the presence of a dilated duct within the mass suggests pancreatitis [9]. Absence of vascular involvement adjacent to a large, diffuse mass should prompt consideration of pancreatitis.

Islet cell tumor is characterized by solid sheets of tumor cells with rich vascularity, therefore it appears characteristically as a hyperattenuating mass [4]. Since functioning islet cell tumor is small and will not deform the pancreatic contour, administration of adequate intravenous contrast material and contiguous thin section are critical for helical CT diagnosis.

Confluent peripancreatic lymphadenopathy in patients with lymphoma or metastatic disease is sometimes difficult to differentiate from pancreatic adenocarcinoma. With helical CT, differential contrast enhancement of pancreatic parenchyma and lymph nodes will often distinguish the two by defining intact fat planes between the pancreas and nodes [9]. Vascular landmarks such as the gastroduodenal artery, the anterior and posterior peripancreatic arcades define the outline of the pancreas, so that peripancreatic process can be distinguished from the lesions arising from the pancreas [12]. The absence of ductal dilatation in the presence of a sizable mass in the region of the head of the pancreas favors peripancreatic adenopathy over ductal cell carcinoma [9].

Staging

The staging of pancreatic adenocarcinoma with abdominal CT involves detecting local tumor extension, major vascular involvement, invasion of contiguous organs, ascites, lymphadenopathy and distant metastasis [16]. All of these are strongly indicative of unresectability. Extrapancreatic local extension, manifested by extrapancreatic mass contiguous with and of similar density to the primary, is present in roughly 40%–70% of patients at initial evaluation [9, 10]. Soft tissue density streaks and strands in the retroperitoneal fat in the region of the mass suggest extension. Helical CT provides superior opacification of peripancreatic vasculatures and shows images similar to angiogram (Fig. 2). Contrast opacification of these peripancreatic vessels provides critical information regarding vascular obstruction or encasement, this in turn will determine tumor resectability [3–5]. Indeed, major peripancreatic arteries and veins are involved in up to 84% of cases of pancreatic carcinoma [10]. Arterial obstruction is seen as a perfusion abnormality during dynamic CT, while venous obstruction is seen as an abrupt occlusion of a major vein or as associated venous collateral vessels or varices [17]. Although the demonstration of venous collateral on routine conventional scanning often implies the existence of venous encasement [18], the actual site of vascular invasion may now be directly visualized with helical technique, increasing the confidence with which we offer both a diagnosis of cancer and the stage of disease. Arterial or venous encasement was seen either as a cuff of tumor tissue surrounding the vessel or as direct contiguity of a major vessel within the tumor mass. The superior mesenteric artery and vein are most commonly involved. The helical technique also provides excellent parenchymal enhancement of the liver which, in turn, improves detection of hepatic metastases.

Helical CT offers an additional distinct advantage to conventional CT because of its potential to provide multiplanar reconstructions based on a volumetric data set without respiratory misregistration [3, 4, 19, 20]. Multiplanar images help to define the local tumor extension, contiguous organ invasion, regional lymph node metastases and vascular involvements. Therefore, this is particularly useful for the accurate staging of pancreatic neoplasms. While axial scans can clearly demonstrate encasement of the superior mesenteric vein and splenic vein, sagittal images are preferable for displaying the superior mesenteric artery as it arises from the aorta at a 90° angle. Coronal scans are then helpful in assessing tumor involvement of the adjacent stomach or duodenum [4]. Recent literature illustrates the value of three-dimensional (3D) rendering of helical CT data in providing useful information for surgical planning and showing the extent of vascular involvement by tumor [21]. However, 3D imaging of the pancreas still has limitations at the present stage and the use of multiplanar reformatting (MPR) is generally preferred.

Relationship of Imaging Modalities

In the past, when cross-sectional imaging methods were not available, plain films and barium studies were the important and major methods for evaluation of the pancreas [2, 8]. However, these studies, now acting as complementary studies to CT, are less diagnostically critical.

Endoscopic retrograde cholangiopancreatographic examination (ERCP) is useful in confirming a suspected diagnosis of carcinoma of pancreas with a specificity reported in successful studies exceeding 88% [10, 22]. Given the high accuracy of noninvasive studies, ERCP is now used primarily as an adjunctive technique to further assess patients with ambiguous CT findings [23].

Angiography had been used for evaluation of major extrapancreatic vascular involvement by the pancreatic tumor, thus indicating peripancreatic tumor extension, and the demonstration of hepatic metastases [16, 17]. In one study [17], CT demonstrated vascular involvement not seen by angiography in 20%, and angiography was superior to CT in only 5%. In these latter cases, however, other CT criteria of unresectability were also present. Now, CT has an advantage over angiography in that it may demonstrate subtle adventitial involvement by tumors which can be missed by angiography. Angiography is currently recommended for preoperative assessment of vascular anatomy ("road map") of patients with pancreatic carcinoma who have resectable tumors by CT criteria [8, 16].

Ultrasonography (US) is probably the best method for screening pancreatic mass and is also an excellent technique for the demonstration of bile duct dilatation and follow up check, because it is the fastest and least costly examination of the pancreas [1, 8]. However, US often is limited in patients who are obese or have a gas-distended abdomen or many abdominal drains and surgical dressings [8]. The recent development of endoscopic ultrasonography (EUS) enables a good display of the anatomy of the pancreas, pancreatic and biliary ducts and peripancreatic vessels [16]. It has been shown to have an accuracy of about 75%–92% in predicting tumor unresectability and will likely play an increasing role in the assessment of tumor resectability if, the future, the technique becomes more widely available [16, 24].

The ability of MR imaging to image the normal and abnormal pancreas has improved with recent technical advances. The most important sequence for imaging the pancreas is fat-suppressed T1-weighted spin echo because of the superior ability of MR to detect non-organ-deforming tumors compared with CT [25–28]. The high aqueous protein content of normal pancreatic tissue results in a relatively high signal intensity (SI) on fat-suppressed images. Pancreatic tumors do not contain aqueous protein and therefore appear as a low-SI focal mass [25]. Conventional T1-weighted spin echo generally yields better contrast between pancreas and peripancreatic fat than fat-suppressed sequence [9]. Gadolinium diethylene triamine penta-acetate (Gd) – (DTPA) enhanced dynamic imaging is particularly important in the investigation of small islet cell tumors and also in detecting liver metastasis [27]. A recent report indicated that manganese dipyridoxaldiphosphate (Mn-DPDP) enhances the pancreatic tissue and postulated that this enhancement could be used for better demonstrating pancreatic pathology [29]. Data from many published reports demonstrated that the specificity and sensitivity of MR for pancreatic tumor identification were superior to those of CT, but the accuracy and sensitivity of CT for predicting tumor resectability and unresectability were superior to those of MR [16, 26]. Despite the favorable results of MR imaging, the relative scarcity and high cost of the technique indicate that it should probably remain a problem-solving modality. Circumstances in which this technique may be useful include: (a) situations in which clinical history and CT findings are discordant; (b) situations in which CT findings are indeterminate in the investigation of pancreatic adenocarcinoma; and (c) situations in which the patient has contrast allergy or renal failure [28].

References

1. Thoeni RF, Blankenberg F (1993) Pancreatic imaging: computed tomography and magnetic resonance imaging. Radiol Clin North Am 31:1085–1113
2. Freeny FC (1988) Radiology of pancreas: two decades of progress in imaging and intervention. AJR 150:975–981
3. Fishman EK, Wyatt SH, Ney DR et al. (1992) Spiral CT of the pancreas with multiplanar display. AJR 159:1209–1215
4. Wyatt SH, Fishman EK (1995) Spiral CT evaluation of the pancreas. In: Fishman EK, Jeffrey RB, ed Spiral CT. New York: Raven Press 57–77
5. Megibow AJ (1992) Pancreatic adenocarcinoma: designing the examination to evaluate the clinical questions. Radiology 183:297–303
6. Federle MP, Goldberg HI (1992) The pancreas. In: Moss AA, ed Computed tomography of the body. 2nd ed. Philadelphia: WB Saunders, 869–932.
7. Wegener OH (1992) In: Whole body computed tomography. 2nd ed Oxford: Blackwell Scientific Publications 289–312
8. Gore RM, Nemcek AA, Vogelzang RL et al. (1994) Pancreas. In: Gore RM, Levine MS, Laufer I ed Textbook of gastrointestinal radiology. Philadelphia: WB Saunders, 2095–2216
9. Friedman AC (1994) Pancreatic neoplasms and cysts. In: Friedman AC, Dachman AH ed. Radiology of the liver, biliary tract, and pancreas. Missouri: Mosby Year Book, 807–934
10. Freeny FC, Marks WM, Ryan JA et al. (1988) Pancreatic ductal adenocarcinoma: diagnosis and staging with dynamic CT. Radiology 166:125–133
11. Hosoki T (1983) Dynamic CT of pancreatic tumors. AJR 140:959–965
12. Kaur H, Park JM, Fenstermacher MJ et al. (1994) Accuracy of diagnosis and staging of pancreatic carcinoma with use of helical CT(abstr). Radiology 193 (p):219
13. Dupuy DE, Costello P, Ecleer CP (1992) Spiral CT of the pancreas. Radiology 183:815–818
14. Schultes J, Baron RL, Teefey SA et al. (1990) CT of the extrahepatic bile ducts: wall thickness and contrast enhancement in normal and abnormal ducts. AJR 154:79–85
15. Neff CC, Simeone JF, Wittenberg J et al. (1984) Inflammatory pancreatic masses: problems differentiating focal pancreatitis from carcinoma. Radiology 150:35–38

16. Nghiem HV, Freeny PC (1994) Radiologic staging of pancreatic adenocarcinoma. Radiol Clin North Am 32:71–79
17. Freeny PC (1989) Radiologic diagnosis and staging of pancreatic ductal adenocarcinoma. Radiol Clin North Am 27:121–128
18. Mori H, McGrath FP, Malone DE et al. (1992) The gastrocolic trunk and its tributaries: CT evaluation. Radiology 182:871–877
19. Heiken JP, Brink JA, Vannier MW (1993) Spiral (helical) CT. Radiology 189:647–656
20. Zeman RK, Fox SH, Silverman PW et al. (1993) Helical (spiral) CT of the abdomen. AJR 160:719–729
21. Zeman RK, Davros WJ, Berman P et al. (1993) Three dimentional model of the abdominal vasculature based on helical CT: usefulness in patients with pancreatic neoplasm. AJR 162:1425–1429
22. Freeny PC, Ball TJ (1981) Endoscopic retrograde cholangio pancreatography(ERCP) and percutaneous transhepatic cholangiography (PTC) in the evaluation of suspected pancreatic carcinoma. Cancer 47:1666–1678
23. Freeny PC, Marks WM, Ball TJ (1982) Impact of high-resolution computed tomography of the pancreas on utilization of ERCP and angiography. Radiology 142:35–39
24. Tio TL, Tytgat GNJ, Cikot RJLM et al. (1988) Ampullopancreatic carcinoma: preoperative TNM classification with endosonography. Radiology 166:409–412
25. Semelka RC, Kroeker MA, Shoenut JP et al. (1991) Pancreatic disease: prospective comparison of CT, ERCP, and 1.5-T MR imaging with dynamic gadolinium enhancement and fat suppression. Radiology 181:785–791
26. Megibow AJ, Walsh SJ, Francis IF et al. (1991) Comparison of CT and MR imaging in evaluation of patients with pancreatic adenocarcinoma: report of the diagnostic radiology oncology group (abstr). Radiology 181 (p):259
27. Semelka RC, Shoenut JP, Kroeker MA et al. (1993) The pancreas. In Semelka RC, Shoenut JP ed. MRI of the abdomen with CT correlation. New York: Raven Press, 59–76
28. Semelka RC, Simm FC, Recht M et al. (1991) MRI of the pancreas at high field strength: a comparison of six sequences. J Comput Assist Tomogr 15:966–971
29. Gehl HB, Vorwerk D, Klose KC et al. (1991) Pancreatic enhancement after low-dose infusion of Mn-DPDP. Radiology 180:337–339

Imaging of Resectable "Periampullary Carcinoma" by Ultrasonography and Computed Tomography

Wei Jia Hu[1], Yu Jing Ying[1], Zhou Cheng[2], and Cao Lian Yi[2]

The term "periampullary carcinoma" includes tumors arising from the distal bile duct, the head of the pancreas, the ampulla of Vater and the papilla of the duodenum. It is well known that resection rate of carcinoma of the head of pancreas is low (9.8%) and the 5-year survival rate is poor (4%); nevertheless, the resection rate of ampullary carcinoma is much better (40%), and the 5-year survival rate is 43.2%.

A total of 37 cases of periampullary carcinoma were resected. Computed tomography (CT) imaging was correlated with Whipple's pathological specimen. Early diagnosis and assessment of origin of tumor and resectability are critical.

The postcontrast CT imaging technique was as follows: injection via the antecubital vein of Ultravist 300 or another 60% nonionic contrast agent (100 ml) at the rate of 2 ml/s, through pressure injection, dynamic incremental mode. For a pancreas of 3-mm thickness, 3-mm spacing was used; from the top of the liver to the pancreas, 10-mm spacing was used for 10-mm thickness.

Carcinoma of the Head of the Pancreas

There were 12 cases of carcinoma of the head of the pancreas (Figs. 1, 2). The appearance on CT was as follows:

1. Head of the pancreas or uncinate process enlarged or deformed ($n=9$)
2. Fuzziness of border of mass ($n=2$)
3. Hypoattenuation and irregular area at center of mass ($n=8$)
4. Dilatation of hepatic and common bile duct, abruptly ended at the head of the pancreas ($n=10$)
5. Atrophy of the body and tail of the pancreas ($n=8$)

On ultrasonography (US), the following was observed:

1. Mass at the head of the pancreas ($n=10$)
2. Dilatation of the common bile duct ($n=11$)

Results for the pathological specimens were as follows:

1. Mass ≤ 3 cm ($n=10$); >3 cm ($n=2$)

[1] Department of Radiology, Beijing Hospital, Beijing, 100730, China.
[2] Department of Radiology, Jiu Xian Qiao Hospital, Beijing, 100016, China.

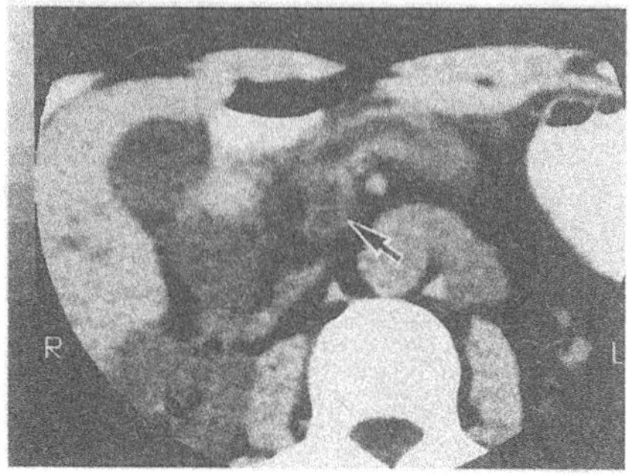

Fig. 1 Adenocarcinoma of the head of the pancreas (3 cm). CT imaging: a hypodense, heterogenous mass at the head of pancreas (*arrow*), associated with dilatation of the pancreatic and common bile duct

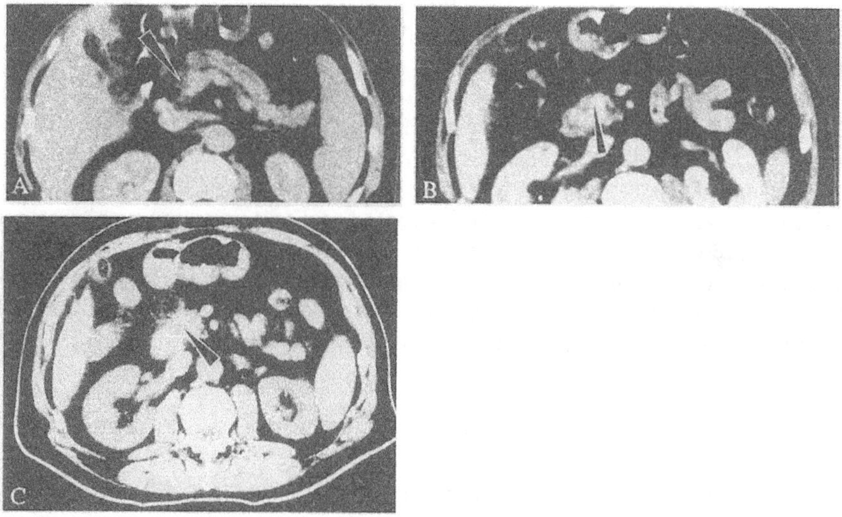

Fig. 2 A–C Ductal adenocarcinoma of the head of the pancreas (2 cm). **A** Contrasted enhanced CT scan. Irregular hypodense mass at the head of the pancreas with dilatation of the pancreatic and biliary duct. **B** Head of the pancreas deformed with heterogenous hypodense area. **C** Infiltrating streaks directed towards peripancreatic fat layer

2. Portal vein invaded ($n=2$)
3. Infiltration into fatty tissue around the tumor in the head of the pancreas ($n=2$)
4. Adjacent duodenum invaded ($n=4$)
5. Metastasis of regional lymph node, <1 cm ($n=1$)
6. Associated with chronic pancreatitis ($n=1$)

On unenhanced CT scan, pancreatic cancer is isodense in most cases. In old people, above 50 years, the presence of interlobular fatty infiltration and fibrosis increases with age, especially above 60–70 years, so that carcinoma could be identified as a mass; after bolus enhancement, the cancer enhanced very little, because of its cirrhotic nature; it becomes hypodense, as compared with the opacified normal parenchyma in arterial phase. An abrupt termination of dilated common bile duct at the head or uncinate process of the pancreas, indicates malignancy.

Follow-up studies after Whipple's operation at 2 months, 6 months, 1 and 2 years, should several any liver metastasis, retroperitoneal lymph node metastasis, ascities etc. After operation, the jejunum occupies the resected area and may mimic a soft tissue mass. One should notice gas inside the small bowel and hepatic duct as a post-operative sign to avoid mistakes.

Carcinoma of the Amullar of Vater

There were 18 cases of ampullar carcinoma (Fig. 3). On CT, the following was observed:

1. Irregular mass at the distal common bile duct or ampullar of Vater ($n=14$)
2. Head or uncinate process of the pancreas derformed ($n=12$)
3. Dilatation of the hepatic and common bile duct, abruptly terminated at the uncinate process ($n=18$)

On US, we observed the following:

1. Mass at the ampulla ($n=4$)
2. Dilatation of the common bile duct ($n=14$)

On ERCP there was a mass at end of the common bile duct in both cases investigated

The pathological specimens of ampullary carcinoma had the following results:

1. Size of tumor
   ≤ 3 cm ($n=14$)
   >3 cm ($n=4$)
2. Head of pancrea invaded ($n=2$)
3. Metastasis to regional lymph node, <1 cm ($n=2$)

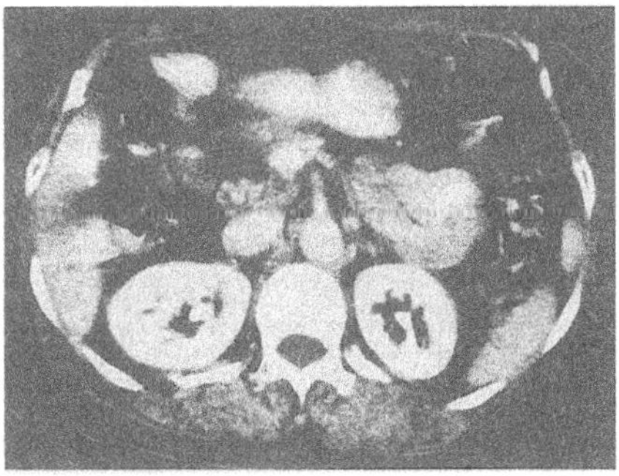

Fig. 3 Papillary carcinoma of the ampulla of Vater. Postcontrast CT: marked enhanced papillary mass in the dilated distal common bile duct

Carcinoma of the Distal Common Bile Duct

There were five cases of carcinoma of the distal common bile duct. On US, the following was observed:

1. Dilatation of the common bile duct ($n=5$)
2. Mass at end of the common bile duct ($n=4$)

On CT, the following was found:

1. Mass at end of the common bile duct or papilla of duodenum ($n=4$)
2. Head of pancreas enlarged ($n=3$)
3. Dilatation of the hepatic and common bile duct, abruptly ended at the head of the pancrease ($n=5$)

Five pathological specimens of carcinoma of the distal common bile duct were inspected:

1. Size of tumor <2.5 cm ($n=4$); 1 cm ($n=1$)
2. Invasion of head of pancreas ($n=2$)
3. Invasion of papilla of duodenum ($n=2$)
4. Associated with chronic pancreatitis ($n=2$)

Adenocarcinoma of the Papilla of the Duodenum

There were two cases of adenocarcinoma of the papilla of the duodenum (Fig. 4). On CT, the following was observed:

1. Head of pancreas enlarged ($n=2$)
2. Mass in papilla of duodenum ($n=2$)
3. Dilatation of the common bile duct ($n=2$)
4. Invasion of the distal common bile duct and pancreas ($n=1$)

On inspection of pathological specimers, invasion of the distal common bile duct and the head of the pancreas was seen in one case and, metastasis to a regional lymph node <1 cm, in one case.

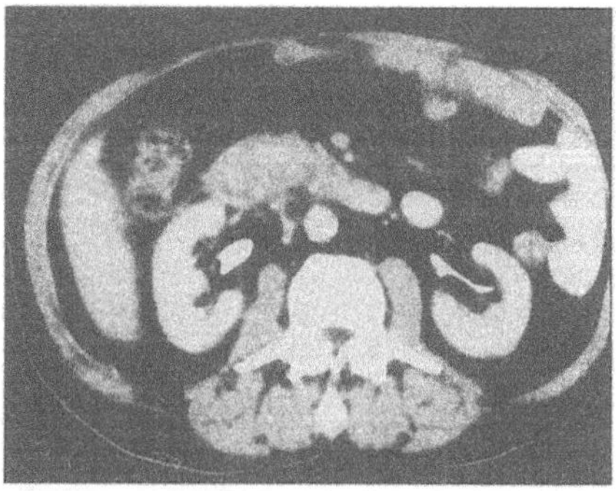

Fig. 4 Mucinous adenocarcinoma of the papilla of the duodenum (3.3 × 5 cm). Postcontrast CT study: an irregular mass inside the duodenum with invasion and obstruction of the distal common bile duct; associated with chronic pancreatitis

Discussion

Precontrast and postcontrast rapid bolus dynamic-enhanced CT, with thin-section 3- to 5-mm pancreas, together with US examination will improve the diagnostic accuracy of periampullary carcinoma to 94.6%. Dynamic contrasted CT reveals pancreatic cancer to be hypoattenuating as compared with the normal pancreatic parenchyma, and this finding reflects the infiltrating and cirrhotic nature of tumors. In elderly people, pancreatic lobules can be seen with fatty infiltration; carcinoma will obliterate this pattern, as an irregular mass.

CT signs of respectability are as follows:

- No signs of extrapancreatic extension or contiguous organ invasion
- No signs of vascular involvement
- No signs of regional or distant metastasis
- No ascitis

The differential diagnosis is as follows:

1. Common duct stone
2. Chronic pancreatitis with focal mass, with the following CT findings suggesting pancreatitis:
   - Irregular and slight dilatation of the pancreatic duct; cancer has more or less smooth and moderate dilatation of pancreatic duct, abruptly ended at the mass in the head of the pancreas
   - Intraductal or parenchmal calcification in the pancreas
   - Gradual, not abrupt, obstruction of the pancreatic and bile duct, rather than sudden transition from a dilated duct to abrupt obstruction by tumor
3. Ampullary carcinoma; irregular intraluminal mass obstructing the dilated distal common bile duct; small defect within the duodenal lumen, ampullary carcinoma enhanced moderately after contrast
4. Lymphoma
5. Metastasis

Conclusion

A total of US/CT imaging of periampullary carcinoma were correlated with Whipple's pathological specimen.

CT precontrast and postcontrast studies with dynamic incremental mode and thin-section pancreas, together with US studies, were able to increase diagnostic accuracy to 94.6%.

Pancreatic carcinoma of the head could be identified as a hypodense irregular mass against the opacified normal parenchyma of pancreas in the arterial phase.

CT assessments of resectibility, diagnosis and differential diagnosis were discussed.

References

1. Lawson TL, Berland LL, and Foley WB (1985) Malignant Neoplasms of the Pancreas, Liver, and Biliary Tract In Oncologic Imaging edited by Bragg D G, Rubin P, Youker JE Pergamon Press Inc. New York, 287
2. Freeny PC, Marks WM, Ryan JA et al. (1988) Pancreatic ductal adenocarcinoma: Diagnosis and staging with dynamic CT. Radiology 166:125-134
3. Megibow AJ (1992) Pancreatic Adenocarcinoma: Designing the Examination to Evaluate the Clinical Questions. Radiology 183:297-303
4. Rezneck PH, Stephens DH (1993) Finding Resectable Pancreatic Carcinoma. Reviews, The Staging of Pancreatic Adenocarcinoma. Clinical Radiology 47:373-381
5. Ni Quan Xin, Wu Shu Qiang, Cao Guo Hai et al. (April, 4, 1994) Pancreatic and Ampullary Carcinoma-diagnosis and treatment, an analysis of 403 cases. In Collected papers, from The First National Conference of Pancreatic Carcinoma. Beijing p 143
6. Zhou Chen, Wei Jia Hu et al. (1993) Problems in Diagnosis of Pancreatic Carcinoma by Computed Tomography, Journal of Chinese Radiology. (27), 846

Chapter 18

Computed Tomography of Solid Splenic Lesions

On Koo Cho[1]

Indications for Computed Tomography scan

Computed tomography (CT) is excellent for evaluating size, shape and position of the spleen, as well as identifying intrasplenic pathology.

The splenic lesions are characterized by their number, size, shape, CT attenuation and pattern of contrast enhancement. Although CT is sensitive in the detection of low attenuation lesions, and most spleen abnormalities presents as relatively low density lesions, the CT findings alone are not helpful in differentiation of different lesions. Associated CT findings in other organs and clinical findings are more helpful than the size, shape and CT attenuation of the lesions.

CT Technique

Splenic CT scans are usually taken 1-cm thick at 1-cm intervals. Precontrast CT scans provide little additional information except in some cases of trauma. Thus, splenic CT can be performed only after administration of intravenous (IV) contrast material.

Dynamic CT scanning during an IV bolus of 100–180 ml contrast medium injected at 1–2 ml/s is useful for accessing splenic vasculature, splenic and parasplenic masses. Dynamic CT scanning of the spleen has not been as useful as the other organs because of the variable patterns of contrast enhancement in normal spleens (Fig. 1). Thus delayed CT images are necessary for the diagnosis of intrasplenic lesions.

By administration of IV liposoluble contrast material (EOE 13), selective enhancement of the liver and spleen parenchyma can be performed.

[1] HanYang University Hospital, Seoul, Korea.

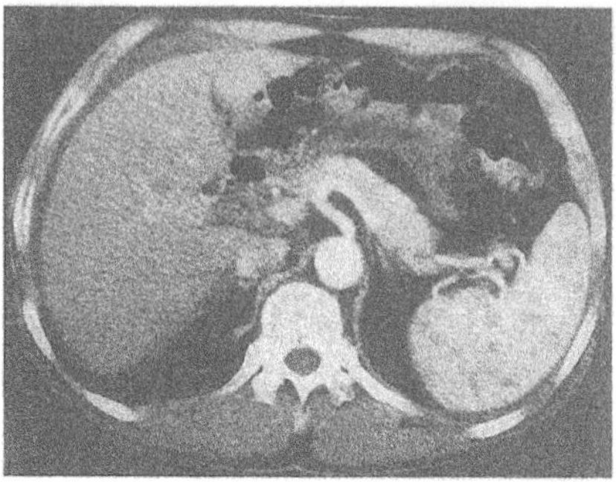

Fig. 1 Early arterial phase of dynamic contrast enhanced CT scan; spleen normally shows heterogeneous enhancement

Low-Attenuation Lesions

1. Splenic cleft
   - Well-defined peripheral low-attenuation lesions
2. During early arterial phase following bolus contrast medium injection
   - Due to variable rate of blood flow through the cord of splenic red pulp
     Transient finding that disappears in delay scan
3. Cystic lesion
   - Splenic cyst or pseudocyst
   - Abscess
   - Infarct
   - Necrotic neoplasms
4. Solid splenic lesion
   - Usually neoplastic
   - Recent infarct or an infarct with scarring

Neoplasms of the Spleen

1. Cysts
   - True epithelial cysts
   - Pseudocysts (post-traumatic or pancreatitis)
2. Benign solid neoplasms
   - Hemangioma
   - Hamartoma
   - Lymphangioma/lymphangiomatosis
3. Malignant solid neoplasms
   - Primary hemangiosarcoma
   - Lymphoma
   - Metastases

Benign Neoplasms

Hemangioma. Although rare, this is the most common benign neoplasm; it occurs in adults aged 35–55 years as an asymptomatic left lower quadrant (LLQ) mass, and rupture occurs in up to 25% of cases. Pathologically, it is homogeneously solid or may contain cystic spaces, it usually occurs as a single lesion and is microscopically similar to other organ hemangioma (proliferated vascular channels lined by endothelium). On CT, it appears as a solid and/or cystic mass (pre-E CT, solid portion is hypo-or isodense; post-E CT, increased attenuation from the periphery to the center). As far as calcification is concerned, it is punctate in the center or has an eggshell rim at the periphery.

Hamartoma. This is a rare benign tumor composed of anomalous mixtures of normal elements of splenic tissue. It appears as an, LLQ mass, with hypersplenism in 8% and rupture in 8% of cases. Pathologically, it is classified as red (vascular) or white pulp (lymphomatous) type; it is usually a solid lesion and may have a cystic component. There is a discrete, circumscribed nodule without encapsulation. On CT, it appears as a cystic or solid mass.

Lymphangioma/lymphangiomatosis. Classically, this lesion is a diffuse process involving almost the entire spleen, but solitary cystic lesions can be found. Pathologically, it appears as a single or as multiple cysts lined by endothelium and filled with proteinaceous fluid. It is usually subcapsular in its location. On CT, an enlarged spleen is observed containing single or multiple cystic areas. It has a thin wall and is sharply marginated, and there is no enhancement.

Malignant Neoplasms

Lymphoma. This is the most common malignant neoplasm of the spleen. It is classified as either primary or as part of systemic lymphoma. Primary splenic lymphoma is rare, while involvement as systemic lymphoma is common. Gross pathological features include the following:

1. Homogeneous enlargement of spleen with no masses
2. Solitary masses measuring 1–5 mm
3. Multiple masses measuring 2–10 cm
4. Large, solitary mass

On CT, it appears as:

1. Homogeneous enlargement without a discrete mass. Although splenomegaly occurs in most patients with non-Hodgkin's lymphoma (NHL) indicates splenic involvement, one third of the patients with splenomegaly have no evidence of splenic involvement have no splenomegaly. Marked splenomegaly can occur when there is extensive bone marrow involvement with resultant hypersplenism.
2. Solitary or multifocal mass (Fig. 2). It is usually observed in NHL and is a low-attenuation mass without contrast enhancement. The margin is well-defined or

ill-defined. The bulky mass may transgress the splenic capsule and extend into adjacent structures. Necrosis is rare and, when present, is similar to an abscess. Calcification before and after treatment is rare.
3. Diffuse infiltration. There is diffuse low-density or diffuse irregular contrast enhancement. Splenic infarction is not uncommon if the spleen is diffusely involved.

Diagnosis of lymphoma should be suggested especially when the masses are accompanied by abdominal lymphadenopathy and prominent splenomegaly (Table 1).

Splenic Metastases. These are relatively uncommon (Fig. 3), occurring in 7.1 % of malignant cases in autopsy. They are, hematogeneous via the splenic artery or vein. There is, generally multiorgan involvement, suggesting that splenic involvement is a late event. The primary lesion commonly occurs in the breast, lung, ovary, stomach and as a melanoma. Pathologically, one third are microscopic nodules and two thirds grossly visible nodules. They occur as a solitary nodule in 31%, as multiple nodules in 60%, and with diffuse infiltration in 9% of cases. On

Table 1 DDx of splenic lymphoma and metastases

	Lymphoma	Metastases
Degree of splenomegaly	+++	+
Splenic contour bulging	+	–
Other organ abnormality (liver)	–	+
Tumor necrosis	–	+
Lymphadenopathy	++	+

2
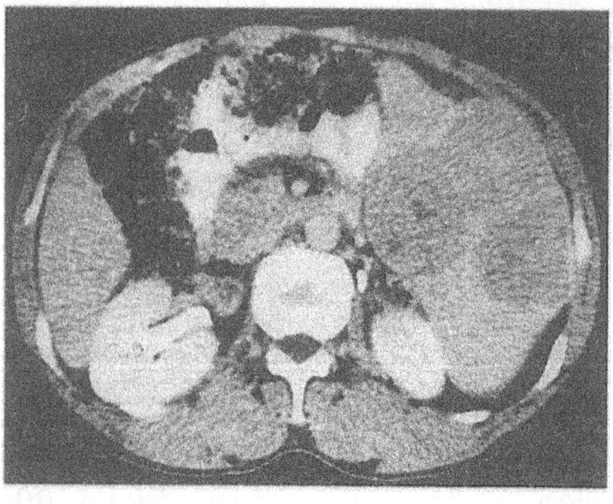
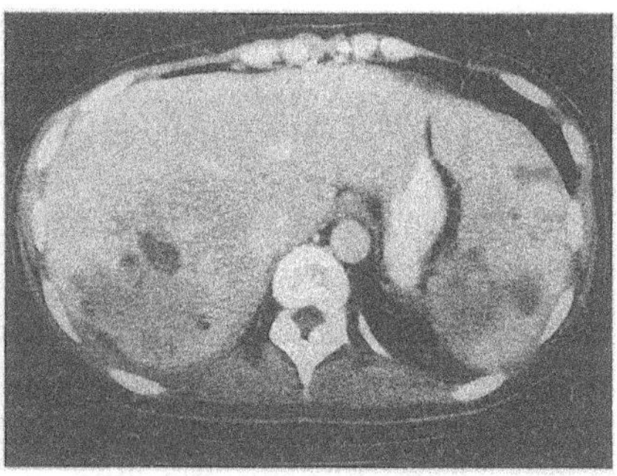
3

Fig. 2 Large cell lymphoma with multiple metastases. The spleen is enlarged with variably sized contour-bulging masses. The nodules are well defined and show relatively homogeneous low attenuation. Splenic hilar lymphadenopathy was seen in an other section

Fig. 3 Metastatic tumor from ovarian cancer. Multiple, scattered, low-attenuation masses in the spleen and liver, consistent with disseminated metastatic disease

CT, they appear as a low-density mass; a necrotic cystic lesion may be present (DDx with cyst, without a well-defined margin). Calcification is rare unless the primary tumor is mucinous adenoma.

Plutoneal implants to the surface of the spleen

Seen with plutoneal carcinomatosis secondary to ovary, GI. tract, appendix and pancreas ca.

CT finding: scalloping of the splenic surface
may intrude into splenic parenchyma from the serosal surface.
DDx: pseudomyonia peritonei.

Direct invasion of the spleen

In general, splenic capsule acts as a barrier against direct invasion. Uncommon but may occur from the adjacent malignant mass (stomach, colon, tail of the pancreas, left kidney, retroperitoneal tumor).

Angiosarcoma. This is a rare pathologic entity which may be associated with toxic exposure or ionizing radiation. It has a poor prognosis with early and widespread metastases. Pathologically, there is formation of vascular channels and a sarcomatous stroma, with either areas of solid tumor surrounding cystic spaces or hemorrhagic nodules. On CT a mass in the spleen is observed, frequently involving the liver as well. The spleen is enlarged, with a hypodense lesion on pre-E scan. The peripheral enhancement is similar to hemangioma, although the pattern of filling is variable. Splenic rupture is a major complication, so in cases of hemoperitoneum with a splenic mass this diagnosis should be considered.

References

1. Rolfes RJ, Ros PR (1990) The spleen: an integrated imaging approach. Crit Rew Diag imaging 30:41–83
2. Rabushka LS, Kawashima AK, Fishman EK (1994) Imaging of the spleen: CT with supplemental MR examination. Radiographics 14:307–331
3. Ros PR, Moser RP, Dachman AH et al. (1987) Hemangioma of the spleen: Radiologic-pathologic correlation in ten cases. Radiology 162:73–77
4. Disler DG, Chew FS (1991) Splenic hemangioma. AJR 157:44–47
5. Strijk SP, Wagener DJ, Bogman MJ et al. (1985) The spleen in Hodgkin's disease: Diagnostic value of CT. Radiology 154:753–757
6. Meyer JE, Harris NL, Elman A et al. (1983) Large cell lymphoma of the spleen: CT appearence. Radiology 148:199–202
7. Marymond JH, Gross S (1963) Patterns of metastatic cancer in the spleen. Am J Clin Pathol 40:58–66
8. Chintapalli K, Thorsen K, Lawson TL (1985) Differential diagnosis of low attenuation splenic lesions on computed tomography. CT 9:311–319

CHAPTER 19

Tissue-Specific Contrast Agents

H.-J. Weinmann, A. Mühler and T. Balzer[1]

Since the early days of diagnostic imaging, one of the main research objectives has been to improve the accuracy and specificity of diagnostic imaging by developing tissue-specific contrast agents. The naturally occurring contrast in classical X-ray studies, modern computed tomography (CT) and even magnetic resonance imaging (MRI) does not always provide a straightforward answer to the diagnostic question. The outcome of the study depens to a great extent on the contrast between the various tissues and the pathologies as well as the skill of the reader and the quality of the equipment.

In 1930, Oka and Rath introduced a stabilized 25% colloidal solution of thorium dioxide, Thorotrast, as a radiodiagnostic contrast medium (Umbrathor, Heyden, München, Germany) for angiography and hepatolienography (Oka 1930; Radt 1930). Because of its long-term toxicity resulting from exposure to radiation, Thorotrast was banned in 1940. In 1938 the first iodinated tissue-specific agent, Hepatoselectan (Schering, Berlin, Germany), was introduced for contrast enhancement of the liver and spleen with standard X-ray techniques. This highly effective suspension was composed of the triiodinated ethyl ester of stearic acid that accumulated in the reticuloendothelial system (RES) after intravenous injection. A dose of about 200–250 mgI/kg body weight produced excellent contrast enhancement of the liver and spleen (Beckermann and Popken 1938). However, the agent was removed from the market because of its high rate of adverse reactions.

Detection Limits and Tolerability

The detection limit of the various contrast agents is quite different in the classical imaging modalities (Table 1). While modern ultrasound modalities and nuclear medicine require concentrations of 1–10 ng/ml or even less, substantially higher concentrations are needed for classical X-ray techniques and modern CT or MRI. To achieve a clinically significant contrast in X-ray film angiography or urography between the area of interest (e.g., a vessel) and the surrounding tissue, an iodine concentration of at least 10–20 mgI/ml is mandatory. Such high concentrations can be achieved only by selective injections (intra-arterial) or by using a physiological concentrating mechanism such as glomerular filtration with reabsorption of water. In man, a concentration of roughly 2–3 mgI/ml, which results from an

[1] Research Laboratories of Schering AG, Müllerstr. 178, 13342 Berlin, Germany.

Table 1 Detection limits of contrast agents used in different diagnostic imaging modalities PET, positron emission tomography; MRI, magnetic resonance imaging; DSA, digital subtraction angiography; CT, computed tomography

Imaging modality	Source of contrast	Detection limit
PET	^{11}C, ^{15}O, ^{18}F etc.	<< ng/ml
Conventional nuclear medicine	^{99m}Tc, ^{123}I, ^{111}In etc.	< 10 ng/ml
Ultrasound	Gas bubbles	100 μg/ml
MRI	Gd, Mn, Fe	1–10 μg/ml
Conventional film X-ray (urography, angiography)	Ba, I	15 mg/ml
Digital X-ray techniques (DSA)	I	10 mg/ml
Digital X-ray techniques (CT)	I	1 mg/ml

intravenous injection of 100 ml (300 mgI/ml) of a contrast agent followed by homogeneous distribution in the extracellular space, does not create enough absorption of X-rays to be detectable by standard equipment.

CT is more sensitive and displays contrast enhancement at much lower iodine concentrations (1 mg I/ml, approximately 25 Hounsfield units, HU). For the liver, for instance, an intravenous bolus injection of about 50–100 ml is sufficient for an improved diagnosis. Detectable contrast occurs in blood during the early perfusion phase when most of the iodinated agent has not yet leaked from the vessels into the interstitial space. Since the duration of iodine peak in blood is very short, only fast CT techniques (spiral CT) are capable of examining the whole liver. Spiral CT allows rapid hepatic imaging during a single breath-hold. This increased imaging speed allows contrast material to be used more efficaciously than with conventional dynamic CT, making it easy to obtain contrast dynamics for evaluation of the portal-venous and arterial vasculature.

However, for accurate diagnosis it is often desirable to have a longer lasting enhancement (i.e., minutes), which can be obtained by selective accumulation of substances in intracellular spaces. Finding liver-specific agents for CT has been a major focus of contrast medium research.

The majority of the liver mass consists of hepatocytes, cells that contain important metabolic functions and properties for substances traveling from the sinusoidal space to the bile. Hepato-biliary contrast agents reach the cytoplasm of the hepatocytes by using one of these transporters.

In one study, water-soluble derivatives of such a cholegraphic agent reached concentrations in the liver detectable by CT (Weinmann et al. 1981). An intravenous dose of 360 mgI/kg (0.47 mmol of the dimeric molecule per kg body weight) increased liver attenuation by 80 HU in dogs. However, this high enhancement was not matched in mini-pigs or man.

Various research groups have tried to target the liver's RES cells. Doppman and coworkers from the National Institutes of Health (Bethesda, MD, USA) achieved good clinical results using the iodinated lipid emulsion EOE-13 (Miller et al. 1984). Other groups worked extensively with other emulsions, suspensions, or liposome-entrapped, water-soluble iodinated contrast agents (Ivancev et al. 1989; Krause et al. 1993; White et al. 1990). None of these experimental contrast formulations were authorized for marketing or reached a sufficiently advanced stage of development due to either low efficacy or a low tolerability profile.

An important property of a tissue-specific agent is the nature of its interaction with receptors, transporters, or other biological structures because any interaction carries the risk of side effects. The more specific the interaction or the smaller the number of receptors, the higher is the likelihood of an exobiotic substance eliciting adverse reactions.

Targeting the hepatocytes or entrapping substances into macrophages of the RES is an effective approach for liver-specific agents since both pathways have a high capacity for handling relatively unspecific bulk amounts of materials. However, experimental studies have shown that, to achieve a significant tissue-specific contrast, CT may require an accumulation of exobiotic substances at levels that produce side-effects.

Because of its higher sensitivity and excellent contrast resolution, contrast enhanced MRI may be the technique of choice for diagnostic imaging, particularly of focal lesions. Most of the investigations in this area have been focused on target-specific agents for the liver, spleen, lymphatic system, and blood pool.

Contrast Agents for Magnetic Resonance Imaging

Liver

The differential diagnosis of focal hepatic lesions continues to be a problem even though many diagnostic methods are available. With the development of faster techniques that reduce artefacts, MRI becomes more sensitive than conventional techniques such as ultrasound and CT in many abdominal areas, including the liver. Despite the high contrast resolution of T2-Weighted techniques, many pathologies are difficult to detect or to differentiate without contrast agents because of their isointensity to normal tissue.

The paramagnetic extracellular contrast agents available today for abdominal imaging (e.g. Magnevist, Schering AG, Berlin, Germany, improves the diagnostic potential after intravenous injection of 0.1 or 0.2 mmol/kg (~10–30 ml per patient) in selected indications. Dynamic Magnevist-enhanced MRI allows a better differential diagnosis of focal liver lesions (Hamm et al. 1994; Mahfouz et al. 1993; Semelka et al. 1992).

MRI for detecting focal liver lesions is at least as sensitive as CT, and is even better suited for specifically determining benign versus malignant etiology. Dynamic contrast enhancement provides a more confident differential diagnosis, and fast imaging procedures such as breath-hold T1-Weighted gradient-echo (GRE) images are superior to spin-echo (SE) techniques. Advances in abdominal MRI, particularly fast scanning techniques and extracellular contrast agents, have improved differentiation but not the detection of small focal liver lesions. Liver-specific agents that increase sensitivity are being developed. Requirements are very high: the new agents must display a greater efficacy than standard imaging procedures and should have a tolerability profile matching that of modern contrast agents including nonionic X-ray agents and even Magnevist (Haustein et al. 1993; Haustein et al. 1992; Niendorf et al. 1991).

Compounds with two different magnetic properties are currently in clinical trial or late preclinical testing phases. These agents include water-soluble paramagnetic chelates with hepatobiliary uptake: Mn-DPDP (manganese(II) N, N′-dipyridoxylethylenediamine-N,N′-diacetate 5,5′-bisphosphate; Nycomed, Oslo, Norway); Gd-BOPTA (gadobenate dimeglumine, Bracco, Milan, Italy); and Gd-EOB-DTPA (gadoxetate disodium, Schering AG, Berlin, Germany) (Fig. 1). Superparamagnetic iron particles sequestered by the RES are also being tested: AMI-25 (Feridex, Advanced Magnetics, Cambridge, USA or Endorem, Guerbet, Paris, France) and Schering's SH U 555A.

Very small superparamagnetic iron particles (e.g., AMI 227; Advanced Magnetics, Cambridge, USA) targeted to the lymphatic system or the asialoglycoprotein receptor (AG-USPIO) are in an early phase of clinical testing.

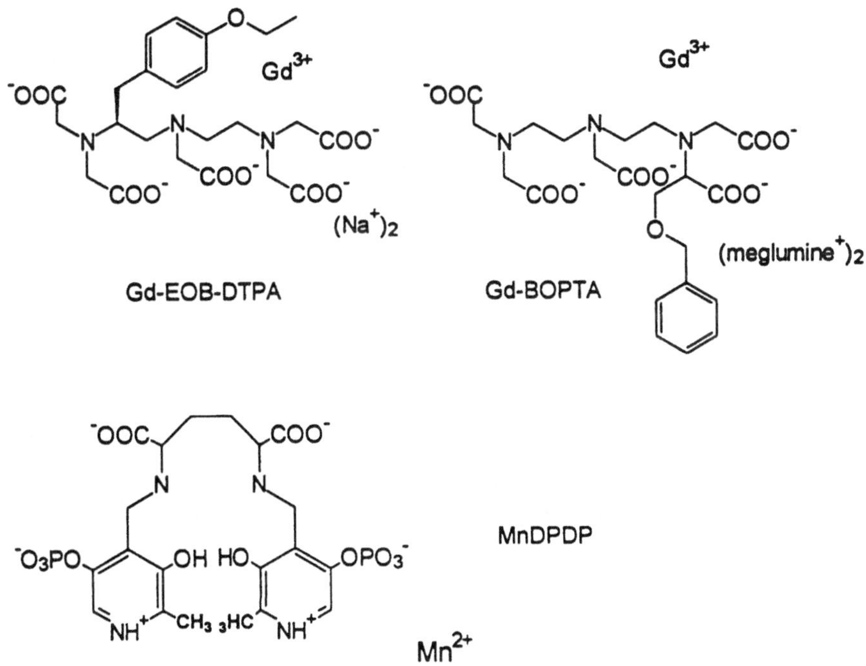

Fig. 1 Chemical structure of the hepatobiliary magnetic resonance (MR) contrast agents which are currently in clinical trials phase II/III

Mn-DPDP

Mn-DPDP is a T1-reducing contrast agent which, after intravenous injection, accumulates predominately in the healthy liver parenchyma, although specific contrast enhancement has also been described for cardiac and pancreatic tissue (Elizondo et al. 1991; Gehl et al. 1993; Gehl et al. 1991; Lim et al. 1991; Liou et al. 1994; Saeed et al. 1989). Published clinical data highlight Mn-DPDP's strong and long-lasting liver enhancement after drip infusion of a very low dose (0.5–1 μmol Mn/kg). Detection of secondary liver tumors was highly improved; no uptake in the malignant cells was reported. However, hepatocellular carcinomas have shown an accumulation of contrast, probably because of some active transport of the complex or manganese in its free form (Marchal et al. 1993b).

In rats, the compound was excreted in the urine and feces in about equal amounts (Elizondoet al. 1991). In some types of liver dysfunction, the use of Mn-DPDP may be a problem because its elimination is strongly impaired in the presence of bile duct obstruction and because manganese has a poor renal glomerular filtration rate (Marchal et al. 1993a). The nonhepatocellular enhancement suggests that free Mn or some Mn-DPDP metabolite is strongly bound to plasma proteins. Recent biodistribution studies demonstrated the poor in vivo stability of the manganese complex (Grant et al. 1994) and explain the related tolerability problems.

Mn-DPDP is an effective agent for liver imaging and provides significant liver enhancement with T1-weighted sequences. Further clinical trials are necessary to assess the risk-benefit of this manganese-containing chelate.

Hepatobiliary Gadolinium Chelates

Magnevist distributes in the extracellular space and is eliminated almost exclusively by the renal route (Hausteinet al. 1992; Schuhmann and Krestin 1991; Weinmann et al. 1984a; Weinmann et al. 1984b). Highly stable gadolinium chelates were synthesized that exhibited remarkably different pharmacokinetic characteristics (Vittadini et al. 1990; Weinmann et al. 1991). Two of them, Gd-BOPTA and Gd-EOB-DTPA, were investigated in more detail and entered clinical trials in Europe (Hamm et al. 1995; Vogl et al. 1992).

Both chelates are ionic DTPA derivatives characterized by lipophilic residues that target the agents to special carriers in the sinusoidal plasma membrane of the hepatocyte. Although the exact transport mechanism is unknown, it is very likely that the agents interact with the organic anion transporter, the same protein that is responsible for bilirubin transport. Both agents enter the intracellular space and are sequestered into the bile by another carrier. According to classical physiology, the first step is driven solely by the concentration gradient between the extra- and intracellular space, whereas the canalicular transport depends on adenosine 5′-triphosphate. Concentration measurements in the plasma and the liver space suggest that the gadolinium chelates exhibit a special liver-uptake mechanism. Although the plasma concentration rapidly decreases after intravenous injection, much higher concentrations remain detectable in the cytosol of the hepatocytes (Fig. 2).

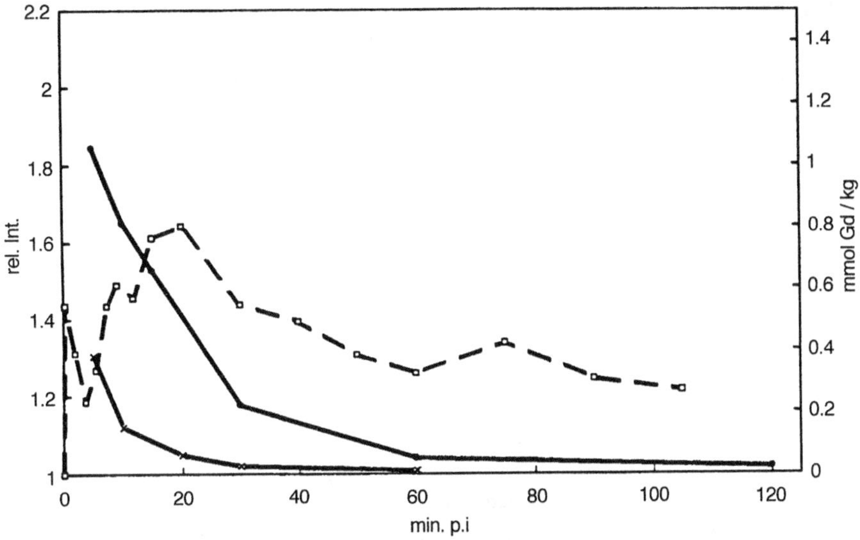

Fig. 2 Gadolinium concentration in plasma and liver tissue after intravenous injection of 0.25 mmol gadoxetate disodium (Gd-EOB-DTPA)/kg in a rat. The *dotted curve* represents the signal intensity of the rat liver measured at 2 T (SISCO, Ca, USA) using a T1-weighted sequence (400 ms/15 ms). The decrease of the signal intensity in the first 5 min after injection is caused by excessive gadolinium concentration

Gd-BOPTA and Gd-EOB-DTPA differ from all other hepatophilic molecules, including cholegraphic X-ray dyes or bilirubin. Both gadolinium chelates exhibit a very pronounced hydrophilic character despite their lipophilic moieties. They are even more hydrophilic than modern nonionic X-ray contrast agents. Unlike bilirubin, Gd-EOB-DTPA demonstrates a relatively weak protein binding of just 10%. In vitro tests have shown that Gd-EOB-DTPA also bind weakly to cytosolic proteins such as ligandin (glutathione-S-transferase). Their high hydrophilicity and low protein binding are responsible for their good acute intravenous tolerability (LD 50) which in rats is about 10 mmol/kg, as good as that of Magnevist (Schuhmann et al. 1992).

Relaxation measurements have shown that the relaxivity of Gd-EOB-DTPA and Gd-BOPTA increased from 5 to about 17 l mmol/s in the liver cell. Intracellular protein binding or the increased microviscosity in the cellular lumen is believed to be responsible for this phenomenon.

In rats receiving up to 100 µmol/kg of Gd-EOB-DTPA, about two-thirds are eliminated by the feces and one-third by the renal route. Gd-BOPTA displays a somewhat weaker hepatobiliary excretion. Because of its hepatocellular uptake and very high relaxivity, as little as 10 µmol of Gd-EOB-DTPA/kg is sufficient for an excellent contrast enhancement of the liver (Marchalet al. 1993b; Muhler et al. 1992; Weinmann et al. 1991).

Gd-EOB-DTPA's half-life in blood is very short because of its renal excretion and hepatocellular uptake. The compound is distributed in the extracellular space throughout the organism except in the liver. After extracellular distribution, Gd-EOB-DTPA is excreted from the organism quantitatively similar to Gd-DTPA. However, in contrast to the latter, the majority of Gd-EOB-DTPA is excreted through the hepatocytes into the bile and feces within the first few hours. No biotransformation or transchelation are apparent.

Because of their rather selective accumulation in the liver, their direct interaction with water protons of the hepatocellular space, and the increased relaxivity of these hepatobiliary agents, the diagnostic dose should be considerably lower than that of Magnevist. In rats, similar to Mn-DPDP and Gd-BOPTA, the effective dose of Gd-EOB-DTPA is on the order of 10–30 μmol/kg body weight, resulting in a margin of safety of about 500.

The bile displays a very short T1-relaxation time which makes contrast-enhanced cholangiography possible by means of a special T1-weighted imaging sequence (saturation inversion projection spin-echo sequence, SIP; Schad et al. 1993). The opportunity for evaluating biliary anatomy offers an advantage over particulate liver contrast agents, which are not subject to biliary excretion.

Despite its specific liver enhancement, Gd-EOB-DTPA can be used as a conventional extracellular MR contrast agent for other abdominal applications or the central nervous system. Gd-EOB-DTPA has better in vivo stability than Mn-DPDP. Studies in rats have shown that much less than 1% of the given dose was detectable in the body 7 days after injection. Since this Gdcomplex is also partially excreted by the kidneys, it may be possible to evaluate renal and hepatocellular functions simultaneously.

Although the chemical structures of Gd-BOPTA and Gd-EOB-DTPA look quite similar, their pharmacokinetics in man differ substantially (Hamm et al. 1995; Rosati et al. 1994). The most striking difference is the relatively poor hepatocellular uptake of Gd-BOPTA. The proportion of biliary excretion represents just 2%–3% of the total dose administered. These pharmacokinetics are almost identical to the data published with Magnevist, demonstrating that Gd-BOPTA behaves like an extracellular chelate and only poorly displays characteristics of a liver-specific substance.

Using the higher dose of 100 μmol/kg, an adequate and longer lasting contrast was obtained between the liver and the blood pool or the focal liver lesion about 60 min after intravenous injection (Vogl et al. 1992). Preclinical investigations have shown that Gd-EOB-DTPA's pharmacokinetics displayed some dose and species dependence. Thus, on the basis of animal experiments, it is not possible to predict what dose will be sufficient for contrast enhancement in man.

The first clinical trials with Gd-EOB-DTPA started in 1993 in Berlin, Germany. The tolerability and pharmacokinetics of the contrast agent were studied in healthy volunteers after intravenous injection of different doses (10, 25, 50, or 100 μmol/kg, and saline) (Hamm et al. 1995; Weinmann et al. 1994). Vital signs, blood chemistry, and urinalysis were monitored at intervals for up to 4 days. Hamm and coworkers investigated the imaging properties of the agent using multiple T1-SE, and T1-FLASH sequences in another group of volunteers (Hamm et al. 1995).

Gd-EOB-DTPA exhibited a dose-independent pharmacokinetic profile. The concentration in blood dropped in a two-exponential curve with a terminal half-life of about 90 min. The pharmacokinetics were comparable to results obtained in animals with a high percentage of fecal excretion. The compound was completely eliminated from the body in equal amounts through renal and biliary excretion. No metabolism of the gadolinium chelate was detectable. It is remarkable that the so-called unspecific organic anion transporter differentiates very clearly between the lipophilic moiety of Gd-BOPTA and Gd-EOB-DTPA.

A dose of 25 μmol/kg was sufficient for selectively enhancing the signal intensity of the healthy liver parenchyma, with an imaging window of 10–120 min after the injection. Shortly after administration, the characteristic perfusion pattern of a lesion can be examined with dynamic imaging techniques. No additional increase of enhancement was observed in the highest dose studied (100 μmol/kg), but a transient decrease of signal intensity was noted which probably resulted from an exceedingly high gadolinium concentration (T2-effect). No adverse reactions or meaningful changes in biological parameters were observed after intravenous injection of up to 100 μmol/kg.

The first use in man showed an excellent profile for Gd-EOB-DTPA as a favorable contrast agent for MRI of the liver with good tolerability, immediate and high contrast enhancement, and complete excretion .

Superparamagnetic Iron Oxide Particles

Special iron oxide aggregates are extremely effective T2-relaxation agents. When placed in a magnetic field they behave like ferromagnetic substances. Outside the magnetic field, superparamagnetic iron oxide particles (SPIO) do not exhibit the magnetic memory of ferromagnetic materials. The diameter of such SPIO is in the nanometer range, as large as proteins such as ferritin.

Such SPIO particles produce a dramatic long-range disturbance in magnetic field homogeneity. The strong T2-effect is especially apparent when the agents distribute inhomogeneously. A magnetic gradient between two separated compartments results in a so-called susceptibility effect. The tiny magnets do not aggregate in the presence of the magnetic field because of their rapid Brownian motion and their special coating, which prevent close direct contact of the iron cores. The iron oxide cores may be monocrystalline or polycrystalline, and they have widely varying relaxivities in the range of 5–200 l mmol/s. These iron particles are coated with polysaccharides (e.g. dextranes) and form a mahogany-colored aqueous solution.

After intravenous administration, SPIO particles are sequestered by normal RES phagocytic Kupffer cells, but they are not retained in tumor tissue (Stark et al. 1988; Weissleder et al. 1988). Some accumulation is also seen in the bone marrow (Seneterre et al. 1991). Unlike the hepatobiliary gadolinium chelates, SPIO particles do not penetrate the plasma membrane of the hepatocytes. Instead, they distribute in a relatively small volume of the target which, in the case of the liver, represents only about 2%–3% of its total cell population. However, their T2-effect is so strong that even a very small dose is sufficient to decrease the signal intensity of the whole liver. This susceptibility effect is especially apparent in T2-Weighted sequences, and some GRE sequences are particularly sensitive. Concentrations as small as 1 μg Fe/m are adequate to significantly reduce the signal intensity of the liver and spleen.

Iron is a biologically important metal that is present in gram amounts in the body and is relatively toxic when not bound to proteins. Biologically, iron is an integral part of important proteins such as myoglobin and hemoglobin and many other proteins that regulate iron metabolism. Since the metal is not subject to renal or biliary excretion, the fate of SPIO particles in the body was of special interest. Nuclear magnetic resonance (NMR) measurements verified that the superparamagnetic iron oxides are metabolized into a soluble – not superparamagnetic – form of iron, probably by lysosomes located in the RES cells. Radio tracer studies show that this iron is incorporated into the normal iron pool (e.g., ferritin, hemosiderin, hemoglobin) in a time- and dose-dependent fashion.

Two different preparations are currently under clinical investigation: Advanced Magnetic's AMI-25 (Feridex) and Schering's SH U 555A. Various clinical trials showed the efficacy of this superparamagnetic material. After slow intravenous infusion of Feridex, a significant increase in contrast-to-noise ratios was observed. SPIO-enhanced images of the liver significantly increased the number of hepatic lesions detected and reduced the threshold size for detection to less than 5 mm. Using T2-Weighted imaging techniques, a dose of 10–20 μmol Fe/kg produced excellent clinical efficacy. The tolerability profile was good, although some adverse reactions such as heat sensation and back pain were reported. AMI-25 was licensed to Guerbet and received marketing authorization in Switzerland in 1994.

Schering's SPIO, named SH U 555A (proposed tradename Resovist), has similar imaging characteristics. However, this drug substance seems to be more stable than Feridex and is available as a ready-to-use formulation. Phase II multicenter clinical trials were conducted in Europe and Japan. Doses in the range of 5–40 μmol Fe/kg were investigated in patients suffering from focal liver lesions. Because of its excellent tolerability profile, a bolus injection was used. Even the very low dose of 5–10 μmol Fe/kg produced a strong decrease in signal intensity that paralleled a significant increase in the contrast-to-noise ratio (Fig. 3). While SH U 555A did not accumulate in metastases, some uptake was observed in FNH. SH U 555A-enhanced images during the early perfusion and retention phases offer improved diagnostic accuracy in the detection and characterization of focal liver lesions.

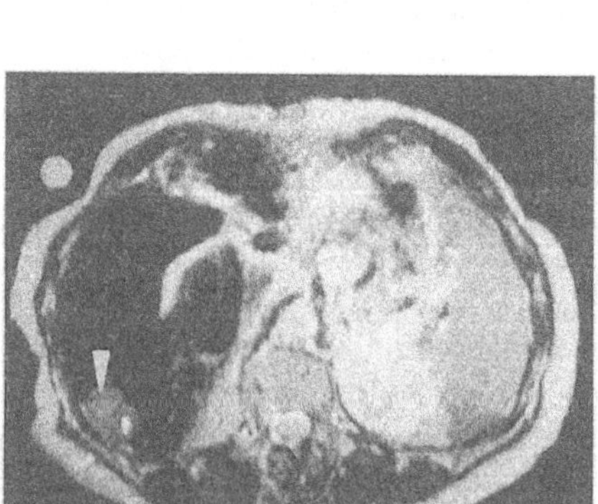

Fig. 3 SH U 555A contrast enhancement of a small hepatocellular carcinoma (*arrow head*). The T2-weighted image was taken 40 min after intravenous bolus injection of 5 μmol Fe/kg. Superparamagnetic iron oxide particles (SPIO) accummulate in the reticuloendothelial system (RES) of the healthy liver but not in the carcinoma. (Photograph kindly made available by Prof. K. Ohtomo, Department of Radiology, University Hospital of Yamanashi, Japan, who conducted the study)

Lymphatic System

The detection of metastases in lymph nodes is still a problem in clinical practice. Highly effective relaxation-enhancing agents combined with T2-weighted techniques may make it possible to develop lymphotropic pharmaceuticals that can be administered interstitially or even intravenously. MR lymphography with an intravenously administered SPIO nanoparticle for distinguishing normal and reactive from tumor-bearing lymph nodes was investigated preclinically and clinically (Hamm et al. 1992; Weissleder et al. 1989; Weissleder et al. 1990). The diameter of such particles measured by laser-light scattering are about 20 nm and exhibit a somewhat reduced T2-relaxivity when compared to SPIO particles. Ultrasmall superparamagnetic iron oxide (USPIO) particles exhibit a longer half-life after intravenous administration because of the less efficient uptake of the RES in the liver and spleen. Weissleder and coworkers demonstrated that USPIO particles travel to the lymphatic system and produce a signal loss. An iron dose of 40–200 μmol/kg body weight produced a distinct signal loss in the various lymph nodes. Although the various lymph nodes were histologically similar, inhomogeneous particle distributions were registered.

Best results, obtained 24 h after administration, show a signal loss in normal but not in metastatic nodes. A single intravenous administration of USPIO particles may allow detection of nodal metastases on the basis of signal intensity characteristics rather than the currently used, insensitive size characteristics. First clinical trials with USPIO (BMS 180549, Squibb, Princetown, USA) enables differentiation of normal from metastatic mediastinal lymph nodes. T2-weighted SE sequences showed better results with histopathology than T1-sequences (Browne et al. 1994; McLachlan et al. 1994).

Receptor and Blood Pool Imaging

USPIO particles were successfully tested for receptor imaging using various molecules chemically linked to the coating material. The magnetic particles were attached to antimyosin Fab and used for immunospecific MRI of cardiac infarcts in rats. A dose of 100 μmol Fe/kg produced a marked decrease in the signal intensity of infarcted myocardium 1 h after intravenous administration (Weissleder et al. 1992). Immunoglobulin-labeled USPIO particles were successfully tested in an animal model to localize inflammatory areas, and arabinogalactan (AG) coupled to USPIO have been directed to proteins located in the plasma membrane of hepatocytes (Schaffer et al. 1993; Weissleder et al. 1991; Weissleder et al. 1990). Gadolinium-labeled monoclonal antibodies were targeted to tumors implanted in a nude mouse (Gohr et al. 1993; Kornguth et al. 1987). Since most of the contrast agents administered do not accumulate in the tumor, the dose necessary to produce an adequate enhancement is still too high. Up to 10 g of a monoclonal antibody, each molecule labelled with dozens of paramagnetic ions, will be required to achieve diagnostically useful enhancement in man. Preliminary preclinical studies indicate the feasibility of receptor imaging in MRI.

Metallo-porphyrins exhibit very interesting imaging characteristics (Bohdiewicz et al. 1990; Ogan et al. 1987; Place et al. 1992; Young et al. 1994). The high relaxivity and claimed avidity of some metallo-porphyrins for divergent tumor histologies support the potential use of these agents for improved diagnostic specificity of MR imaging for neoplastic masses. However, because of their poor tolerability, clinical trials have not been initiated.

Higher molecular compounds exhibit a prolonged rotational correlation time and, hence, increased relaxivity. In addition, larger molecules display a unique distribution characteristic: they do not diffuse into the extravascular space and thus are useful as blood-pool contrast agents that demonstrate the perfusion characteristics of the area of interest.

Several macromolecular, polymeric gadolinium chelates have been studied in animals, including Gd-DTPA-albumin, Gd-DTPA-dextran, and Gd-DTPA-polylysine (Adam et al. 1994; Berthezene et al. 1991; Bock et al. 1994; Gibby et al. 1990; Lim et al. 1993; Schmiedl et al. 1990; Schuhmann et al. 1991; Wiener et al. 1994).

A Gd-DTPA-polylysine derivative with a relative molecular weight of approximately 40000 results in a plasma relaxivity of about 14 l mmol/s at 0.47 T, which is three to four times greater than that of Magnevist.

After distribution in the vascular system, the agent does not leak significantly and is finally eliminated by renal filtration. The blood-pool agent Gd-DTPA-polylysine is fundamentally suitable as an angiographic contrast agent. It even allows the demonstration of tiny structures less than 1 mm in diameter and perfusion studies of the myocardium and pulmonary MRI.

In combination with highly T1-weighted imaging techniques the T2-effect of USPIO particles does not dominate, and the iron particles can be used as positive contrast enhancers for MR angiography (Canet et al. 1993).

Special attention must be focused on the tolerability to those materials to ensure that the diagnostic benefits are not obtained at the cost of a higher incidence of adverse reactions. However, it is very likely that clinical diagnostic imaging will be further improved by well-tolerated, tissue-specific MRI contrast agents.

References

1. Adam G, Neuerburg J, Spuntrup E, Muhler A, Scherer K, Gunther RW (1994) Gd-DTPA-cascade-polymer: potential blood pool contrast agent for MR imaging. J Magn Reson Imaging 4:462–6
2. Beckermann F , Popken C (1938) Kontrastdarstellung der Leber und Milz im Röntgenbild mit Jodsolen. Fortschritte auf dem Gebiet der Röntgenstrahlen 58:519–535
3. Berthezene Y, Vexler V, Jerome H, Sievers R, Moseley ME, Brasch RC (1991) Differentiation of capillary leak and hydrostatic pulmonary edema with a macromolecular MR imaging contrast agent. Radiology 181:773–7
4. Bock JC, Pison U, Kaufmann F, Felix R (1994) Gd-DTPA-polylysine-enhanced pulmonary time-of-flight MR angiography. J Magn Reson Imaging 4:473–6
5. Bohdiewicz PJ, Lavallee DK, Fawwaz RA, Newhouse JH, Oluwole SF, Alderson PO (1990) Mn (III) hematoporphyrin. A potential MR contrast agent. Invest Radiol 25:765–70
6. Browne G, Stanford W, Thompson B, Kern J, Lanza L (1994) Use of an Iron Oxide MR Contrast Agent for the Detection of Metastatic Mediastinal Lymph Nodes

7. Canet E, Revel D, Forrat R, Baldy PC, de LM, Sebbag L, Vallee JP, Didier D, Amiel M (1993) Superparamagnetic iron oxide particles and positive enhancement for myocardial perfusion studies assessed by subsecond T1-weighted MRI. Magn Reson Imaging 11:1139–45
8. Elizondo G, Fretz CJ, Stark DD, Rocklage SM, Quay SC, Worah D, Tsang YM, Chen MC, Ferrucci JT (1991) Preclinical evaluation of MnDPDP: new paramagnetic hepatobiliary contrast agent for MR imaging. Radiology 178:73–8
9. Gehl HB, Urhahn R, Bohndorf K, Klever P, Hauptmann S, Lodemann KP, Matern S, Schumpelick V, Gunther RW (1993) Mn-DPDP in MR imaging of pancreatic adenocarcinoma: initial clinical experience. Radiology 186:795–8
10. Gehl HB, Vorwerk D, Klose KC, Gunther RW (1991) Pancreatic enhancement after low-dose infusion of Mn-DPDP. Radiology 180:337–9
11. Gibby WA, Billings J, Hall J, Ovitt TW (1990) Biodistribution and magnetic resonance imaging of cross-linked DTPA polysaccharides. Invest Radiol 25:164–72
12. Gohr RS, Schmitt WH, Ebert W, Conrad J (1993) The demonstration of human tumors on nude mice using gadolinium-labelled monoclonal antibodies for magnetic resonance imaging. Invest Radiol 28:789–95
13. Grant D, Zech K, Holtz E (1994) Biodistribution and In Vivo Stability of Manganese Dipyridoxyl Diphosphate in Relation to Imaging Efficacy. Invest Radiol 29:S249–S250
14. Hamm B, Staks T, Mühler A, Bollow M, Taupitz M, Frenzel T, Wolf K-J, Weinmann H-J, Lange L (1995) Phase I Clinical Evaluation of Gd-EOB-DTPA as a New Hepatobiliary MR Contrast Agent: Safety, Pharmacokinetics and MR Imaging. Radiology (in press)
15. Hamm B, Taupitz M, Hussmann P, Wagner S, Wolf KJ (1992) MR lymphography with iron oxide particles: dose-response studies and pulse sequence optimization in rabbits. Am J Roentgenol 158:183–90
16. Hamm B, Thoeni RF, Gould RG, Bernardino ME, Luning M, Saini S, Mahfouz AE, Taupitz M, Wolf KJ (1994) Focal liver lesions: characterization with nonenhanced and dynamic contrast material-enhanced MR imaging. Radiology 190:417–23
17. Haustein J, Laniado M, Niendorf HP, Louton T, Beck W, Planitzer J, Schoffel M, Reiser M, Kaiser W, Schorner W et al. (1993) Triple-dose versus standard-dose gadopentetate dimeglumine: a randomized study in 199 patients. Radiology 186:855–60
18. Haustein J, Niendorf HP, Krestin G, Louton T, Schuhmann GG, Clauss W, Junge W (1992) Renal tolerance of gadolinium-DTPA/dimeglumine in patients with chronic renal failure. Invest Radiol 27:153–6
19. Ivancev K, Lunderquist A, Isaksson A, Hochbergs P, Wretlind A (1989) Clinical trials with a new iodinated lipid emulsion for computed tomography of the liver. Acta Radiol 30:449–57
20. Kornguth SE, Turski PA, Perman WH, Schultz R, Kalinke T, Reale R, Raybaud F (1987) Magnetic resonance imaging of gadolinium-labeled monoclonal antibody polymers directed at human T lymphocytes implanted in canine brain. J Neurosurg 66:898–906
21. Krause W, Leike J, Sachse A, Schuhmann GG (1993) Characterization of iopromide liposomes. Invest Radiol 28:1028–32
22. Lim KO, Stark DD, Leese PT, Pfefferbaum A, Rocklage SM, Quay SC (1991) Hepatobiliary MR imaging: first human experience with MnDPDP. Radiology 178:79–82
23. Lim TH, Lee DH, Kim YH, Park SW, Park PH, Seo DM, Kim ST, Lee TK, Mun CW (1993) Occlusive and reperfused myocardial infarction: detection by using MR imaging with gadolinium polylysine enhancement. Radiology 189:765–8
24. Liou J, Lee JK, Borrello JA, Brown JJ (1994) Differentiation of hepatomas from nonhepatomatous masses: use of MnDPDP-enhanced MR images. Magn Reson Imaging 12:71–9
25. Mahfouz AE, Hamm B, Taupitz M, Wolf KJ (1993) Hypervascular liver lesions: differentiation of focal nodular hyperplasia from malignant tumors with dynamic gadolinium-enhanced MR imaging. Radiology 186:13–8
26. Marchal G, Ni Y, Zhang X, Yu J, Lodemann KP, Baert AL (1993a) Mn-DPDP enhanced MRI in experimental bile duct obstruction. J Comput Assist Tomogr 17:290–6

27. Marchal G, Zhang X, Ni Y, Van HP, Yu J, Baert AL (1993b) Comparison between Gd-DTPA, Gd-EOB-DTPA, and Mn-DPDP in induced HCC in rats: a correlation study of MR imaging, microangiography, and histology. Magn Reson Imaging 11:665–74
28. McLachlan SJ, Morris MR, Lucas MA, Fisco RA, Eakins MN, Fowler DR, Scheetz RB, Olukotun AY (1994) Phase I clinical evaluation of a new iron oxide MR contrast agent. J Magn Reson Imaging 4:301–7
29. Miller DL, Vermess M, Doppman JL, Simon RM, Sugarbaker PH, O'Leary TJ, Grimes G, Chatterji DG, Willis M (1984) CT of the liver and spleen with EOE-13: review of 225 examinations. Am J Roentgenol 143:235–43
30. Muhler A, Clement O, Vexler V, Berthezene Y, Rosenau W, Brasch RC (1992) Hepatobiliary enhancement with Gd-EOB-DTPA: comparison of spin-echo and STIR imaging for detection of experimental liver metastases. Radiology 184:207–13
31. Niendorf HP, Dinger JC, Haustein J, Cornelius I, Alhassan A, Clauss W (1991) Tolerance data of Gd-DTPA: a review. Eur Radiol 13:15–20
32. Ogan MD, Revel D, Brasch RC (1987) Metalloporphyrin contrast enhancement of tumors in magnetic resonance imaging. A study of human carcinoma, lymphoma, and fibrosarcoma in mice. Invest Radiol 22:822–8
33. Oka AM (1930) Klinische Anwendung der „Lienographie", einer neuen Methode zur röntgenologischen Darstellung von Milz und Leber. Fortschr Röntgenstr 41:892–898
34. Place DA, Faustino PJ, Berghmans KK, van ZP, Chesnick AS, Cohen JS (1992) MRI contrast-dose relationship of manganese(III)tetra(4-sulfonatophenyl) porphyrin with human xenograft tumors in nude mice at 2.0 T. Magn Reson Imaging 10:919–28
35. Radt P (1930) Eine neue Methode zur röntgenologischen Sichtbarmachung von Leber und Milz durch Injektion eines Kontrastmittels (Hepatolienographie). Med Kl 26:1888–1891
36. Rosati G, Pirovano G, Spinazzi A (1994) Interim Results of Phase II Clinical Testing of Gadobenate Dimeglumine. Invest Radiol 29:S183–S185
37. Saeed M, Wagner S, Wendland MF, Derugin N, Finkbeiner WE, Higgins CB (1989) Occlusive and reperfused myocardial infarcts: differentiation with Mn-DPDP-enhanced MR imaging. Radiology 172:59–64
38. Schad LR, Semmler W, Knopp MV, Deimling M, Weinmann HJ, Lorenz WJ (1993) Preliminary evaluation: magnetic resonance of urography using a saturation inversion projection spin-echo sequence. Magn Reson Imaging 11:319–27
39. Schaffer BK, Linker C, Papisov M, Tsai E, Nossiff N, Shibata T, Bogdanov AJ, Brady TJ, Weissleder R (1993) MION-ASF: biokinetics of an MR receptor agent. Magn Reson Imaging 11:411–7
40. Schmiedl U, Brasch RC, Ogan MD, Moseley ME (1990) Albumin labeled with Gd-DTPA. An intravascular contrast-enhancing agent for magnetic resonance blood pool and perfusion imaging. Acta Radiol Suppl 374:99–102
41. Schuhmann G, Krestin G (1991) Pharmacokinetics of Gd-DTPA in patients with chronic renal failure. Invest Radiol 26:975–9
42. Schuhmann G, Schmitt WH, Press WR, Negishi C, Weinmann HJ, Speck U (1992) Preclinical evaluation of Gd-EOB-DTPA as a contrast agent in MR imaging of the hepatobiliary system. Radiology 183:59–64
43. Schuhmann GG, Schmitt WH, Frenzel T, Press WR, Weinmann HJ (1991) In vivo and in vitro evaluation of Gd-DTPA-polylysine as a macromolecular contrast agent for magnetic resonance imaging. Invest Radiol 26:969–74
44. Semelka RC, Shoenut JP, Kroeker MA, Greenberg HM, Simm FC, Minuk GY, Kroeker RM, Micflikier AB (1992) Focal liver disease: comparison of dynamic contrast-enhanced CT and T2-weighted fat-suppressed, FLASH, and dynamic gadolinium-enhanced MR imaging at 1.5 T. Radiology 184:687–94
45. Seneterre E, Weissleder R, Jaramillo D, Reimer P, Lee AS, Brady TJ, Wittenberg J (1991) Bone marrow: ultrasmall superparamagnetic iron oxide for MR imaging. Radiology 179:52–33
46. Stark DD, Weissleder R, Elizondo G, Hahn PF, Saini S, Todd LE, Wittenberg J, Ferrucci JT (1988) Superparamagnetic iron oxide: clinical application as a contrast agent for MR imaging of the liver. Radiology 168:297–301

47. Vittadini G, Felder E, Musu C, Tirone P (1990) Preclinical profile of Gd-BOPTA. A liver-specific MRI contrast agent. Invest Radiol
48. Vogl TJ, Pegios W, McMahon C, Balzer J, Waitzinger J, Pirovano G, Lissner J (1992) Gadobenate dimeglumine – a new contrast agent for MR imaging: preliminary evaluation in healthy volunteers. Am J Roentgenol 158:887–92
49. Weinmann H, Mützel W, Souchon R, Wegener OH (1981) ed. Experimental water-soluble contrast media for computed tomography of the liver. Vol 561 Contrast media in computed tomography. Intern congress series. Amsterdam-Oxford-Princeton: Excerpta Medica
50. Weinmann H-J, Staks T, Frenzel T, Mühler A, Hamm B, Lange L, Wolf K-J. "Gd-EOB-DTPA: first use in man." In European Society for Magnetic Resonance in Medicine and Biology, 11th Annual Scientific Meeting in Vienna, Austria, Year
51. Weinmann HJ, Brasch RC, Press WR, Wesbey GE (1984a) Characteristics of gadolinium-DTPA complex: a potential NMR contrast agent. Am J Roentgenol 142:619–24
52. Weinmann HJ, Laniado M, Mutzel W (1984b) Pharmacokinetics of GdDTPA/dimeglumine after intravenous injection into healthy volunteers. Physiol Chem Phys Med Nmr 16:167–72
53. Weinmann HJ, Schuhmann GG, Schmitt WH, Vogler H, Frenzel T, Gries H (1991) A new lipophilic gadolinium chelate as a tissue-specific contrast medium for MRI. Magn Reson Med 22:233–7
54. Weissleder R, Elizondo G, Josephson L, Compton CC, Fretz CJ, Stark DD, Ferrucci JT (1989) Experimental lymph node metastases: enhanced detection with MR lymphography. Radiology 171:835–9
55. Weissleder R, Elizondo G, Wittenberg J, Lee AS, Josephson L, Brady TJ (1990) Ultrasmall superparamagnetic iron oxide: an intravenous contrast agent for assessing lymph nodes with MR imaging. Radiology 175:494–8
56. Weissleder R, Hahn PF, Stark DD, Elizondo G, Saini S, Todd LE, Wittenberg J, Ferrucci JT (1988) Superparamagnetic iron oxide: enhanced detection of focal splenic tumors with MR imaging. Radiology 169:399–403
57. Weissleder R, Lee AS, Fischman AJ, Reimer P, Shen T, Wilkinson R, Callahan RJ, Brady TJ (1991) Polyclonal human immunoglobulin G labeled with polymeric iron oxide: antibody MR imaging. Radiology 181:245–9
58. Weissleder R, Lee AS, Khaw BA, Shen T, Brady TJ (1992) Antimyosin-labeled monocrystalline iron oxide allows detection of myocardial infarct: MR antibody imaging. Radiology 182:381–5
59. Weissleder R, Reimer P, Lee AS, Wittenberg J, Brady TJ (1990) MR receptor imaging: ultrasmall iron oxide particles targeted to asialoglycoprotein receptors. Am J Roentgenol 155:1161–7
60. White C, Slifkin M, Seltzer SE, Blau M, Adzamli IK, Adams DF (1990) Biodistribution and clearance of contrast-carrying MREV liposomes. Invest Radiol 25:1125–9
61. Wiener EC, Brechbiel MW, Brothers H, Magin RL, Gansow OA, Tomalia DA, Lauterbur PC (1994) Dendrimer-based metal chelates: a new class of magnetic resonance imaging contrast agents. Magn Reson Med 31:1–8
62. Young SW, Sidhu MK, Qing F, Muller HH, Neuder M, Zanassi G, Mody TD, Hemmi G, Dow W, Mutch JD et al. (1994) Preclinical evaluation of gadolinium (III) texaphyrin complex. A new paramagnetic contrast agent for magnetic resonance imaging. Invest Radiol 29:330–8

CHAPTER 20

Computed Tomography and Magnetic Resonance Imaging of the Female Pelvis

Bernd Hamm[1]

Examination Technique

Computed Tomography

Computed tomography (CT) of the pelvis requires good contrasting of the gastrointestinal tract; this is achieved by oral application of about 1000 ml of an appropriate contrast medium solution, which the patient starts drinking about 1 hour before the examination. Retrograde contrasting of the rectosigmoid is normally not required, but is recommended for evaluating a possible infiltration of the colon in patients with suspicion of an advanced ovarian carcinoma (in such cases about 250 ml of the contrast solution are sufficient). The bladder should be well filled with urine. Since a precontrast examination is not required, CT starts directly with the intravenous bolus enhanced contrast study. It is important to ensure adequate contrast enhancement of both the arteries and the veins in order to facilitate the differentiation of suspicious lymph nodes from vascular structures. A digital radiogram for adjustment of the first scanning plane is not required. When conventional CT is used (i.e., without spiral technique), scanning should proceed from the floor of the pelvis in a cranial direction to make optimal use of the strong contrast enhancement of the uterus and ova ries in the early phase after application of the contrast agent. For staging or follow-up of ovarian carcinomas, the entire abdomen should be scanned to identify possible lymphomas, liver metastases or subdiaphragmatic metastases. In such cases, however, scannin g should start at the diaphragm and continue caudad, since the reversed order (i.e., from the floor of the pelvis in a cranial direction) might lead to obscuring of potential liver metastases in the late phase of contrast enhancement.

Magnetic Resonance Imaging

Magnetic resonance imaging (MRI) is typically performed with the patient supine (a knee cushion ensures a relaxed positioning of the patient for longer examinations). It is also recommended to use an "abdominal belt" applied with slight

[1] Institut für Röntgendiagnostik, Universitätsklinikum Charité, Medizinische Fakultät der Humboldt-Universität, Schumannstraße 20/21, 10098 Berlin, Germany.

pressure above the symphysis. This belt helps to reduce motion artifacts produced by the abdominal wall and also reminds the patient to breathe smoothly and regularly and avoid deep respiratory excursions (reduction of respiratory artifacts). The bladder should be moderately to well filled with urine, intruding bowel loops can thus be displaced from the pelvis. For reduction of peristalsis-related artifacts, application of a spasmolytic is recommended (i.m. or protracted i.v. application). It is furthermore advisable to administer an oral contra stagent, since it might otherwise be difficult to differentiate bowel loops from liquid ovarian masses. Oral MRI contrast agents have already undergone clinical trials and will soon be available for routine application. Diagnostic evaluation of the female pelvis by MR imaging always requires a combination of T1- and T2-weighted pulse sequences. T1-weighted sequences yield images with a good anatomical resolution and a high contrast between lesions and neighboring fatty tissue. Furthermore, they offer a good characterization of hemorrhagic and fatty lesions. T1-weighted images should cover the region between the floor of the pelvis and the hilum of the kidneys (retroperitoneal lymphomas!), while T2-weighted imaging may focus on the true pelvis or the lesion itself. The section thickness for T2-weighted imaging should be 5–8 mm. T2-weighted images are highly suitable for assigning a lesion to the uterus or the ovaries and additionally provide important information for tissue characterization and for evaluating a possible infiltration of the pelvic wall. In addition to conventional spin-echo (SE) sequences, so-called "fast SE" or "turbo SE" sequences have recently proved effective. They provide the same diagnostic information at a considerably shorter examination time [4, 11, 14]. Fat-suppression pulse sequences improve the differentiation of teratomas and hemorrhagic cystic lesions [16]. Paramagnetic extracellular contrast agents, e.g., gadolinium-DTPA (diethylene triamine pentaacetate), improve the visualization of the intratumoral architecture on T1-weighted images and facilitate the diagnosis of peritoneal carcinosis. A markedly better spatial resolution with improved visualization of anatomic details can be achieved with the multicoil technique [15]. MRI of the uterus should be performed in the sagittal and transverse plane, wh ile the latter alone is normally sufficient for evaluating ovarian tumors.

Normal Pelvic Anatomy

Uterine Corpus

The normal position of the uterus varies widely. It is typically anteflexed and located centrally on the roof of the urinary bladder. The CT appearance of the uterus depends on the filling of the bladder. Its size and perfusion (enhancement after application of contrast material) vary during the menstrual cycle. The diameter of the uterus in women of reproductive age should not exceed 6 cm [21]. After intravenous application of a contrast agent, the uterine cavity may be visualized as a ring- or T-shaped hypointense structure. Differentiation of the myometrium and endometrium by CT is not possible.

At MRI, the corpus of uterus is characterized by a relatively low signal intensity on T1-weighted images. On T2-weighted images, the high-signal-intensity endometrium can be distinguished from the myometrium, which has an intermediate signal intensity. On these images, the two layers are separated by a hypointense band, the so-called junctional zone, for which there is no clear histomo rphologic correlate. The appearance of this zone on MR images is accounted for by the reduced water content of the inner portion of the myometrium, which is assumed to attenuate the signal [8]. The size of the endometrium varies between 1 and 7 mm through the menstrual cycle [9].

After intravenous administration of Gd-DTPA, the myometrium of the premenopausal corpus uteri demonstrates early strong enhancement and the endometrium late moderate enhancement on dynamic sequences [22], while the junctional zone shows markedly less enhancement. This results in the characteristic zonal anatomy of the uterus as it is also seen on T2-weighted images [18]. In the postmenopausal uterus, these three zones are no longer discernible on T2-weighted images. Rather, the myometrium is characterized by a homogeneous signal intensity, which is lower than that of the premenopausal uterus. The postmenopausal endometrium has a maximal thickness of 3 mm [2].

Cervix and Vagina

On CT scans, the cervix/corpus junction is discernible only at the isthmus of the organ. The cervix appears as a roundish to transverse oval structure with a maximum diameter of 3 cm. The cervix or cervical canal is occasionally seen as a central hypointense zone.

At MRI, the cervix is characterized by a low signal intensity on T1- and T2-weighted images due to its high proportion of fibrous tissue. A central high-signal-intensity layer on T2-weighted images corresponds to the epithelial and mucosal coat of the cervical canal. T2-weighted sequences allow a clear identification of the anterior and posterior vaginal layers, which are both of low signal intensity, as well as of the ventrally located urethra and the dorsally situated rectum. Intravenous application of contrast medium leads to a pronounced signal enhancement of the cervical and vaginal epithelium, the cervical wall and paracervical tissue, while the cervical stroma shows only little enhancement.

Occasionally, a delicate, central ring structure of low signal intensity becomes visible after contrast application, which is assumed to correspond to the internal vaginal epithelial layer.

Parametrium

The parametria are the spaces between the layers of the broad ligament extending from the side of the uterus to the wall of the pelvis. CT only visualizes the round and broad ligaments and occasionally the adnexa and ovaries.

With MR imaging, the normal parametrial connective tissue can best be evaluated on T1-weighted axial images, on which it is distingu ished from the hyperintense surrounding fatty tissue by its intermediate signal intensity. It shows moderate enhancement after application of Gd-DTPA.

Ovaries

The ovaries in women of reproductive age have a size of about 3–5 cm × 1.5–3 cm × 0.6–1.5 cm. Due to physiological atrophy, the postmenopausal ovaries are difficult to differentiate from surrounding structures.

The advantages of CT include its high spatial resolution and the absence of motion artifacts, while the radiation exposure is a major drawback, particularly in younger women. CT allows a good differentiation of cystic and solid tumors. The densities of cysts containing serous fluid correspond to those of urine. Hemorrhagic cysts may reach rather high densities, but it is not always possible to differentiate them from solid lesions [13], whereas fat-containing teratomas (dermoid cysts) are easy to diagnose. The differentiation of benign from malignant ovarian tumors by both CT and MRI is based on morphologic criteria. Due to its high spacial resolution, CT offers good visualization of these morphologic features. On T1-weighted images, the normal ovary is characterized by a low signal intensity and isointensity with muscle or uterine tissue. On T2-weighted images, the ovaries have a signal intensity equivalent to that of fatty tissue and show areas of higher signal intens ity corresponding to small cysts. With MRI, the intratumoral architecture can best be evaluated on T1-weighted images obtained after intravenous contrast application. The main advantage of MRI in the diagnostic evaluation of ovarian tumors is the high soft tissue contrast, while the ability to freely orient the imaging plane is less important. Both cystic and solid lesions of the ovaries can be reliably delineated from the uterus, since the latter is distinguished by the high signal intensity endometrium and the low signal intensity myometrium on T2-weighted images. Especially large masses in the true pelvis may be difficult to differentiate by CT.

Carcinoma of the Uterus

Since MRI is superior to CT in the T-staging of uterine cancer, the following presents the different stages of cervical and endometrial carcinomas together with their corresponding features on MR images.

Carcinoma of the Cervix

Stage I. Stage I tumors are those that are confined to the cervix. High signal intensity tumor tissue is seen against the dark background of the cervical stroma on T2-weighted sagittal or axial images. The depth of cervical stroma infiltration corresponds to the area of increased signal intensity on T2-weighted images. Application of Gd-DTPA makes it possible to differentiate viable tumor from necrotic areas, but it does not improve tumor detection [5, 20].

Stage II. Tumors extending beyond the uterus with infiltration of the upper and middle third of the vagina are classifie d as stage IIa. This stage is characterized on MR imaging by the loss of the normally low signal intensity in the upper third of the vagina on T2-weighted images. Stage IIb is defined as parametrial involvement without infiltration of the pelvic wall. Evaluation of the parametrium can best be done with axial T2-weighted images in combination with T1-weighted images, which will show either a symmetry as an indication of parametrial infiltration or direct tumor extension along the parametrial vascular ligaments. Reports in the literature suggest that parametrial evaluation is not [5] or only slightly [20] improved by application of Gd-DTPA.

Stage III. Deep vaginal invasion without tumor extension to the pelvic wall is classified as FIGO stage IIIa disease. T2-weighted axial MR images show the high-intensity tumor to extend into the lower part of the vagina. Involvement of the pelvic wall or hydronephrosis is present in stage IIIb tumors, which are characterized on axial images by disappearance of the fatty layer medial to the muscular pelvic wall or by macroscopic infiltration of pelvic wall structures.

Stage IV. Stage IVa is defined as tumor infiltration of the bladder and/or rectum. On axial or sagittal T2-weighted ima ges, the high signal intensity tumor masses are seen to involve the wall of the bladder or rectum. For the evaluation of advanced stages with infiltration of the bladder, rectum or pelvic wall, Gd-DTPA has been shown to improve the delineation of tumor tissue from soft-tissue structures in the pelvis [5, 18]. Presence of distant metastases is defined as stage IVb disease irrespective of the local tumor stage.

Carcinoma of the Endometrium

Stage Ia. Isointense tumors confined to the endometrium do not always have a clear correlate on MR images. A slight increase in the size of the endometrium or inhomogeneity of its internal structure may be indicative of a stage Ia tumor. Tumors that are hypointense relative to the normal endometrium, on the other hand, are easy to discern. However, the changes depicted by MRI are unspecific and may be due to blood clots or hormone replacement therapy. The junctional zone should be intact at this tumor stage, though it may sometimes be difficult to delineate in postmenopausal women.

Stage Ib. This stage is defined by superficial myometrial infiltration (< 50% of myometrial wall). The MR appearance is characterized by disruption of the junctional zone with increased signal intensity on T2-weighted images or a relative decrease in signal intensity on contrast-enhanced T1-weighted images, since normal myometrium shows a more pronounced uptake of contrast material than the tumor.

Stage Ic. This stage is characterized by involvement of the outer muscular layer (> 50% infiltration) without tumor growth extending beyond the organ. The area of higher signal intensity on T2-weighted images or the relatively lower enhancement of the tumor may extend to the subserous layer.

Stage II. Infiltration of the cervix can easily be depicted on sagittal images. The high signal intensity tumor is clearly delineated from the low signal intensity normal cervical stroma on T2-weighted sequences.

Stage III. Extension beyond the serosa of the uterus or adnexal involvement is defined as stage IIIa, growth of the tumor into the vagina as stage IIIb. Visualization of these changes on T2-weighted images is unproblematic in the majority of cases.

Stage IV. Invasion of adjacent organs (rectum, bladder) by stage IVa tumors is indicated by intramural areas of contrast uptake or increased signal intensity in these organs on T2-weighted images. Disappearance of the interposed fatty layer is likewise highly suggestive of infiltration. Stage IVb disease is characterized by the presence of distant metastases.

Ovarian Tumors

The diagnostic value of CT and MRI in the characterization of ovarian tumors can only be assessed in comparison to ultrasound (US). In one study comparing CT and transabdominal US in 130 patients with a total of 170 epithelial tumors of the ovaries, Buy et al. [1] found the two procedures to have identical sensitivity in the detection of these lesions (CT, 87%; US, 86%). In the differentiation of benign and malignant tumors, CT was even superior to transabdominal US with an accuracy of 94% versus 80% [1]. Another study by the same group comparing CT and MR imaging in 40 patients with 23 benign and 27 malignant ovarian tumors found CT to be slightly, but not significantly, superior to MR imaging in differentiating benign and malignant lesions (accuracy of 92% versus 86%) [3].

Mature cystic teratomas (dermoid cysts) are reliably identified by CT as well as MRI on the basis of their fatty tissue components. The absence of radiation exposure has to be considered an advantage of MRI, especially since these tumors occur predominantly in younger women. MRI is likewise superior in the detection of hemorrhagic lesions and thus in the diagnosis of end ometrial cysts. However, the results of a study by Outwater et al. [12] should be mentioned here. In this study, 74 hemorrhagic lesions were evaluated by three blinded assessors and the MR criteria for endometrial cysts were found to have a diagnostic accuracy of only 76%. The authors therefore concluded that MRI has only a limited reliability in differentiating endometrial cysts from other hemorrhagic lesions of the ovaries.

Transvaginal US has almost completely replaced transabdominal US in the diagnostic evaluation of ovarian tumors. However, there are only a few studies comparing transvaginal US with CT or MRI [6, 7, 10]. In one of these studies, 32 patients with suspected ovarian masses were prospectively examined by transvaginal US and MRI [6]. The authors found tranvaginal US to be superior to MRI in the characterization of ovarian tumors (accuracy 83% versus 70%). The authors conclude that the superiority of transvaginal US results from the better visualization of the internal tumor structure, particularly if the lesions are small. The use of intravenous contrast agents in combination with surface coils will in the future improve the evaluation of internal tumor structures by MRI [15, 17, 19].

Tumor staging of ovarian carcinomas by imaging procedures is primarily performed for planning surgery. CT is at present the technique of choice for staging ovarian carcinomas, in particular in advanced disease with tumor extension beyond the true pelvis. The role of MRI remains to be defined, especially in view of newly developed imaging techniques, but there is a tendency that it will improve the diagnostic evaluation of peritoneal carcinosis.

References

1. Buy J-N, Ghossain MA, Sciot C, Bazot M, Guinet C, Prévot S, Hugol D, Laromiguiere M, True JB, Poitout P, Vadrot D, Ecoiffier J (1991) Epithelial tumors of the ovary: CT findings and correlation with US. Radiology 178:811
2. Demas BE, Hricak H, Jaffe RB (1986) Uterine MR imaging: effects of hormonal stimulation. Radiology 159:123
3. Ghossain M, Buy J-N, Lignères C, Bazot M, Hassen K, Malbec L, Hugol D, True JB, Decroix Y, Poitout P, Vadrot D (1991) Epithelial tumors of the ovary: comparison of MR and CT findings. Radiology 181:863
4. Haldemann RC, Krestin GP, Duewell S, Marincek B, von Schulthess GK, Saadi-Elamandjra M, Fuchs WA (1993) Verkürzung der MRT-M eßzeiten im weiblichen Becken mit Hilfe der T2-gewichteten Fast-Spinecho(FSE)-Technik. RöFo 158:127
5. Hricak H, Hamm B, Semelka RC, Cann CE, Nauert T, Secaf E, Stern JL, Wolf KJ (1991) Carcinoma of the uterus: use of gadopente tate dimeglumine in MR imaging. Radiology 181:95
6. Jain KA, Friedmann DL, Thomas W, Pettinger W, Alagappan R, Jeffrey RB, Sommer FG (1993) Adnexal masses: comparison of specif icity of endovaginal US and pelvic MR imaging. Radiology 186:697
7. Kombächer P, Hamm B, Becker R, Hese S, Weitzel H-K, Wolf K-J (1992) Tumoren der Adnexe – Vergleich von Magnetresonanztomographie, Endosonographie und histologischen Befunden. RöFo 156:303
8. McCarthy S, Scott G, Majumdar S, Shapiro B, Thompson S, Lange R, Gore J (1989) Uterine junctional zone: MR study of water content and relaxation properties. Radiology 171:241
9. McCarthy S, Tauber C, Gore J (1986) Female pelvic anatomy: MR assessment of variations during the menstrual cycle and with use of oral contraceptives. Radiology 160:119
10. Mitchell DG, Mintz MC, Spritzer CE, Gussmann D, Arger PH, Coleman BG, Axel L, Kressel HY (1987) Adnexal masses: MR imaging observations at 1.5 T, with US and CT correlation. Radiology 162:319
11. Nghiem HV, Herfkens RJ, Francis IR, Sommer FG, Jeffrey RB, King CP, Steiner RM (1992) The pelvis: T2-weighted fast spin-echo MR imaging. Radiology 185:213
12. Outwater E, Schiebler ML, Owen RS, Schnall MD (1993) Characterization of hemorrhagic adnexal lesions with MR imaging: blinde d reader study. Radiology 186:489
13. Sawyer RW, Vick CW, Walsh JW, McClure PH (1985) Computed tomography of benign ovarian masses. JCAT 9:784
14. Smith RC, Reinhold C, Lange RC, McCaulex TR, Kier C, McCarthy S (1992) Fast spin-echo MR imaging of the female pelvis. Radio logy 184:665
15 Smith RC, Reinhold C, McCauley TR, Lange RC, Todd RT, Kier R, McCarthy S (1992) Multicoil high-resolution fast spin-echo MR imaging of the female pelvis. Radiology 184:671
16. Stevens SK, Hricak H, Campos Z (1993) Teratomas versus cystic hemorrhagic adnexal lesions: Differentiation with proton-selective fat-saturation MR imaging. Radiology 186:481

17. Stevens SK, Hricak H, Stern JL (1991) Ovarian lesions: Detection and characterization with gadolinium-enhanced MR imaging at 1.5 T. Radiology 181:481
18. Thurnher SA (1992) MR imaging of pelvic masses in women: contrast enhanced vs unenhanced images. AJR 159:1243
19. Thurnher S, Hodler J, Baer S, Marincek B, von Schulthess GK (1990) Gadolinium-DOTA enhanced MR imaging of adnexal tumors. JC AT 14:939
20. Thurnher S, McPhillips M, von Schulthess K, Marincek B (1991) Staging des Zervixkarzinoms mit der magnetischen Resonanztomog raphie: Anwendung von Gadolinium-DOTA bei 31 Patientinnen. RöFo 154:643
21. Walsh JW, Goplerud DR (1982) Computed tomography of primary, persistent, and recurrent endometrial malignancy. AJR 139:1149
22. Yamashita Y, Harada M, Sawada T, Thakahashi M, Miyazaki K, Okamura H (1993) Normal uterus and FIGO stage I endometrial carcinoma: dynamic gadolinium-enhanced MR imaging. Radiology 186:495

CHAPTER 21

Computed Tomography Diagnosis and Staging for Cancer of Urinary Bladder

Cheng Zhou, Jiahu Wei, and Guozhen Li[1]

In recent years computed tomography (CT) has been used not only for diagnosis but also for staging of bladder tumors, because staging is very important in accessing prognosis and in therapy planning [1–3]. The aim of this study is to investigate thin-section CT imaging for the detection of bladder cancer and increase the accuracy of staging by CT.

Material and Methods

A total of 45 cases of bladder tumor were studied: 42 of transitional cell carcinoma (TCC), one of adenocarcinoma, one of ectopic bladder pheochromocytoma and one of lymphoma. The common clinical symptom was hematuria. All cases were proved by operation and pathology.

Oral 1.5% contrast agent (800 ml) was administered 2 h before the CT scan to fill the intestine in order to distinguish it from soft tissue around the bladder. As the configuration and wall thickness of the urinary bladder varies with the state of filling, we always asked the patient to fully fill the bladder.

All scans were obtained with a slice thickness of 5 mm from the neck to the dome of the bladder continuously. A 3-mm thickness and spacing is recommended for smaller lesions.

The bladder wall is well seen as its medium density is in contrast to low density perivesical fat on one side and urine on the other. Intravenous (IV) contrast was used in only five cases.

Six patients underwent 1.5 T magnetic resonance imaging (MRI) study after CT. T1- and T2-weighted axial, sagittal and coronal views were performed, using the spin-echo technique.

Results

A papillary mass protruding into the cavity with or without thickening of the wall is the most common appearance in TCC (Fig. 1). Thickening of the bladder wall without tumor nodule was seen in only one case. The pathology is adenocarcinoma (Fig. 2). A total of 25% of TCC tumors were multiple, 14 cases with

[1] Department of Radiology, Beijing Hospital, Beijing, 100730 China.

1 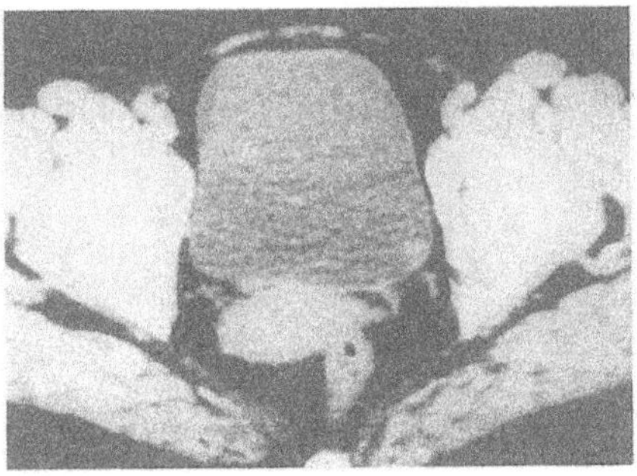 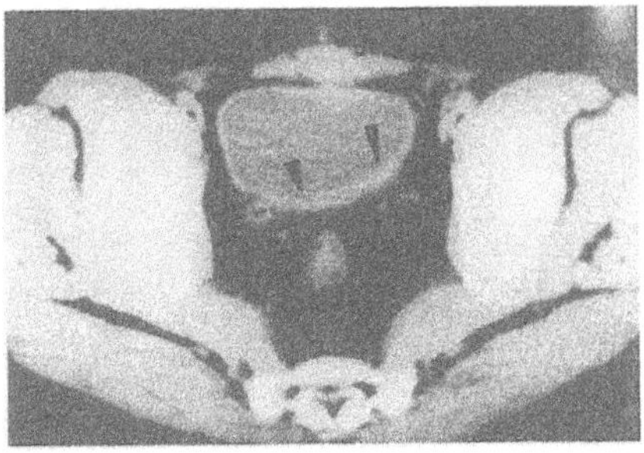 2

Fig. 1 Transitional cell carcinoma (TCC) of the bladder. Papillary tumor protruding into the cavity, without thickening of the bladder

Fig. 2 Adenocarcinoma of urinary bladder. Thickening of the bladder wall (arrowheads) without tumor nodule

tumor penetrating the urinary bladder wall to invade perivesical fat even extending to the pelvis. Two cases showed multiple dot calcification inside the tumor and ring-like calcification around the tumor.

Ectopic pheochromocytoma of the urinary bladder appeared as a broad-based, soft tissue mass with smooth margin protruding into the bladder (Fig. 3). One case of lymphoma was also encountered. The appearance of these two cases was not significantly different from TCC.

A total of 42 cases of TCC were staged according to TNM system and the Jewett-Marshall-Strong system.

Stage Tis or 0, carcinoma in situ is negative in CT scan, and stage Ta, non-invasive papillary carcinoma is impossible for CT staging.

Stage T1 or A. With tumor invasion limited to mucosa and submucosa appears on CT as nodular mass that can be separated from the bladder wall. The bladder wall, which appears as a white line, is intact (Fig. 4).

Stage T2 or B1 and Stage T3a or B2. In cases with tumor invasion of superficial and deep muscular wall, it is impossible for CT to distinguish superficial from deep muscles these merged into the same stage B. It appears on CT that there is thickening of the urinary bladder wall and the tumor mass cannot be separated from the bladder wall. However, the outer margin of the wall is regular and smooth (Fig. 5).

Stage T3b or C. With tumor invasion of perivesical fat, this appears on CT as disruption of the bladder wall. The outer margin of the bladder wall becomes irregular and fuzzy. The low-density perivesical fat is obliterated (Fig. 6).

Stage T4 or D. In our patients with tumor invasion of adjacent organs, we demonstrated tumor invasion of the prostate gland, seminal vesicle, uterus, vagina, pelvic and abdominal wall. Pelvic lymph node involvement was seen in three cases (Fig. 7).

3 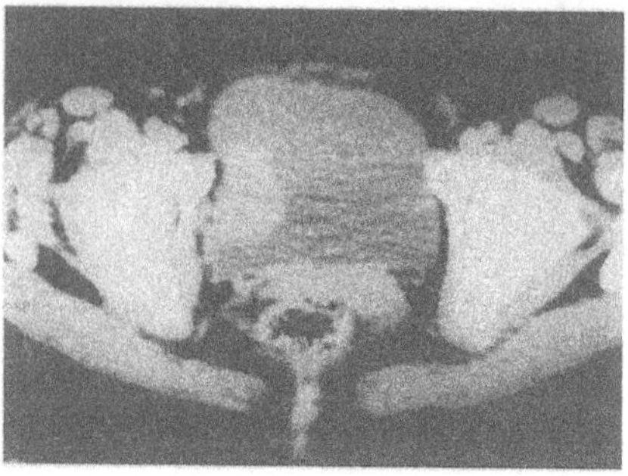 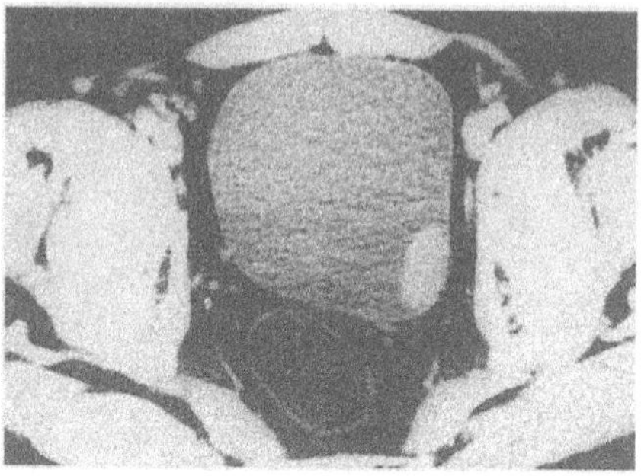 4

Fig. 3 Ectopic bladder pheochromocytoma. Broadbased mass with smooth margin protruding into the bladder

Fig. 4 Transitional cell carcinoma (TCC) stage T1 or A. Tumor invasion limited to submucosa can be distinguished from the bladder wall. The wall appears as a *white line*

5 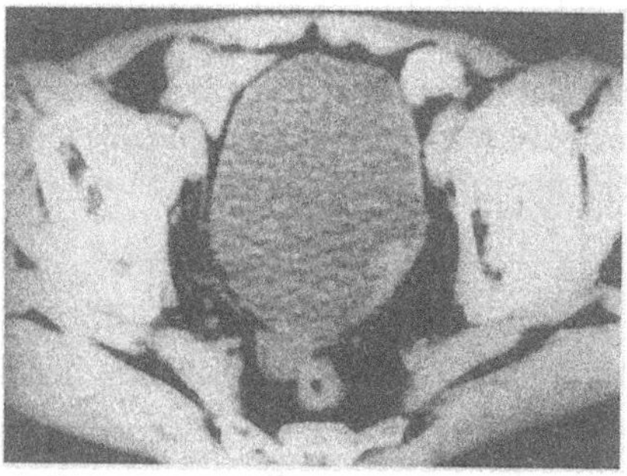 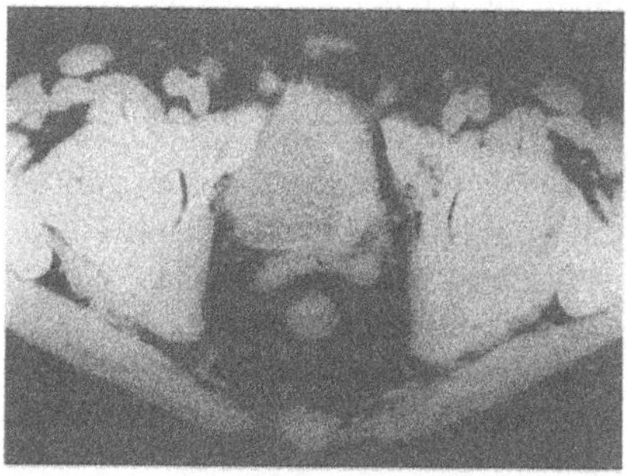 6

Fig. 5 Transitional cell carcinoma (TCC) stage T3a or B2. Tumor invasion of deep muscle. Bladder wall thickening; tumor cannot be distinguished

Fig. 6 Transitional cell carcinoma (TCC) stage T3b or C. Tumor disrupts the wall and invades the perivesical fat

Fig. 7 Transitional cell carcinoma (TCC) stage T4 or D. Tumor invades to the lower abdominal wall; metastasis to lymph nodes (*arrowheads*)

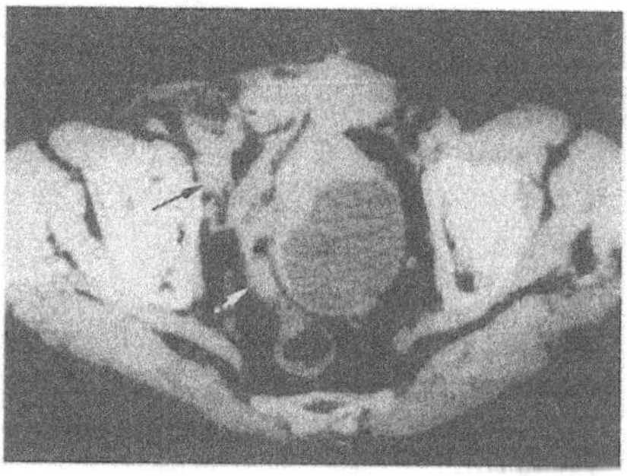

Table 1 Staging of 42 cases of transitional cell carcinoma (TCC)

Stage	Pathologic (*n*)	CT	
		Correct (*n*)	Overstaged (*n*)
A	9	2	–
B	19	17	7
C	11	10	2
D	3	3	1

Table 2 Staging of six cases of transitional cell carcinoma (TCC) examined by computed tomography (CT) and magnetic resonance imaging (MRI)

Stage	Pathologic (*n*)	MRI (*n*)	CT	
			Correct (*n*)	Overstaged (*n*)
A	2	2	1	–
B	4	4	3	1
C	–	–	–	1

In Table 1, there were seven cases of stage A by pathology overstaged to B by CT, two cases of stage B by pathological overstaged to C by CT, and one case of stage C by pathology overstaged to D by CT.

In Table 2, the staging by MRI is correct, but the number of cases is too limited. One case each of stages A and B by pathology were overstaged to B and C by CT.

Discussion

Role of CT in the Diagnosis and Differential Diagnosis of Bladder Tumor. CT is a noninvasive technique with high-density resolution and cross-section scanning ability, suitable as a routine examination for hematuria patients. As there is very good contrast between soft tissue of bladder wall and urine [4], intraluminal tumors can be well detected even if less than 1 cm in diameter using a thin-section scan. CT has difficulty in detecting small tumors located on the dome or neck of the urinary bladder. The bladder cancer presented as a nodular papillary soft tissue mass and thickening of bladder wall. However, the CT appearance are not specific [5]. Even in retrospective review, ectopic pheochromocytoma and lymphoma can mimic TCC. In our experiences, one case of amyloidosis and one case of malacoplakia of the bladder also appeared as a solid mass. Therefore cystoscopy and biopsy are necessary.

Accuracy of CT Staging for Bladder Tumors. The staging of bladder tumors depends on the state of tumor invasion of the wall. On conventional clinical staging, including urography, cystoscopy and transurethral resection, the extension of tumor could not be determined. Therefore, the major rule of CT is to stage the tumor. As individual layers of the bladder wall cannot be visualized, CT is not accurate in the early stages [4, 6]. In this study, out of nine of cases stage A by pathology, seven cases were over staged to stage B; accuracy was only 22%. However, in clinical practice, the important point is to separate stage AB from stage CD to decide on the operation to be performed [7], and CT is highly accurate in this aspect. From the literature the accuracy of CT staging for AB and CD is 60%–90% [2, 4, 8]. In our series it is 89%.

Role of MRI in the Staging of Bladder Tumors. From the literature, there is no significant difference between MRI and CT in the accuracy of staging of bladder tumor [9]. In our group, six cases were examined both by MRI and CT. The staging by MRI is correct, but this numbers are too limited. However, we should point out that in one case stage B by pathology, MR staging is correct and CT overstaged because CT misinterprets perivesical edema as a tumor.

MRI has direct multiplanar capacity and several different scan parameters, so that we can get more information, especially better delineation of tumors on the bladder base and dome, by using direct sagittal and coronal views [2, 3, 9, 10]; it also provides improved demonstration of the seminal vesicles, prostate gland, and perivesical fat.

Conclusion

CT as a noninvasive imaging modality is highly sensitivity for detecting bladder tumors. It can be used as a routine examination for hematuria patients.

The major role of CT is the staging of bladder tumors as staging is important for patient management.

CT can reliably differentiate stage AB from CD. The accuracy in our series is 89%.

MRI has direct multiplanar imaging capability and hence is able to demonstrate lesions in locations that are obscure even for CT, such as dome of the bladder.

References

1. Sager EM, Talle K, Fossa S et al. (1983) The role of CT in demonstrating perivesical tumor growth in the preoperative staging of carcinoma of the urinary bladder. Radiology 146:443
2. Amendola MA, Glazer GM, Grossman HB et al. (1986) Staging of bladder carcinoma: MRI-CT-surgical correlation. AJR 146:1179
3. Bryan PJ, Bulter HE, Lipuma JP et al. (1987) CT and MR imaging in staging bladder neoplasms. JCAT 11:96
4. Hricak H. (1990) Imaging of the Urinary bladder and prostate gland. Monographs in Urology 11:70
5. Koss JC, Arger PH, Coleman BG et al. (1981) CT staging of bladder carcinoma. AJR 137:359

6. Husband JE (1985) Staging of bladder and prostate cancer, in Walsh JW Computed tomography of the pelvis. New York, Churchill Livingstone P135
7. Wood DP, Lorig JR Pontes JE, et al. (1988) The role of magnetic resonance imaging in the staging of bladder carcinoma. J Urology 140:741
8. Kraus W, Schild HH (1992) Urinary Bladder, in Schild HH, Computed tomography in urology. New York, Georg Thieme Verlag Stuttgart, P226
9. Hricak H, (1991) MRI of the pelvis. London, Martin Dunitz, P417
10. Fisher MR, Hricak H, Tanagho EA (1985) Urinary bladder MR imaging. Radiology 157:471

CHAPTER 22

Computed Tomography of the Prostate

Jong Chul Kim[1]

Indication for Computed Tomography in Prostatic Diseases

The major role of computed tomography (CT) in prostatic diseases is staging of prostatic carcinoma (not diagnosis) and evaluation of therapy in prostatic diseases. CT can estimate prostatic volume accurately. CT is also useful for demarcating optimal radiation treatment portals and determining the geometry of radioactive implants.

CT Technique and Contrast Medium Administration

All patients are scanned with a full bladder, and dilute oral contrast medium is given at least 1 hour before the scan. Contrast opacification of the distal small bowel and the colon is essential, so about 500–800 cc Gastrografin or dilute barium is usually administered 45–60 min prior to the scan. Rectal contrast medium (optional 200 cc dilute contrast enema immediately prior to scanning) is also helpful in patients with prostate carcinoma with suspicious invasion to recto-sigmoid or perirectal areas. A scout view is taken in all patients for preliminary localization. This view is also used after the examination to relate the position of a tumor to anatomic bony landmarks for radiotherapy planning.

Intravenous contrast medium (e.g., a 50-cc bolus of 60% contrast medium followed by a rapid drip infusion of 300 cc 30% contrast medium) is routinely used for evaluating prostate tumors because it delineates the bladder lumen with positive contrast and shows the position of the ureters. Precontrast scans are also useful for comparison with postcontrast scans. In patients with prostate carcinoma, the most important slices for assessing extraprostatic spread are both below and above the bladder base. To differentiate the lymphadenopathy from blood vessels, dynamic scans with rapid table incrementation and large bolus injection of contrast media may be useful. Percutaneous biopsy of suspicious enlarged pelvic lymph nodes may be done under CT guidance.

High-dose scanning technique may provide us with the best quality images of the prostate. A small field of view further improves spatial resolution. Contiguous slices of 4-mm or 5-mm collimation may be useful. Contiguous thin slices can be

[1] Department of Diagnostic Radiology, Chungnam National University School of Medicine, Taejeon, Korea.

used to produce reconstructions in the coronal, sagittal, or oblique planes. This is particularly important for the precise delineation of a tumor prior to surgery or radiotherapy.

Scanning is commenced 1 cm below the lower border of the symphysis pubis and continued through the prostate gland and seminal vesicles in patients with prostate cancer. After the tumor has been covered using thin slices the remainder of the pelvis is scanned at 1-cm intervals using 8- to 10-mm collimation to the mid-fifth lumbar vertebra. Scans through the abdomen (from the diaphragm to the mid-bladder) are usually taken at 8- to 10-mm thickness or 1.5- to 2-cm intervals. Where available, this is best done with a power injector and dynamic (or rapid) imaging mode.

Spiral CT may help to limit patient dose in CT examination of the prostate. The dosage of radiation exposure varies widely with the selection of scan parameters and type of scanner used. For example, we may use 16-cm scan range, 3-mm slice width, 165-mA tube current and 120 kVp in the examination of the prostate or urinary bladder.

Standard supine scans are adequate for the majority of studies. The prone or lateral position may be useful for distinguishing tumor invasion of the rectum, posterior bladder wall or pelvic sidewalls from a tumor that is contiguous but not fixed. The images should be filmed with soft tissue window settings and also with bone window settings in cases of advanced disease.

For an advanced tumor that is to be treated by radiation therapy, reference markers should be placed on the patient's skin delineating the superior to inferior as well as the anterior to posterior extent of the suspected disease defined for radiation planning.

CT Anatomy of the Prostate

The prostate appears on CT as a homogeneous, smoothly marginated, elliptical, round or triangular infravesical soft tissue with a density approaching that of skeletal muscle. Slight contrast enhancement is evident. In men of 30 years old and younger, the aver age craniocaudal diameter measures 3 cm; the anteroposterior diameter, 2.3 cm; and the lateral diameter, 3.1 cm. In the 60- to 70-y ear-old group, these average measurements increase to 5 cm for the craniocaudal diameter, 4.3 cm for the anteroposterior diameter, and 4.8 cm for the lateral diameter. The lateral contours of the prostate are usually masked by the contiguous ligament of the levator ani muscle, but can sometimes be demarcated when thin sections are scanned. Unlike ultrasound and magnetic resonance imaging (MRI), CT can not depict the internal prostatic architecture. The border of the prostate oriented towards the urinary bladder is either virtually horizontal or it rises slightly cranial from the supine aspect. Partial volume artifacts arising from these structures can mask slight irregularities on the bladder wall or contours of the prostate. The parenchymal density is about 40–65 HU. Peripheral calcifications on the capsule of the prostate usually correspond to phleboliths within the periprostatic plexus.

General Pathology

The prostate should not be considered enlarged if a scan 1 cm above the symphysis does not visualize the prostate. Prostatic enlargement can be diagnosed if the prostate is seen 2–3 cm or more above the symphysis, in which instance it is usually surrounded by the bladder. The actual volume of prostatic tissue can be calculated by summating prostatic volumes on sequential CT scans.

Prostatic calcifications (small calculospherules within the prostatic ductules) are detected by CT more frequently with increasing patient age, reaching 60% in the 50- to 70-year-old group. The calcifications usually appear as punctate, scattered, rounded densities that may not be identified on plain radiographs. An increase in the number of calcifications is seen in chronic or granulomatous prostatitis. Large foci of calcification with irregular margins also are demonstrable. Calcifications in the prostate and seminal vesicles can be found in diabetes mellitus (DM), tuberculosis, and shistosomiasis, and calcification in vas deferens may be found in DM.

The margins of different prostatic lobes cannot be distinguished by CT, and prostatic gland tissue cannot be differentiated from the prostatic capsule; thus CT is a reliable indicator of prostatic disease only when the prostate is either grossly enlarged or contains gas, fluid, or calcium.

Prostatic Cysts

Prostatic cysts may be congenital or acquired. Midline cysts include congenital utricular cysts, müllerian duct cysts, or true prostatic cysts. Lateral cysts consist of acquired parasitic cysts, cysts associated with prostatic carcinoma or BPH, or retention cysts.

Utricular cysts with dome-shaped bases are usually associated with genitourinary anomaly such as hypospadia, cryptorchidism, renal agenesis, etc., so are usually found in patients younger than 20 years. Patients with utricular cysts may present ejaculatory dysfunction such as hematospermia, oligospermia, or pain on ejaculation. If excision of the utricular cyst is necessary, it is generally less difficult to do than an excision of a müllerian duct cyst.

Müllerian cysts, which arise from the müllerian ducts, arise behind the verumontanum, lie in the midline posterior to the prostate, and extend above the base of the prostate. They occasionally communicate with the urethra at the verumontanum, where a typical beaked projection appears at the inferior edge of the cyst. They are shaped like inverted pears. They may become larger than 5 cm in diameter and thereby compromise the urinary bladder and rectum. Patients with müllerian cysts have normal external genitalia, and do not usually present clinically until they are over 20 years of age.

Prostatic Infections

Intracanalicular, blood and lymph-borne infection of the prostate leads to diffuse inflammation. Depending on the pathogen, phlegmon s or abscesses may develop. The most common complications of chronic prostatic infection include the formation of fibrous tissue and scar tissue and, ultimately, atrophy of the prostate.

Genital tuberculosis is frequently accompanied by prostatitis. The ulcerous, cavernous type of this disease can lead to fistulization of the urethra, rectum, and perineum. Calcification of tuberculous necrosis is sometimes also found. Because of their compact, amorphous nature, these secondary prostatic calculi can usually be easily differentiated from primary prostatic calculi (products of prostatic secretion).

In the acute stages of prostatitis, there is uniform enlargement of the prostate that does not displace the urethra. Prostatic adenomas cannot be diagnosed on the basis of attenuation differences. Inflammatory liquefaction leads to the appearance of areas of hypodensity. When these areas increase in size, the contours of the organ may protrude and the capsule may, ultimately, be breached. Periprostatic infection results in temporary, ill-defined masking of surrounding fat. After the administration of contrast medium, these zones are demarcated as hypodense, often loculated zones which display the type of rim enhancement typical of abscesses.

Benign Prostatic Hyperplasia or Hypertrophy or Prostatic Adenoma

As the most common urologic disease and the most common cause of infravesical obstruction among men of middle old age, benign adenomatous hyperplasia (BPH) of the prostate usually involves the transition zone (95%) and periurethral glandular tissue (5%). About 50% of men up to the age of 60 and 80% of men up to the age of 80 are affected by BPH.

The only visible sign of prostatic adenoma is enlargement of the prostate, the borders of which are sharply delineated from surrounding fat and the ligaments of the levator ani muscle. In the presence of an enlarged prostate with sharp, smooth borders, it is impossible to distinguish on CT between BPH and a small focal adenocarcinoma of the prostate. CT usually cannot reveal the internal architecture of the prostate in detail. Not infrequently, asymmetry and curved polycyclic protrusions into the base or floor of the urinary bladder are found in BPH.

A bolus of contrast medium creates homogeneous enhancement and allows for reliable differentiation between adenomas and peripheral, compromised prostatic tissue.

Like ultrasound or MRI, CT can estimate prostatic volume accurately. However, because of its cost, the radiation it produces, and th e medical resources consumed, it is used infrequently as an imaging modality for BPH. In the absence of frank tumor invasion, CT is of little value in determining the cause of prostatic enlargement. MRI on T2-weighted image is readily able to display the zonal anatomy of the prostate. The central zone (25% of gland) has intermediate to low signal intensity, in contrast to high signal intensity of the peripheral zone (70% of gland). The anterior fibromuscular band has a very low signal intensity. The transitional zone (5% gland volume) has signal intensity characteristics close to those of the central zone in young men. As BPH develops, this zone enlarges and signal intensity becomes more variable. BPH changes are best seen on T2-weighted, endorectal coil and/or phased-array coil images. BPH nodules contain varying amounts of stromal and glandular elements that may influence the MRI appearance. Stromal BPH generally has an intermediate signal intensity, while glandular BPH has a high signal intensity.

Sonographically, BPH presents as symmetric enlargement having a homogeneous texture and sharp margination. The accuracy of transrectal ultrasonography TRUS in detecting BPH ranges from 91% to 97% and TRUS is 89% accurate in detecting prostatitis.

Prostatic Carcinoma

The prostatic carcinoma is the second most common malignant tumor in men of western countries. Like BPH, it most often occurs very late in life. It develops in the peripheral zone (70%), transition zone (20%), and central zone (10%).

The diagnosis of prostatic carcinoma is usually made by physical examination and biopsy under the guidance of ultrasonography or digital rectal examination. Depending on the clinical and surgical findings, prostatic carcinoma is placed in one of four stages (Table 1).

In addition to enlargement of the prostate, an eccentric, fine nodular protrusion on the contours of the prostate is also an important, but nonspecific, sign of prostatic carcinoma. These findings are suggestive of stage T2 tumors, but may be difficult to differentiate from incipient periprostatic infiltration of stage T3 tumors.

Table 1 Staging of prostatic cancer

Stage	Description
A (Microscopic)	Occult; incidentally found
A1	Focal; <5% of tissue examined; low grade
A2	Diffuse (>5%) or high grade
B (Macroscopic)	Palpable; confined to capsule
B1	Nodules (<1.5 cm)
B2	Nodules (>1.5 cm)
C (Extracapsular)	Localized clinically
C1	Periprostatic, not fixed to sidewall (<70 g)
C2	Fixed to sidewall (>70 g)
D (Metastatic)	
D1	Confined to pelvis
D2	Extrapelvic spread

The major role of CT and MRI in prostatic carcinoma is not diagnosis, but staging and evaluation of therapy. CT can neither diagnose stage A disease nor detect stage B carcinoma unless the tumor mass alters the contour or the focally altered margin suggests the presence of a carcinoma, and a smooth contour in an enlarged gland suggests BPH, but the separation is imprecise. CT can neither differentiate benign from malignant causes of prostatic enlargement nor depict the internal architecture of the prostate.

Clear organ invasion can be recognized as irregular, sometimes streaklike, masking of periprostatic or perirectal fat. Asymmetrical dilatation of the seminal vesicle is suggestive of tumor invasion, especially when there is visible obliteration of the angle between the urinary bladder and seminal vesicles. Only in tumors that extend cranially and grow rapidly can the border facing the urinary bladder be reliably assessed for a possible early diagnosis of bladder wall infiltration. Proper filling of the urinary bladder is, therefore, important for good results. Infiltration (T4) of the rectum, pelvic wall, and ureter can usually be diagnosed with confidence.

Since a bolus of contrast medium enhances tumor tissue to the same extent as normal prostatic tissue, intracapsular tumors (T1, T2) will not be identifiable. In extensive tumors (T3, T4), the bladder wall or walls of other hollow organs are enhanced, which makes it possible to determine the extent of infiltration. When necrotic regions are delineated, tumor regression and lymph node enlargement can be better distinguished from ectatic vessels.

MRI usually enables easy differentiation of BPH from prostate carcinoma. Extraprostatic extension of prostatic carcinoma (stage C or D) can be accurately assessed by CT, MRI, or transrectal ultrasonography. Extension of prostatic carcinoma most frequently involves the seminal vesicles and the urinary bladder, producing loss of tissue fat planes. Invasion of the seminal vesicles is found in 17% of patients with newly diagnosed prostatic carcinoma, whereas bladder and rectal invasion occurs less frequently. Stage D prostatic carcinoma is diagnosed when metastatic lesions in the pelvis, spine, long bones, liver, lung, or retroperitoneal lymph nodes are demonstrated. Bone metastases occur most frequently in the bony pelvis, lumbar vertebrae, and proximal femur and appear as osteoblastic (80%), mixed osteolytic-osteoblastic (10%–15%), or osteolytic (5%) lesions.

The CT criteria pertaining to evaluation of possible lymph node involvement are similar to those of other pelvic tumors. Metastases can be concluded only if the lymph nodes have reached a size of about 1.5 cm or larger (specificity, 70%–90%). Multiple smaller lymp h nodes and localized streaks in fatty tissue may also raise the suspicion of malignant infiltration. If pelvic lymphadenopathy is n ot present, the CT scan need not be carried out above the aortic bifurcation, since abdominal adenopathy without pelvic adenopathy is very uncommon in carcinoma of the prostate.

The reported accuracy of CT in detecting pelvic and retroperitoneal nodal metastases from prostatic carcinoma ranges from 33% to 93% (80–90%), whereas that of MRI ranges from 44% to 69%. Both CT and MRI detect nodal metastases on the basis of nodal enlargement, and thus metastatic deposits that do not produce lymphadenopathy go undetected. Therefore a negative CT or

MRI examination does not exclude lymph node metastasis, and pelvic lymphadenectomy must be performed if optional staging of prostatic carcinoma is required.

Percutaneous needle biopsy can be used to document metastasis in patients with abnormal or suspicious lymph nodes seen on lymphangiography, CT, or MRI.

The overall accuracy of CT for staging prostatic carcinoma is 67%–75%. Most errors are results of the inability of CT to recognize depth of tumor within the gland and to detect microscopic invasion of surrounding fatty tissues or metastatic foci in normal-sized lymph nodes.

The exquisite resolution provided by endorectal coil MRI makes it the ideal technique for evaluating the prostatic capsule, the neurovascular bundles, and the seminal vesicles. At the present time it is the imaging modality of choice for staging carcinoma of the prostate. Distinguishing stage B from C or D on MRI appears possible in approximately 80–90% of cases.

Postoperative Complications

Following prostatic surgery, CT is useful for evaluating the pelvis for postoperative changes and a variety of complications such as pelvic lymphoceles (usually located anterolateral to the bladder and within 3 cm of the anterior abdominal wall), hematoma, and/or abscesses that may follow pelvic lymphadenectomy.

Evaluation of Therapy

CT has proven to be a useful method for assessing the adequacy of portals for external beam radiation and for calculating the volume and average dimensions of the prostate (especially in stages A and B prostate carcinoma) for correct dosimetry of iodohippurate sodium ^{125}I seeds. Optimal therapy is given when there is even distribution of seeds, and CT has been capable of assessing precisely the distribution of seeds within the prostate and of determining whether extraprostatic radioactive seeds have been placed. Depending on clinical and CT findings, external radiation may be directed to areas that are not adequately treated by the ^{125}I seeds.

Prostatic Sarcoma

Prostatic sarcomas are much rarer than carcinomas, and they usually affect younger men. Sarcomas are usually diagnosed after they have already become rather extensive. Rabdomyosarcomas develop in children, whereas leiomyosarcomas usually present in middle-aged patients. In addition to aggressive growth, they are further characterized by hematogeneous metastases in the lungs, liver, and skeleton.

Conclusion

The major role of CT and MRI in prostatic carcinoma is not diagnosis, but staging and evaluation of therapy. CT and MRI can also provide an accurate estimation of prostatic volume. CT can demarcate the optional radiation therapy portals and determine the geometry of radioactive implants. But CT can neither differentiate benign from malignant causes of prostatic enlargement nor depict the internal architecture of the prostate. Ultrasonography can be used as a screening tool of palpable or nonpalpable prostatic lesion and can provide the guidance of biopsy. Ultrasonographic measurement can be used to assess the response of the prostate to various treatment modalities for benign and malignant disease. MRI provides us with the zonal anatomy of the prostate, usually enables easy differentiation of BPH from carcinoma and has a high degree of accuracy in distinguishing intracapsular carcinoma (surgically curable stage B carcinoma) from extracapsular (stage C, D) carcinomas. At the present time endorectal coil MRI with or without pelvic array coil MRI is the imaging modality of choice for staging carcinoma of the prostate.

References

1. Kalender WA (1994) Technical foundations of spiral CT. Semin Ultrasound CT MR 15:81–89
2. Scoutt LM, McCarthy SM, Moss AA (1992) Computed tomography and magnetic resonance imaging of the pelvis, in Moss AA, Gamsu G, Genant HK (eds): Computed tomography of the body with magnetic resonance imaging. Philadelphia, WB Saunders Co, 1203–1210
3. Wegener OH (1993) Whole body computed tomography. Boston, Blackwill Scientific Publications 423–430
4. Yang A, Yang S (1990) MRI and CT of the prostate gland, in Goldman SM, Gatewood OMB (eds): CT and MRI of the genitourinary tract. New York, Churchill Livingstone 157–184
5. Lee JK, Marx MV (1989) Pelvis, in Lee KT, Sagel SS, Stanley RJ (eds): Computed Tomography with MRI Correlation. New York, Raven Press, 859
6. Salo JO, Kivisaari L, Ranniko S et al. (1987) Computerized tomography and transrectal ultrasound in assessment of local extension of prostatic cancer before retropubic prostatectomy. J Urol 137:435–438
7. Platt JF, Bree RL, Schwab RE (1987) Accuracy of CT in the staging of carcinoma of the prostate. Am J Roentgen 149:315–318
8. Demas BE (1988) Computed tomography of the prostate gland. Semin Ultrasound CT MR 9:339–342
9. Hricak H, Thoeni RF (1989) Neoplasms of the prostate gland, in Pollack HM(ed): Clinical urography. Philadelphia, WB Saunders Co, 1381–1403
10. Weinerman PM, Arger PH, Coleman BG et al. (1993) Pelvic adenopathy from bladder and prostate carcinoma: detection by rapid sequence computed tomography. Am J Roentgen 140:94–99
11. Hricak H, Dooms GC, Jeffery RB et al. (1987) Prostatic carcinoma: Staging by clinical assessment, CT and MR imaging. Radiology 162:331–336
12. Husband JE (1985) Staging of bladder and prostate cancer, im Walsh JW (ed): Computed tomography of the pelvis. New York, Churchill Livingstone, 135–163

13. Schnall MD, Imai Y, Tomaszewski JE et al. (1991) Prostate cancer : local staging with endorectal surface coil MR imaging. Radiology 178:797–802
14. McCarthy P, Pollack HM (1991) Imaging of patients with stage D prostatic carcinoma. Urol Clin North Amer 18:35–53
15. Chelsky MJ, Schnall MD, Seidmon EJ (1993) Pollack HM. Use of endorectal surface coil magnetic resonance imaging for local staging of prostate cancer. J Urol 150:391–395
16. Schiebler ML, Schnall MD, Pollack HM et al. (1993) Current role of MR imaging in the staging of adenocarcinoma of the prostate. Radiology 189:339–352

CHAPTER 23

Computed Tomography After Nephrectomy for Renal Cell Carcinoma

Mulan Shi and Jing-rui Dai[1]

Renal cell carcinoma is a tumor which is frequently unpredictable, with peculiar tumor behavior and remains poorly understood. Surgical procedure, according to the staging of the tumor, including radical nephrectomy, partial nephrectomy or tumor enucleation, is the choise of treatment. Renal cell carcinoma might recur late after more than 10 years or might be dormant for as long as 35 years when untreated [1]. Once treated for renal cell carcinoma, there is always the risk of recurrence. With the use of multimodality treatment, survival after recurrence might hopefully be improved, although the outcome is still undetermined, and further studies are necessary [2, 3]. Since clinical application of imaging techniques, more small renal cell carcinomas have been detected; therefore, more attention should be paid to their outcome, in order to have a greater understanding of renal cell carcinoma and to improve survival after treatment.

CT, due to the outstanding resolution, wide-ranging availability, and affordability, is the most preferred imaging technique for the staging as well as follow-up [4, 5]. Ultrasonography and MRI are complimentary and are good at detecting lesions in soft tissue of abdominal wall or blood vessels. If only one kidney remains half of the dosage of contrast medium should be used for enhancement. In our department, non-ionic contrast medium (Ultravist 300, 50 ml, 15 gm I) is usually used. Early postoperation complications, such as local hematoma or abscess, are usually absorbed or reduced in size after treatment within 2–4 months. Baseline CT is recommended 2-4 months after nephrectomy.

Local recurrence occurs in 2%–4% of cases after radical nephrectomy of renal cell carcinoma, and in approximately 10% after partial resection of the kidney. Clinical symptoms appear in 80% of recurrences [6, 7] but mostly in advanced stage. Regular follow-up might be helpful for earlier detection of recurrence.

CT of the retrepteritoneum in 70 patients (98 scans) who had undergone nephrectomy for renal cell carcinoma at the Cancer Hospital, Chinese Academy of Medical Sciences were reviewed [8]. 84% of the scans were performed within the first 2 years. In 15 cases, local recurrences or metastases were detected, of which, 67% were found within 2 years. Recurrences were revealed at the excision site [5], renal fossae [6], adrenal gland [4], retroperitoneal lymph node [7] and contralateral kidney [1]. Seven patients had silitary lesions and 8 had multiple recurrences (Figs. 1, 2). In two patients, local recurrences were detected by routine follow-up

[1] Department of Diagnosis Radiology, Cancer Hospital, Chinese Academy of Medical Sciences, Beijing, China.

Fig. 1 Renal fossae recurrence. A 35-year-old patient, 4 months after right nephrectomy for renal cell carcinoma. A large (8 cm) irregular tumor mass (*arrows*) involving Riedel's lobe (*arrowhead*)

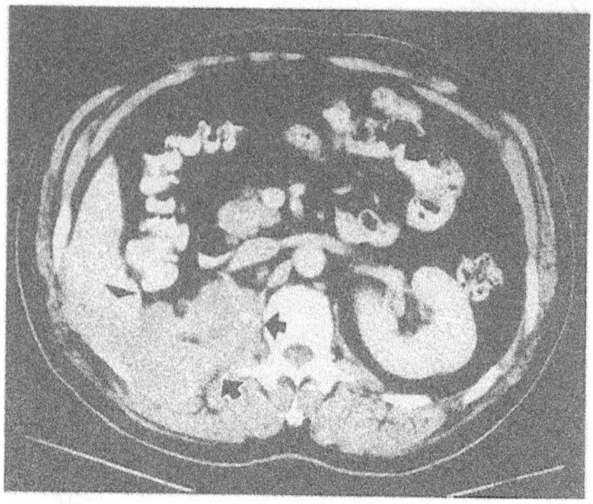

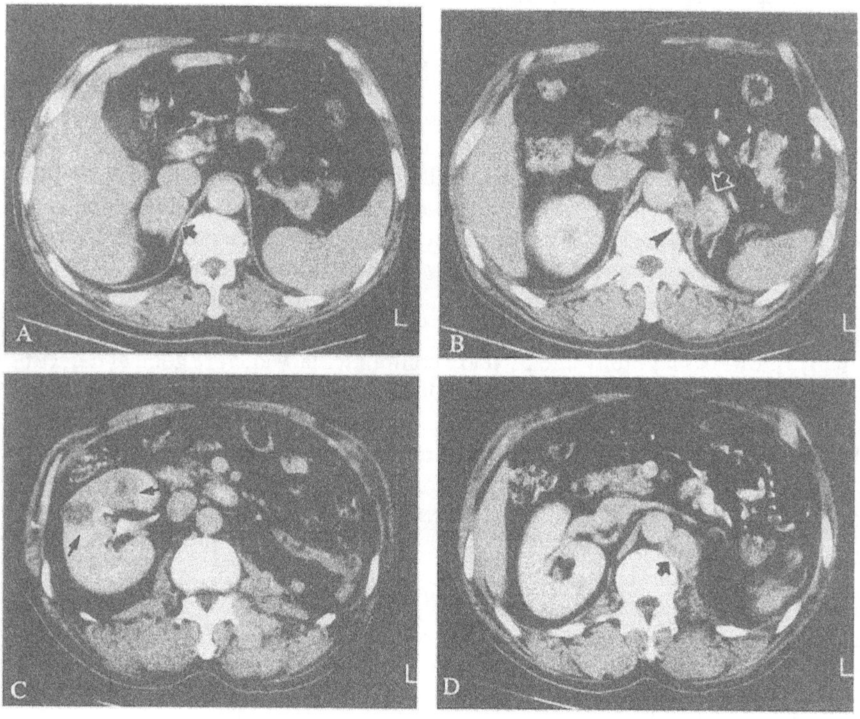

Fig. 2 A–D Retrocrual lymph node, bilateral adrenal gland and contralateral kidney metastases. A 65-year-old patient. Postcontrast CT 11 years after left nephrectomy for renal cell carcinoma and 4 years after resection of left axillary lymph node metastases. **A** Nodular enlargement (4 cm) of the right adrenal gland (*arrow*). **B** A more caudal section reveals left nonhomogenous adrenal enlargement (2.5 cm *arrow*); and left retrocrual lymph node enlargement (arrowhead). **C** Section at the level of left renal vein, left retrocrual lymph node metastases (*arrow*). **D** Section at the level of right renal hilum. Two nonhomogenous metastatic nodules at the ventral portion of right kidney (*arrows*)

CT scanning. In four cases, recurrences were found by surgery, and others by clinical follow-up. Nine patients had venous thrombus (inferior vena cava, IVC, nine; renal vein, three), the size of which was reduced after radiotherapy in one case (Fig. 3). Sites of metastases in decreasing order of frequency are intrathorax, bone, liver and brain. About 10%–25% of cases of renal cell carcinoma metastases might precede the primary tumor. Apart from the most common venacaval route, the route of metastases is often by way of the lymphatics.

Cancer cells may metastasize via lymphatics of renal hilar, para-aortic area, then furter to pulmonary hilar and mediastinal lymph nodes. It can also be via cisterna chyli, thoracic duct to supraclavicular lymph nodes. Direct communication might present between intra-abdomen and pulmonary hilum via inferior pulmonary ligament, therefore, lymph node enlargement of right inferior hilum might indicate metastases of renal cell carcinoma. Rarely, bilateral hilar lymph node metastases mimics X-ray manifestation of sarcoidosis [9–11].

The third route of metastases is via Batson's venous plexus. In Batson's plexus, there are profound anastomoses communicating with other systemic veins such as azygous vein, hemiazygous vein, lumbar vein, bronchical vein, intercostal vein etc. Miscellaneous sites of metastases such as ear, nose, larynx, eye, tongue, breast, diaphragm, gall bladder might occur.

The classic appearance of lung metastases is well demarcated multiple nodules or masses that look like cannon balls. Solitary pulmonary metastases as well as pulmonary lymphagitis carcinomatosa can occur (Figs. 4, 5). Solitary pulmonary metastases account for 2% of secondary renal carcinoma. After resection, the 3-year and 5-year survival rates are 45% and 34%, respectively.

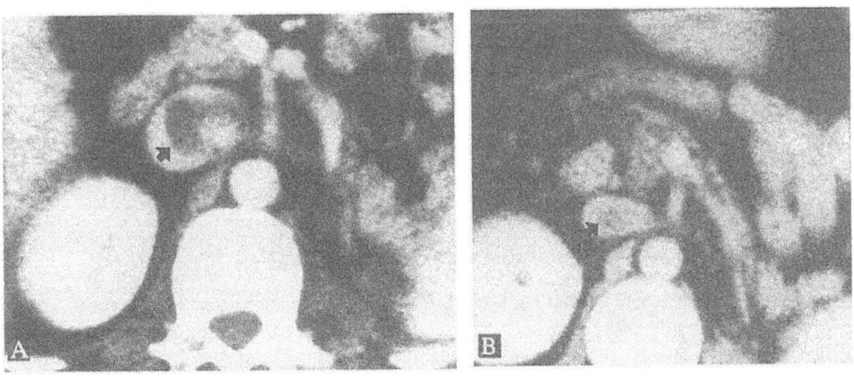

Fig. 3 A, B Tumor thrombus in inferior venal cava. A 58-year-old patient with stage III renal cell carcinoma resected. Postcontrast CT. **A** One month after nephrectomy. Filling defect in venal cava (*arrow*). Radiotherapy (50 Gy) was performed. **B** One year after the first scan. Filling defect reduced in size and stayed stable for 6 years. The patient then developed lung metastases. After LAK cell treatment, the patient is still alive

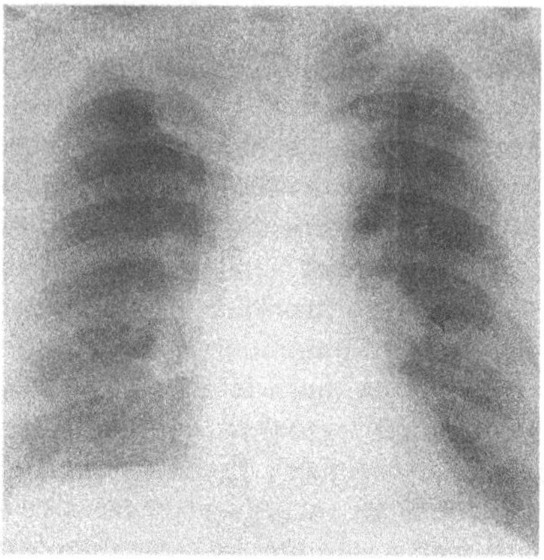

Fig. 4 Solitary pulmonary metastases. A 57-year-old patient 11 years after right nephrectomy and prevention radiotherapy. Solitary mass (3.5 cm) in left lower lobe (*arrow*). After lobectomy, it proved to be metastatic renal cell carcinoma. The patient had left kidney metastases 17 years after the first nephrectomy, and partial resection was done. He died 22 years after the first nephrectomy (11 years after lobectomy for lung metastases) as a result of widespread metastases

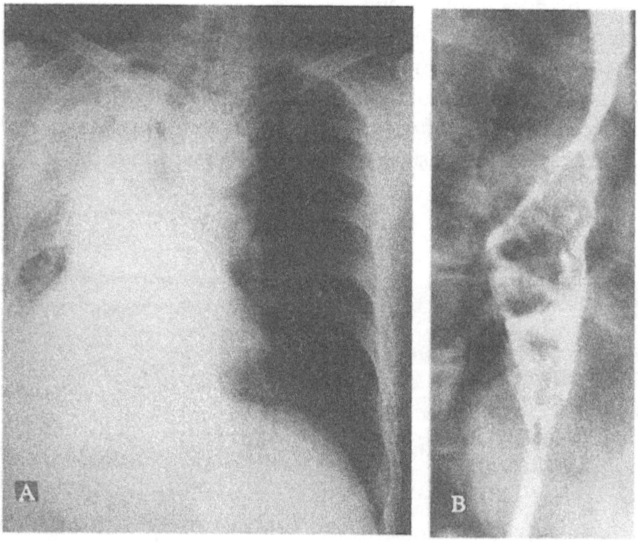

Fig. 5. A, B Intratracheal and intra-esophageal metastases. A 53-year-old patient 4 years after right nephrectomy for renal cell carcinoma. Patient had a cough and hemotypsis for 2 months. **A** Atelectasis was revealed by chest X-ray film. Metastasis from renal cell carcinoma was proved by fiberoptic bronchoscopy (FOB). Improved after radiotherapy (47 Gy). Recurred one year later with same signs and symptoms and improved after second course of radiotherapy treatment. **B** One year later, patient had dysphagia. Intraluminal mass appeared on esophagogram. Renal cell carcinoma was proved by FOE and biopsy. Improved after radiotherapy. The patient died one year later due to widespread metastases

It is well known that the bone metastases from kidney and thyroid carcinoma mimic primary bone tumor, with solitary, lytic, expansile lesion with soft tissue mass (Fig. 6). Sometimes it may precede the primary tumor. In elderly patients, metastases should be kept in the gamut of differential diagnosis when this kind of bone lesion is encountered, and ultrasonographic examination of kidney and thyroid should be done.

There is a peculiar tendency of renal cell carcinoma to have late recurrence, which is defined as 10 years after nephrectomy. Metastases could be observed in 22% after 5 years, and 11% of those patients after nephrectomy [1, 12]. Late recurrences mostly occur in lung, but other sites can also be found (Fig. 7).

In conclusion, renal cell carcinoma is an unpredictable tumor. Lifetime follow-up is necessary. Baseline CT of abdomen 2–4 months after nephrectomy, chest X-ray film and abdominal CT for every year are recommended for follow-up. Hopefully, early recurrence can be detected and better outcome can be obtained. Ultrasonography and MRI are complimentary imaging techniques.

Physicians need to be aware of unusual patterns of recurrence, i.e., solitary metastases, late recurrence, and unusual sites of metastases.

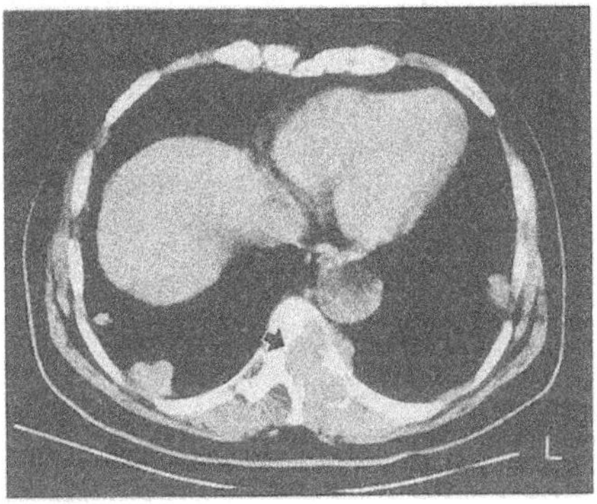

Fig. 6 Bone metastases. A 56-year-old patient 4 years after nephrectomy for left renal cell carcinoma. CT scan. Multiple lung metastases and T10 metastases with expansile, lytic lesion (*arrow*)

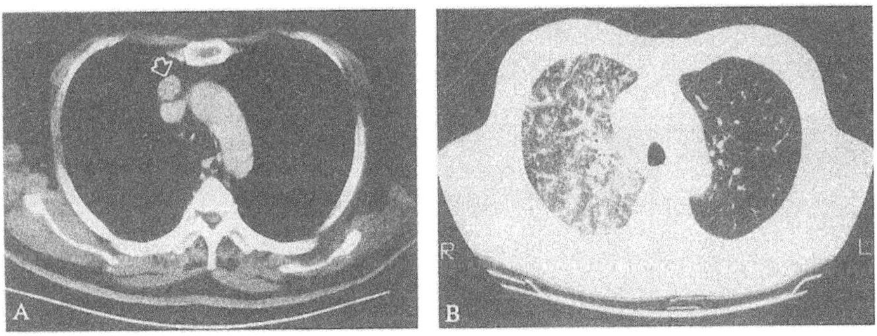

Fig. 7 Late intrathoracic recurrence. A 62-year-old patient, postcontrast CT of thorax. Right nephrectomy for a 6 cm renal cell carcinoma and prevention radiotherapy was performed 14 years previously. A mass in the scalp and in the right supraclavicular lymph node were found. **A** Mediastinal lymph node metastases (*arrow*). **B** Right pulmonary lymphagitis carcinomatosa

References

1. McNichols DW, Segura JW, de Weerd JH (1981) Renal cell carcinoma, long-term survival and late recurrence. J Urol 126:17
2. Lemmers M, Ward K, Hatch T et al. (1989) Renal adenocarcinoma with silitary metastasis to the contralateral adrenal gland: report of 2 cases and review of the literature. J Urol 141:1177
3. Morgan WR, Zincke H (1990) Progression and survival after renal conserving surgery for renal cell carcinoma: Experiance in 104 patients and extended follow-up. J Urol 144:852
4. Alter AJ, Uehling DT, Zwiebel WJ (1979) Computed tomography of the retroperitoneum following nephrectomy. Radiology 133:663
5. Bernadino ME, De Santos LA, Johnson DE et al. (1979) Computed tomography in the evaluation of post-nephrectomy patients. Radiol 130:187
6. Schweden FJ, Schild HH, Riedmiller H (1992) Chapter 9, Renal tumors in adults. Computed tomography in urology. Vol 2, pp 135–147. Ed by Schild HH, Schweden JK, Lang EK. Georg Thieme Verlag, Thieme Medical Publishers Inc. New York
7. Parienty RA, Richard F, Pradel J et al. (1984) Local recurrence after nephrectomy for primary renal cancer, Computerized tomography recognition. J Urol 132:246
8. Dai JR, Shi ML, Li YP (1994) Computed tomography of the retroperitoneum following nephrectomy for renal cell carcinoma. Chin J Oncol 16:144
9. Wright FW (1977) Enlarged hilar and mediastinal nodes (and especially lower right hilar node enlargement) as a sign of metastasis of a renal tumor. Clin Radiol 121:43
10. Arkless R (1965) Renal carcinoma: How it metastases? Radiol 84:496
11. Latour A, Shulman HS (1976) Thoracic manifestations of renal cell carcinoma. Radiol 121:143
12. Shi ML, Zheng MZ (1979) X-ray manifestations of intrathoracic metastases of renal cell carcinoma. Cancer Prevention and Treatment (in Chinese) 4:22

CHAPTER 24

Computed Tomography in the Diagnosis of Cystic Renal Diseases

Shyh-Jye Chen and Yiu-Wah-Li[1]

Cystic renal diseases are usually asymptomatic and found incidentally. They are classified according to genetic factors, clinical course as well as pathological and radiological findings. The classification of renal cysts from Kissane (1967), Spence and Singleton (1972) and Fanre (1977) is satisfactory in this condition. The classification presented in Table 1 is modified from Bernstein (1973). Conventional plain abdominal film and intravenous urography are performed as a screening procedure. Sonography and computed tomography (CT) demonstrate more detail and are able to make the accurate diagnosis. This chapter describes these cystic renal diseases and focuses on the findings of CT.

Table 1 Classification of cysts of the kidney

Cysts associated with renal dysplasia
Multicystic kidney
Renal cystic dysplasia
Polycystic disease
Infantile polycystic disease
Adult polycystic disease
Cortical cysts
Multilocular cyst
Simple cysts
Glomerulocystic disease
Cysts in syndromes of multiple defects
Medullary cysts
Medullary sponge kidney
Juvenile nephronophthisis (medullary cystic disease)
Microcystic disease
Pyelogenic cyst (calyceal diverticulum)

[1] Department of Medical Imaging. Medical College and Hospital, National Taiwan University, Taipei, Taiwan.

Cysts Associated with Renal Dysplasia

Multicystic Kidney

Multicystic kidney is a common cause of an abdominal mass in neonates. The incidence is about one in 10000 livebirths and is more common among infants of diabetic mothers. This disease is not hereditary and is more common in men [1].

Histologically, numerous immature glomeruli and a reduction in the number of renal tubules are found. The proposed cause is external obstruction of the collecting duct, before 8–10 weeks of fetal life, leading to aberrant development and cystic expansion of these renal tubules with failed development of the nephrons. Muticystic kidney is usually unilateral and rarely bilateral. The ureter is almost always atretic in the uppermost portion and the renal vessels slender or absent [2].

In infants, multicystic kidney is the most common form of cystic disease. Bilateral multicystic dysplastic kidney occurs in the presence of severe obstruction in utero from the posterior urethral valve or urethral atresia. Oligohydramnios and pulmonary hypoplasia present in cases involving bilateral kidneys which lead to the cause of death. Unilateral multicystic kidney may be asymptomatic and detected in adult life incidentally, or during evaluation for infection or hematuria. Abdominal mass, intermittent abdominal pain or failure to thrive are other symptoms appearing in children. Spontaneous regression of a multicystic kidney has been reported [3].

Association with renal anomalies of the contralateral side are frequently identified [4] as ureteropelvic junction obstruction, horseshoe kidney, ureteral anomalies, renal hypoplasia, vesicoureteral reflux and malrotation.

The radiological findings are variable since there is a spectrum of involvement on multicystic kidney. No function of the kidney is noted during intravenous urography (IVU) study if the whole kidney is affected. Retrograde pyelography shows an atretic or dysplastic ureter.

Sonography reveals random cysts of varying size (cluster of grapes) with the largest one in the peripheral location. Absence of parenchymal rim, corticomedullary differentiation and central renal sinus complex is recognized. These cysts do not communicate with each other and are separated by septa. Rim-like calcifications are occasionally found in adults [5].

The CT diagnosis is as follows [6, 7] (Fig. 1):

- Multiple, varying-sized cysts replace the renal parenchyma or have segmental involvement.
- There is no enhancement after intravenous contrast medium administration.
- Compensatory hypertrophy of the contralateral kidney with possible associated anomalies.

Renal Cystic Dysplasia

Renal cystic dysplasia is very rare. Multiple tiny (1–2 mm) cortical cysts are recognized with preserved calyces, renal pelvis and ureter. The entire kidney ist

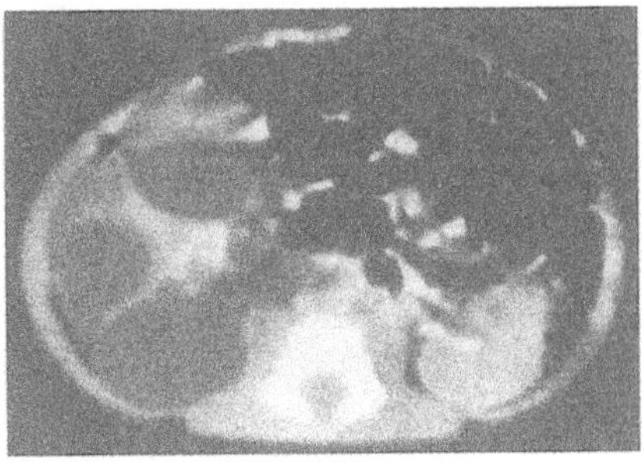

Fig. 1 Multicystic kidney. Multiple cysts replace the right kidney, without enhancement after intravenous contrast medium administration

usually involved and has become small. Generally, the renal outline is smooth though some accentuation of normal fetal lobulation is found.

Bilateral involvement of the kidneys results in chronic renal failure within the first year of life. Increased incidence of vesicoureteral reflux is recognized in renal cystic dysplasia. Focally affected dysplasia to the upper pole has been described.

IVU reveals the small renal shadow with poor nephrogram. Bilateral vesicoureteral reflux may be identified on voiding cystourterography.

Sonography demonstrates loss of differentiation between the renal cortex and medulla. Increased echogenicity, higher than that of the liver, is found. The affected kidney reduces in size.

The CT diagnosis is as follows:

- Tiny renal cortical cysts
- Poor corticomedullary differentiation
- Small kidney, unilateral or bilateral
- Normal preserved renal calyces, renal pelvis and ureter if no versicoureteral reflux

Polycystic Disease

Infantile Polycystic Kidney Disease

Most cases of infantile polycystic kidney disease have autosomal recessive heredity. It is found in 1 in 6000–150000 live births [8]. Bilateral renal involvement is noted with massively large size. Normal renal parenchyma is replaced by numerous small cysts. Four forms of this disease are classified: antenatal, neonatal, infantile and juvenile.

Infantile polycystic kidney disease is associated with different degrees of periportal fibrosis and abnormal proliferation of dilated bilary ducts. The less severe the renal findings, the more severe the hepatic findings.

Pathologically, abnormal proliferation and dilatatiion of the collecting tubules resulting in multiple 1–2 cysts are recognized in bilateral kidneys. In liver, periportal fibrosis is noted, often combined with abnormal proliferation and dilatation of the bile ducts. Fibrosis ot the pancreas has also been described.

The antenatal and neonatal forms of this disease are most severe; patients affected may die within days or months from renal failure or respiratory insufficience. The infantile form has about 20% of renal tubules involved and mild to moderate periportal fibrosis. The disease appears 3–6 months of age and results in death from chronic renal failure. In the juvenile form, only about 10% of the renal tubules are involved, renal function is preserved. Portal hypertension and hepatosplenomegaly are the leading clinical presentations [1, 9].

IVU show faint nephrogram on the initial images and increasing density with persistency later. Accumulation of the contrast medium in the dilated collecting ducts leads to a "sunburst" appearance (persistent radiating opaque streaks to the capsular surface). Bilateral renal enlargement, faint opacification of the collecting systems and prominent fetal lobulation are the other findings.

Sonography shows large kidneys with diffuse increased echogenicity (ectatic dilatation of numerous renal tubules increases the number of acoustic interfaces) and loss of cortiomedullary differentation. Small (1–2 mm) individual cystic lesions are not usually seen but occasionally, discrete macroscopic cysts may be recognized. Associated hepatic changes can also be checked by sonography. Poor visualization of the renal contour and sinus have been described.

The CT diagnosis is as follows [10, 11] (Fig. 2):

- Bilateral large kidneys with pronounced lobulation
- Prolonged corticomedullary phase after intravenous contrast medium administration (evidencing increasing renal failure)
- Stripes in cortex radiating to the capsular surface (elongated cylindrical cysts representing dilated collecting ducts)
- Signs of periportal fibrosis and dilated bile ducts recognized in elderly patients

Adult Polycystic Kidney Disease

Adult polycystic kidney disease is an autosomal dominant hereditary disease with nearly 100% penetration but is slowly progressive and of variable expression. One in 1000 people carry the mutant gene (short arm of chromosome 16); this makes it the third most prevalent cause of chronic renal failure. Bilateral renal involve-

Fig. 2 Infantile polycystic disease. Bilaterally enlarged kidneys with multiple dilated collecting ducts are noted in radiating pattern

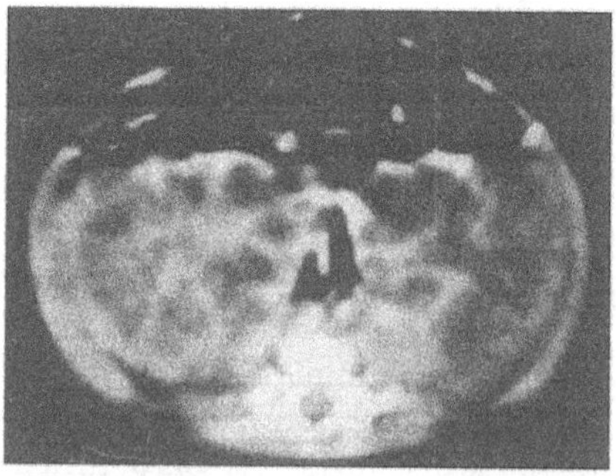

ment is noted with enlarged size and containing many cysts of various sizes [12].

Histologically, these cysts represent dilatations of various parts of the tubuli, e.g., Bowman capsule, loop of Henle, proximal convoluted tubule. This is the reason why the contents of these cysts are varied (urine, serous or gelatinous fluid).

Gradual obstruction of the dilated tubuli by hyperplasia of tubular mocosal epithelium increases the size of cysts [13]. Because of the pathophysiology, typically the disease presents symptoms (hematuria, proteinuria, flank pain, azotemia, hypertension, urinary infection and palpable abdominal mass) in the third of fourth decade with 100% manifestation if the person affected survives long enough. Pressure atrophy effect of the surrounding normal renal parenchyma by the gradually enlarged cysts correlates with the progressive renal insufficiency.

IVU demonstrates the characteristic "Swiss cheese" nephrogram indicating multiple round non-perfusion masses embedded in the normal renal parenchyma. Mass effect of these cysts leads to elongation and distortion of the attenuated collecting system. Cysts may calcify in curvilinear rim- oder ring-like irregular amorphous patterns. In the early stage, bilateral kidneys are enlarged but shrink after the beginning of renal failure, renal transplantation or on chronic renal hemolysis.

Sonography demonstrates increased echogenicity when the cysts are small (less than 5 mm) and in children, particularly if the kidneys are not enlarged. In adult patients multiple cortical cysts with hypoechoid internal and poor demarcated renal contour are noted. Sonography is also useful as a screening tool for other solid organs (e.g., liver, pancreas) for checking for the presence of cysts.

Associated findings with adult polycystic kidney disease are as follows:

- Cysts in the liver (25%–50%), pancreas (10%) and rarely in other organs, e.g., lung, spleen, ovaries, uterus, testis, seminal vesicle, epididymis, bladder [14, 15]
- Berry aneurysm of the Willis circle [16]
- Mitral valve prolapse

Increased incidence of occurrence of bilateral renal cell carcinoma in patients with adult polycystic kidney disease has been reported [17].

The CT diagnosis is as follows [12, 14, 15] (Fig. 3):

- Bilaterally large kidneys with lobulation
- Multifocal round lesions of various size

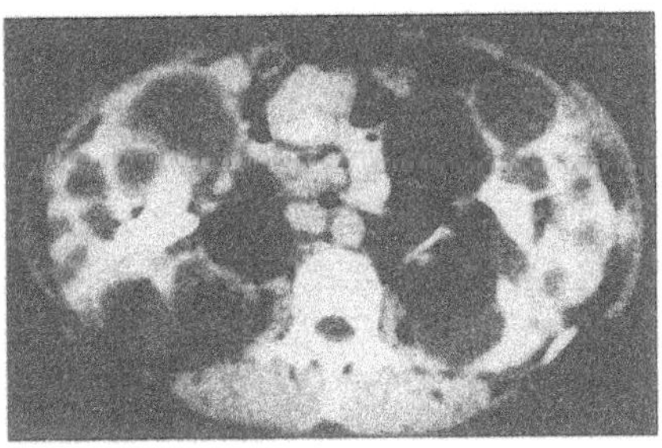

Fig. 3 Adult polycystic disease. Multifocal round cysts are noted in bilateral kidneys without enhancement after intravenous contrast medium administration

- No enhancement of these cysts but the compressed functioning part of the renal parenchyma enhances after intravenous contrast medium administration
- Cysts in other organs
- Shrinkage of kidneys at the later stage

Cortical Cysts

Multilocular Renal Cysts

Multilocular renal cysts are rare and are nonhereditary benign neoplasms. Synonyms of this disease include: multilocular cystic nephroma, cystic adenoma, cystic lymphangioma, cystic hamartoma, cystadenoma, multilocular cystadenoma, cystic Wilms' tumor, polycystic nephroblastoma, Perlmann tumor, benign cystic nephroma and adenomatous polycystic tumor.

Histologically, they arise from undifferentiated mesenchymal and primitive glomerulotubular elements [18]. Malignant potential has been described [19]. The content of these cysts is clear fluid in most cases, but sometimes mucous material is found. These cysts are lined by a typical eosinophilic epithelium. They predipose to affect the low pole of kidney; bilateral or diffuse renal involvement is occasionally seen. This disease is typically noted in children between the age of 3 months and 4 years and men predominates. In adults, women in the fourth to eighth decade are more commonly affected [18, 19]. Multilocular renal cysts are frequently asymptomatic. Herniation of the tumor into the collecting system, with resulting necrosis and ulceration, is found with hematuria.

IVU demonstrates the irregular renal outline and mass effect by these cysts. Distorsion of the calyces or hydronephrosis are frequently seen [19]. Herniation of the tumor into the renal pelvis is a suggestive finding for diagnosis.

Sonography is a good modality for showing a cluster of different sized cysts separated by thick septa as the characteristic pattern of this disease. Sometimes, solid character (fine cystic structure with jelly-like contents and solid components) is recognized.

The CT diagnosis is as follows [18, 19] (Fig. 4):

- Unilateral unifocal well-delineated mass, usually in lower pole
- Cluster of noncommunicating cysts of various sizes separated by thick septa
- Thick fibrous capsule
- Enhancement of the septations and capsule after intravenous contrastmedium administration
- Calicification (central, peripheral, granular, eggshell-like, or amorphous) uncommon

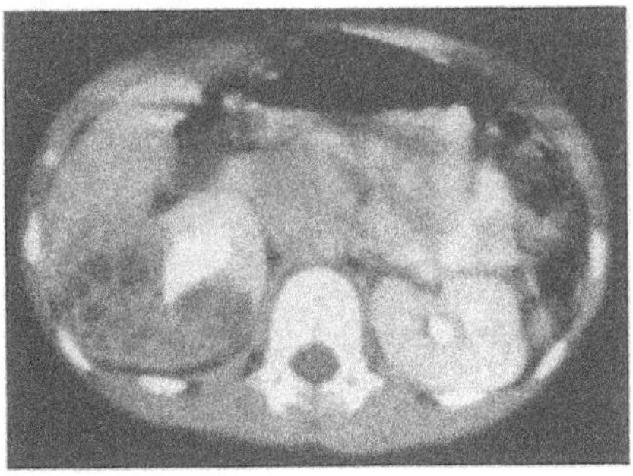

Fig. 4 Multilocular cyst. Cluster of non-communicating, various-sized cysts are found in the right kidney. There is enhancement of the septa

Simple Renal Cysts

Simple renal cysts are rare in the pediatric age-group, and their frequency increases with age [20]. The incidence is about 0.22% in children age and about 50% of patients are over the age of 50. It is assumed to be an acquired disease and the proposed cause of these simple renal cysts are that they are possibly secondary to tubular obstruction [21].

Pathologically findings usually reveal that they have very thin walls, with flat epithelium and thin septation. They are most commonly located at the renal cortex. The content of these simple renal cysts is a clear or yellow fluid; with low fat, protein, LDH and amylase concentrations [22].

Simple renal cortical cysts may be associated with the following diseases: tuberous sclerosis, von Hippel-Lindau disease, Caroli disease and neurofibromatosis.

Small, uncomplicated cysts are usually asymptomatic and do not need any treatment. Large cysts will displace the collecting system leading to urinary obstruction. Large, symptomatic cysts can be treated by puncture, drainage and sclerosing. Infection, hemorrhage (1%–11.5%), rupture or even tumor within the cyst (<1%) are the possible complications [23].

IVU reveals focally replaced nephrogram with smooth margin and "beak" sign on the edge to suggest a space occupied mass. The collecting system may show the pressure effect with some displacement. The displacement condition depends on the size and location of the cysts; if cysts are small, especially those located ventrally or dorsally, they may not be diagnosed at all.

Sonography is very accurate (90%–100%) in the diagnosis of simple renal cysts. These are typically spherical or ovoid in shape and are anechoic lesions without internal echoes and with smooth, clearly demarcated walls and dorsal echo enhancement.

The CT diagnosis is as follows [7, 21, 22, 24–26] (Fig. 5):

1. Uncomplicated simple renal cysts.
   - Sharply defined, round lesion
   - Homogeneous low density (–10 to +20 HU)
   - Indistinguishable, very thin wall
   - No enhancement after contrast

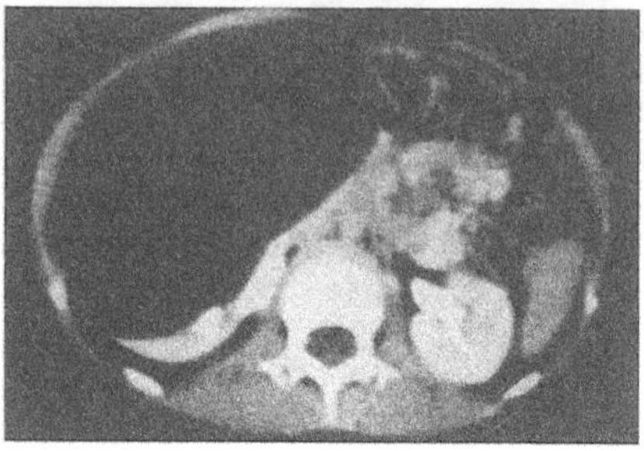

Fig. 5 Simple renal cyst. There is a huge low-attenuation cyst in the right kidney. No enhancement is found after intravenous contrast medium administration. The renal parenchyma and calyces are displaced dorsally

2. Complicated, infected or hemorrhaging renal cysts have a higher density than uncomplicated cysts. In acute hemorrhage, the density of these cysts may increase to 40–90 HU.

Medullary Cysts

Medullary Sponge Kidney

Medullary sponge kidney is a congenital disease with sporadic occurence. The incidence is about one in 5000 people; there is no definite sex bias. The cause of this disease is dysplastic cystic dilatation of the papillary and medullary portions of collecting ducts in one or more pyramids of one or both kidneys [27].

Histologically, cysts of 1–3 mm in diameter are recognized in the pyramids, resulting from dilatation of the collecting ducts. Stone formation after long term urinary stasis is found within the parenchyma.

Generally, patients with medullary sponge kidney are asymptomatic. The become symptomatic if complications arise from stones, such as colic, hematuria, obstruction or infection. These symptoms lead to diagnostic studies usually at a young age or in middle age.

Plain abdominal film reveals multiple small opaque calcification spots in the portion of pyramids and may sometimes be negative. Typical striped picture, representing the ectatic ducts or papillary cysts of the renal parenchyma appears after intravenous contrast medium administration

Sonography only detects large cysts. The kidneys are of normal size or only slightly enlarged. Small calcifications (up to 5 mm) in the pyramids are the reason for increased echogenicity of the pyramids.

Medullary sponge kidney may be associated with Ehlers-Danlos syndrome, parathyroid adenoma and Caroli disease.

The CT diagnosis is as follows [28] (Fig. 6):

- Medullary nephrocalcinosis, although plain abdominal film may be negative
- "Bunch of flowers" appearance, thick dense streaks of contrast medium radiating from pyramids peripherally

Fig. 6 Medullary sponge kidney. Dilated tubules are noted in bilateral kidneys with radiating pattern. Dense streaks of contrast material radiating peripherally are also noted

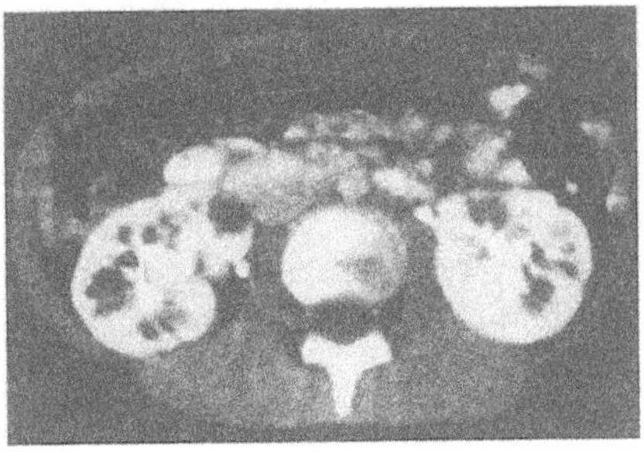

- Enlargement of the pyramid calculi due to stasis of the contrast medium in the stone-containing collecting ducts
- Small cysts filled with contrast medium in delay scan
- Unilateral in 25%

Calyceal Diverticulum

The synonyms of calyceal diverticulum include pyelocalyceal diverticulum, renal pelvic diverticulum, calyceal cyst, pyelorenal cyst, pericaliceal cyst and pyelogenic cyst. The incidence is about 2.1–4.5 per 1000 people [29].

Their cause may be congenital or acquired. In the congenital cases, developmental origin from the ureteral bud remnant or obstruction of the peripheral aberrant minicalyx is the underlying pathogenesis. Acquired cases are believed to originate from infection, inflammatory fibrosis, achalasia or dysfunction of the sphincter at the infundibulum of a minor calyx [30].

Histologically, a pouch extending from a peripheral point of the collecting system into adjacent renal parenchyma with transitional epithelium lining indicates the diagnosis. Two types of calyceal diverticulum are classified. Type I (or calyceal type) is more common and connects to the calyceal cup (usually at the fornix) with bulbous shape. They are located in the polar region, especially at the upper pole. Their narrow connecting infundibulum of varying length is a few millimeters in diameter. Type II (or pelvic type) is located at the interpolar region and is usually larger and rounder. The necks are short and not easily identified, with communication directly with the pelvis.

Calyceal diverticula are usually detected incidentally. If complications (hematuria, hemorrhage, infection or calculus formation) occur, the become symptomatic. Flank pain, recurrent infection and stone-related problems are the most common clinical presentations [31]. Xanthogranulomatous pyelonephritis has also been described [30].

Plain abdominal film may reveal single or multiple stones, sometimes "milk of calcium" can be found by fluid-calcium level. After intravenous contrast medium administration, the diverticula are opacified on the delay film and persist over a long period. Mass effect on the surrounding pelvocaliceal system is observed if the diverticulum is large enough.

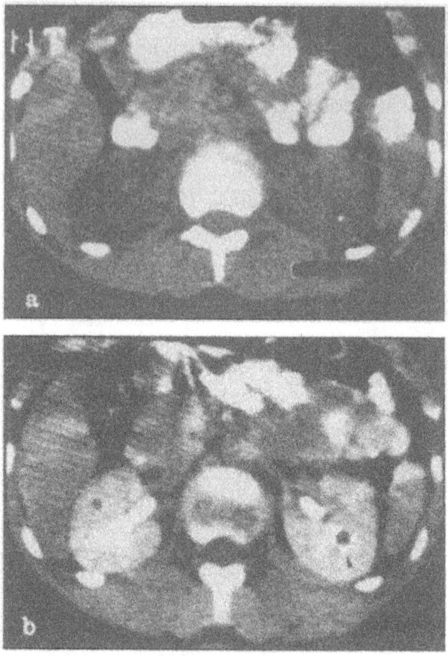

Fig. 7 a, b Calyceal diverticulum. **a** A round, low-attenuation lesion with a tiny calculus in the dependent portion is noted at the dorsal part of left kidney before contrast medium study. **b** The postcontrast image shows the urine-contrast level (*arrowhead*) within this lesion connecting with the renal calyx

Sonography can detect the large diverticula but is unable to differentiate them from renal cysts. Fluid-calcium level or movable calculi in a hypo- or anechoic diverticulum is recognized easily with acoustic shadows.

The CT diagnosis is as follows [29, 32, 33] (Fig. 7):

- Diverticulum communicates with pelvicaliceal system in the polar region
- Fluid-calcium level in diverticulum before contrast
- Diverticulum filled with contrast-laden urine after contrast medium administration
- Isolated, thick-walled cyst if the diverticulum seals off
- Mass effect on adjacent collecting system

References

1. Madewell JE, Hartmann DS, Lichtenstein JE (1979) Radiologic-pathologic correlations in cystic disease of the kidney. Radiol Clin N Amer 17:261
2. Beckmann CF, Abrams HL (1980) Renal venography: anatomy, technique, applications, analysis of 132 venograms and a review of the literature. Cardiovasc Intervent Radiol 3:45
3. Pedicelli G, Jequir S, Bowen AD et al. (1986) Multicystic dysplastic kidneys: spontaneous regression demonstrated with US. Radiology 160:23
4. Green LF, Feinzaig W, Dahlin DC (1971) Multicystic dysplasia of the kidney, with special reference to the contralateral kidney. J Urol 105:482
5. Stuck KJ, Koff SA, Siver TM (1982) Ultrasonic features of multicystic dysplastic kidney: expanded diagnostic criteria. Radiology 143:217
6. Diard F, Le Dosseur P, Cardier L, Calabet A, Bondonny JM (1984) Multicystic dysplasia in the upper component of the complete duplex kidney. Pediatr Radiol 14:310

7. Fishman MC, Pollak HM, Arger PH et al. (1983) High protein content: another cause of CT hyperdense benign renal cyst. J Comput Assist Tomogr 7:1103
8. Cussen LG, Stephens FD (1983) Renal dysgenesis: a urologic classification. In Stephens FD: Congenital malformations of the urinary tract. Praeger, New York
9. Gang DL, Herrin JT (1986) Infantile polycystic disease of the liver and kidneys. Clin Nephrol 25:28
10. Rabinowitz R, Segal AJ, Rao HKM et al. (1978) Computed tomography in diagnosis of infantile polycystic kidney disease. J Urol 120:616
11. Kuhn JP, Berger PE (1981) Computed tomography of the kidney in infancy and childhood. Radiol Clin AN Amer 19:445
12. Parfrey PS, Bear JC, Morgan J, Cramer BC, McManamon PJ et al. (1990) The diagnosis and prognosis of autosomal dominant polycystic kidney disease. N Engl J Med 323:1085
13. Evan AP, Gardner KD, Jr. Bernstein J (1979) Polypoid and papillary epithelial hyperplasia: a potential cause of ductal obstruction in adult polycystic kidney disease. Kidney Int 16:743
14. Hartnett M, Bennett W (1976) Extrarenal manifestations of cystic renal disease. In Gardner KD: Cystic diseases of the kidney. Wiley, New York
15. Milutinovic J, Fialkow PJ, Rudd TG et al. (1980) Liver cysts in patients with autosomal polycystic kidney disease. Amer J Med 68:741
16. Wakabayashi T, Fujita S, Ohbora Y et al. (1983) Polycystic kidney disease and intracranial aneurysm: early angiographic diagnosis and early operation for the unruptured aneurysm. J Neurosurg 58:488
17. Lippert MC (1988) Renal cystic disease. In Gillenwater JY et al. Adult and Pediatric Urology. Year Book Medical, Chicago
18. Banner MP, Pollak HM, Chatten J et al. (1981) Computed tomography of multilocular cystic nephroma. Radiology 140:135
19. Madewell JE, Goldman SM, Davis CJ et al. (1983) Multilocular cystic nephroma: a radiographic-pathologic correlation of 58 patients. Radiology 146:309
20. McHugn K, Stringer DA, Herbert D, Bablak CA (1991) Simple renal cysts in children: diagnosis and follow-up with US. Radiology 178:383
21. Tada S, Yamagishi J, Kobabyahi H et al. (1983) The incidence of simple renal cyst by computed tomography. Clin Radiol 437
22. Lang EK (1980) Roentgenologic approach to the diagnosis and management of cystic lesions of the kidney: in cyst exploration mandatory? Urol Clin N Amer 7:677
23. Siegel MJ, AcAlister WH (1980) Simple cysts of the kidney in children. J Urol 123:75
24. Bosniak MA (1986) The current radiological approach to renal cysts. Radiology 158:1
25. Zirinsky K, Auh YH, Rubenstein WA et al. (1984) CT of the hyperdense renal cyst: sonographic correlation. Amer J Roentgenol 143:151
26. Sussman S, Cochran ST, Pagani JJ et al. (1984) Hyperdense renal masses: a CT manifestation of hemorrhagic renal cysts. Radiology 150:207
27. Yendt ER (1982) Medullary sponge kidneys and nephrolithiasis. N Engl J Med 306:1106
28. Boag G, Nolan SR (1988) CT visualization of medullary sponge kidney. Urol Radiol 9:220
29. Mosli H, MacDonald P, Schillinger J (1986) Calyceal diverticula developing into simple renal cyst. J Urol 136:658
30. Siegl MJ, McAlister WH (1979) Calyceal diverticula in children: unusual features and complications. Radiology 131:79
31. Wulfsohn MA (1980) Pyelocaliceal diverticula. J Urol 123:1
32. Bejjani B, Faddoul A, Constantinople NL, Edson M (1981) Pyelocaliceal diverticulum presenting as a disappearing renal mass. J Urol 190:980
33. Yachiro N, Yoshida H, Araki T (1555) Bilateral "milk of calcium" r, nl cysts CT findings. J Comput Assist Tomogr 9:199

CHAPTER 25

Computed Tomography in Acute Renal Infection

Kyoung-Sik Cho[1]

Introduction

Acute bacterial infection of the kidney is a common disease that occurs in patients of all ages. The organisms causing the inflammatory reaction arrive in the kidney either through the hematogenous route or ascend in the ureter and into the renal-collecting system from the bladder. Hematogenous spread infection from Staphylococcus aureus has become less frequent, whereas fungal and opportunistic infections have become more frequent. The great majority of renal infections, however, are still caused by gram-negative enteric organisms that ascend to infect the kidney after bladder infection. Pathologically, it spans a continuum of severity from uncomplicated acute pyelonephritis through a progressively worsening stage of interstitial inflammation to abscess formation. Knowing the pathogenesis of the various acute disease subgroups make it easier to understand the imaging features that characterize the specific entities.

The initial acute phase of interstitial nephritis caused by microorganisms is characterized by purulent inflammation featuring a neutrophilic infiltrate. On gross examination of the kidney there are small, yellow-white abscesses in the cortical lesion. Microscopic examination reveals the presence of interstitial edema, hyperemia, and infiltrates of neutrophilic leukocytes between tubules. This uncomplicated condition is termed *acute pyelonephritis*. The disease process may then follow one of three potential courses. First, it may gradually improve as a result of antibiotic therapy and/or the immune response of the host. Second, it may progress in localized form or generally throughout the kidney as an increasingly suppurative process with focal areas of tissue necrosis. The generalized form of acute pyelonephritis has been called acute bacterial nephritis and the localized form has been called *acute focal bacterial nephritis*. Third, multiple small suppurative foci may coalesce into a large focal collection of pus localized in a portion of the kidney. This complicated acute pyelonephritis is called an *acute renal abscess*. The abscess may break out into the perinephric space and become a perinephric abscess. If the acute pyelonephritis occurs in the hydronephrotic kidney with obstruction to urinary outflow, the purulent exudate also collects in the dilated renal-collecting system. This condition is called *pyonephrosis*.

Most patients with renal infections have some predisposing factor, such as renal calculi, anatomic anomalies, neuropathic bladder or diabetes mellitus.

---

[1] Department of Diagnostic Radiology, Asan Medical Center, University of Ulsan.

Imaging Diagnosis of Renal Infection

Typical clinical symptoms such as flank pain and tenderness, fever, and chills are accompanied by laboratory findings of bacterial infection including leukocytosis, bacteriuria, pyuria and sometimes bacteremia and hematuria. Most adult patients with renal infection are easily diagnosed by such clinical symptoms and laboratory findings that do not ordinarily require imaging diagnosis. Quick response to antibiotic therapy is the rule, and patients usually improve without complications. However, in children or with complicated infections such as frank renal abscess or pyonephrosis, the clinical findings are nonspecific and the response to antibiotic therapy is sluggish or suboptimal. In these cases, imaging diagnostic tools play an important role. Intravenous urography (IVU) is insensitive and nonspecific in detection and characterization of acute renal infection [1]. The two most reliable imaging diagnostic tools for diagnosing acute renal infection are ultrasonography (US) and computed tomography (CT). Recent experience from the literature suggests that CT offers some advantages over US particularly in distinguishing degree and type of involvement of the renal parenchyma and in more accurate diagnosis of acute abscess [2]. Some authors suggest that cortical scintigraphy, such as Tc-99m DMSA (dimercaptosuccinic acid) is the most sensitive imaging technique for the detection and localization of renal parenchymal lesion in acute pyelonephritis of children [3] or experimental animals [4]. However, CT is almost as sensitive as cortical scintigraphy in detecting focal abnormalities in patients with clinical and laboratory evidence of acute pyelonephritis [5].

CT examination technique in acute pyelonephritis is the same as for other lesions in the kidney. The entire kidney is routinely scanned using contiguous CT sections 1 cm thick during suspended respiration with the patient supine. Oral contrast medium is administered to ensure that the gastrointestinal tract is adequately opacified. Scanning of the kidneys before and after administration of intravenous contrast media ensure the greatest diagnostic yield, but the patient receives twice the radiation exposure, the examination is longer, and frequently the precontrast scans provide no unique information. The majority of cases of acute pyelonephritis are expected to show some parenchymal abnormality on contrast-enhanced CT. Thus, contrast-enhanced CT is obtained as the initial scan procedure in acute pyelonephritis. Intravenous contrast medium is given as a drip infusion, a bolus injection, or as a combination of the two methods. Most commonly, either 100–120 ml ionic agent (Rayvist 300) or a nonionic agent (Ultravist 300) is administered as a bolus injection at a rate of 1.5–2 ml per s by a mechanical injector

CT Diagnostic Criteria

Acute Diffuse Bacterial Nephritis (Pyelonephritis)

In some patients early with acute pyelonephritis in the early stages, CT is normal. However, in many patients not responding to treatment, CT will reflect the pathologic findings of diffuse interstitial edema, hyperemia, and infiltrates of

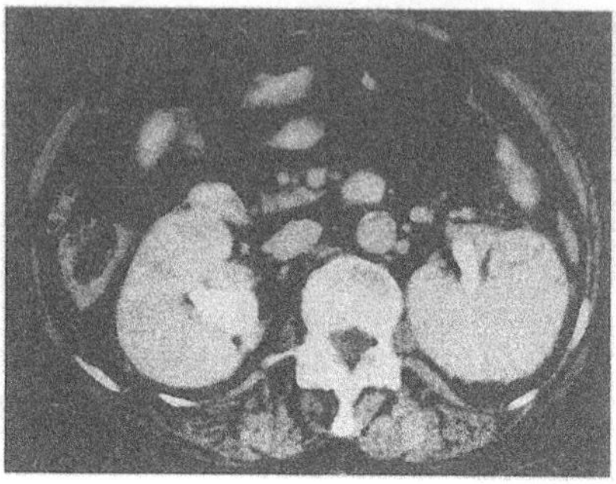

Fig. 1 Acute diffuse bacterial nephritis (pyelonephritis). Both kidneys are enlarged. Wedge-shaped decreased enhancement and striated area of mottled enhancement are observed in both kidneys

leukocytes between the tubules. The most common finding in contrast-enhanced CT is wedge-shaped or striated areas of decreased or mottled enhancement of the renal parenchyma [2, 6]. The wedge-shaped areas emanate from the renal hilum and correspond to the lobular architecture of the kidney (Fig. 1). These areas are usually sharp at the edges in the acute infection but become indistinct during the healing process. In noncontrast CT, these areas are occasionally higher in density than the surrounding uninvolved renal parenchyma (hemorrhagic pyelonephritis) [7], but in most cases, noncontrast CT are nondiagnostic. A striated pattern of alternating submillimeter lines of increased and decreased density is another common manifestation of pyelonephritis. This is presumed to result from capillary stasis or hyperdense concentration of urine within tubules plugged by pus. The ancillary findings of the acute diffuse bacterial nephritis are global renal enlargement, inflammatory changes in the perinephric fat, and thickening of Gerota's fascia [2].

CT appears to be very sensitive and relatively specific for the diagnosis of acute diffuse bacterial nephritis, and patients who exhibit such findings generally have resolution of symptoms and signs and radiographic abnormalities within a few days of institution of appropriate antibiotic therapy. Patients with pyuria and bacteria with normal contrast-enhanced CT findings probably have cystitis or pyelitis. Patients with the above-described CT findings, but no pyuria or bacteria, may be suffering from renal ischemia or noninfectious nephritis.

CT appears to be more sensitive than US and cortical scintigraphy in diagnosing of acute diffuse bacterial nephritis. One published study found that US failed to detect acute bacterial nephritis in three of five patients with both CT and US [2].

Acute Focal Bacterial Nephritis

The inflammatory process of the renal parenchyma may be limited to a focal area. However, this condition represents a severe infection of the kidney. Acute focal bacterial nephritis may produce a mass effect on imaging study. The terminology of this condition has been confusing. "Lobar nephronia," "focal bacterial nephritis," "carbuncle," "cellulitis," and "renal phlegmon" are some of more frequently used terms. The Society of Uroradiology recommends that all these

Fig. 2 Acute focal bacterial nephritis. A round mass with mottled enhancement in the left kidney. Mild thickening of Gerota's fascia is observed

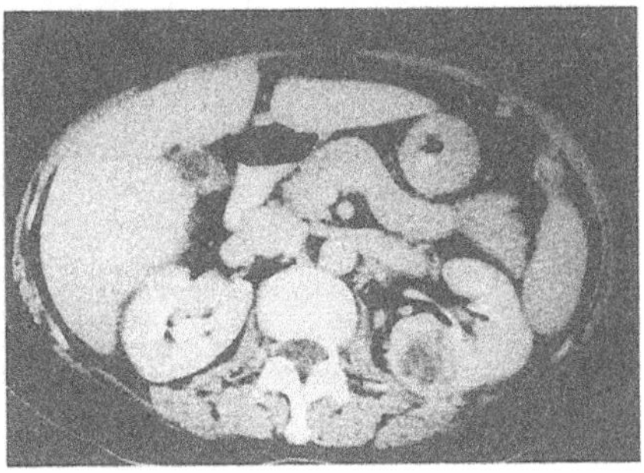

terms be dropped in favor of the simpler "acute pyelonephritis," with or without focal swelling [8].

CT demonstrates a rounded mass of mottled enhancement that is not encapsulated or liquefied [2]. The masses may be single or multiple. The perinephric fat and fascia are often infiltrated and the radiographic findings closely resemble those of a renal neoplasm (Fig. 2). Clinical presentation of the patients may differentiate focal nephritis from neoplasm. Other helpful CT features are compression of adjacent renal parenchyma, causing rim enhancement, and delayed persistent enhancement on CT scans repeated some hours after contrast administration [9]. The uptake of gallium- or indium-labeled white cells has been reported as an additional helpful sign in distinguishing focal infection from neoplasm. Serial examinations are often necessary to see whether focal acute bacterial nephritis evolves into an abscess or heals with antibiotic therapy.

Abscess

An abscess is an encapsulated liquefied or necrotic collection of pus and tissue debris that may be limited to the kidney itself or extend into the perinephric space. The clinical presentation usually mimics that of acute pyelonephritis. However, in up to 20% of patients urine cultures will be negative. Abscesses commonly occur after surgery or instrumentation in immunocompromised patients or in those with congenital anomalies or ureteral obstruction. CT demonstrates nonenhancing fluid collections in a spherical mass with an enhancing rim that is particularly evident where it abuts perinephric fat (Fig. 3). Other CT findings of renal abscesses are inflammatory perinephric fat changes, thickening of Gerota's fascia and direct extension of disease into the spaces around the kidney [2].

CT is more effective than US in distinguishing abscess from focal bacterial nephritis and in revealing the total extent of the renal and perinephric abscess.

Pyonephrosis

This condition is the accumulation of pus within a hydronephrotic-obstructed kidney. The purulent process involves the urine in the dilated collecting system, as

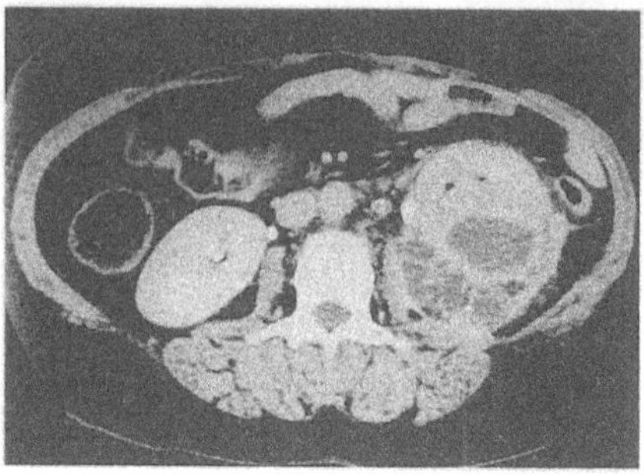

Fig. 3 Renal abscess extends to perinephric space. An elliptical fluid collection mass and perinephric fluid collection in the left kidney. Rim enhancement is observed in the perinephric abscess

well as the thinned renal parenchyma. Pyonephrosis is often associated with severe urosepsis and is a urologic emergency, requiring urgent drainage. US is the method of choice, although the differentiation of uncomplicated hydronephrosis from pyonephrosis may be difficult [10]. Fluid-debris levels or low-amplitude echoes within the dilated collecting system indicates pyonephrosis.

CT is a second line study for pyonephrosis. CT findings of pyonephrosis are an enlarged kidney with a grossly dilated collecting system containing higher than usual fluid attenuation [2]. The next step is percutaneous aspiration and nephrostomy treatment.

References

1. Morehouse HT, Weiner SN, Hoffman-Tretin JC (1986) Inflammatory disease of the kidney. Semin Ultrasound CT MR 7:246–258
2. Soulen MC, Fishman EK, Goldman SM, Gatewood OMB (1989) Bacterial renal infection: role of CT. Radiology 171:703–707
3. Sty J, Wells R, Starshak R, Schoeder B (1987) Imaging in acute renal infection in children. AJR 148:471–477
4. Rushton HG, Majd M, Chandra R, Yim D (1988) Evaluation of 99 m technetium-demercapto-succinic acid renal scan in experimental acute pyelonephritis in piglets. J Urol 140:1169–1174
5. Fraser I, Whitworth J, Birch D et al. (1989) Parenchymal involvement in cases of acute pyelonephritis in patients with normal IVP (abstr). Kidney Int 36:1178
6. Goldman SM (1988) Acute and chronic urinary infection: present concepts and controversies. Urol Radiol 10:17–24
7. Rigsby CM, Rosenfield AT, Glickman MG, Hodson J (1986) Hemorrhagic focal bacterial nephritis: findings on gray scale sonography and CT. AJR 141:343–349
8. Talner LB, Davidson AJ, Lebowitz RL, Dalla Palma L, Goldman SM (1994) Acute pyelonephritis: can we agree on terminology? Radiology 192:297–305
9. Ishigawa I, Saito Y, Onouchi Z et al. (1985) Delayed contrast enhancement in acute focal bacterial nephritis: CT features. J Comput Assist Tomogr 9:894–897
10. Jeffrey RB, Laing FC, Wing VW, Hoddick W (1985) Sensitivity of sonography in pyonephrosis: a reevaluation. AJR 144:71–73

CHAPTER 26

Computed Tomography of Osteogenic Tumors

Heung Sik Kang[1]

The roles of imaging in the diagnosis of bone tumors are correct diagnosis, accurate staging for the proper management and post treatment follow-up monitoring. Conventional radiography can provide much information in establishing a specific diagnosis. Tumor position, pattern of bone destruction, presence of visible tumor matrix, presence and type of periosteal reaction, and other characteristics are important clues to the nature of the lesion. However, computed tomography (CT) is better to reveal the osseous and soft tissue extent of the process. Intraosseous extension of the tumor leads to the conversion of fatty marrow to marrow-containing tumorous tissue with higher attentuation. The ability of CT to delineate the soft tissue extent of a bone tumor is the consequence of its excellent contrast resolution. The relationship between the tumor and major neurovascular bundles can be demonstrated effectively by CT, especially if intravenous contrast material is administered.

CT is more important in staging for the surgical planning than in the actual diagnosis of primary bone tumors. However, in anatomically complex areas, such as the spine, pelvis, scapula, cross-sectional imaging obtained by CT may identify lesions that are obscured on the conventional radiography. CT allows differentiation of a fatty, cystic and fibrous lesion. Matrix calcification or ossification, indicative of a cartilagenous or a osteogenic tumor, is better demonstrated by CT than conventional radiography.

CT represents an excellent technique for monitoring the effects of radiation therapy or chemotherapy on bone tumors. Tumor regression, growth, or recurrence can be defined by CT. Also, the ability of CT to monitor biopsy or aspiration procedure provides additional advantages.

CT is superior to magnetic resonance imaging (MRI) for detecting subtle cortical erosions and periosteal reaction. If the conventional radiographs suggest cortical destruction and soft tissue mass, MRI would be the preferred modality since it provides an excellent soft tissue contrast and can determine the extraosseous extension of the tumor much better than CT.

[1] Department of Diagnostic Radiology, Seoul National University College of Medicine, Seoul, Korea.

Osteoma

Osteoma is a slow growing osteoblastic lesion which arises from membranous bones such as the outer table of the calvarium and in the frontal and ethmoid sinuses. Osteoma is an asymptomatic lesion and its importance lies in its common association with intestinal polyposis in the condition known as Gardner syndrome. The radiographic features consist of a mass of dense bone of variable size with a sharply defined and homogeneously dense bony structure on CT.

Osteoid Osteoma

Osteoid osteoma is a benign but painful bone tumor usually identified by means of its clinical and radiographic features. The pain arising from osteoid osteoma is classically worse at night and strikingly responsive to aspirin. Use of conventional radiography, radioisotope bone scan and CT provides a definite preoperative diagnosis and precise localization. The long tubular bones of the lower extremity are most frequently affected, although any bone may be affected. The lesion is characterized by a nidus may be purely radiolucent or have a sclerotic center, measuring up to 1.5 cm in diameter and showing variable degrees of ossification and is often surrounded by a zone of reactive bone formation. Four types of osteoid osteoma - cortical, medullary, subperiosteal and periarticular(intracapsular) - can be distinguished depending on the location of the lesion in the bone. The degree and extent of the sclerotic reaction surrounding an osteoid osteoma are variable. When the tumor occurs in cortical bone, the lesion is surrounded by dense sclerosis and periosteal new bone. Lesions arising in subperiosteal, trabecular bone or within joints may evoke limited sclerotic response. Osteoid osteoma arising in an intra-articular location deserve special emphasis. Clinical manifestations may be attributed falsely to a primary articular disorder, so that accurate diagnosis is commonly delayed. Osteoid osteomas arising in the spine also represent a diagnostic challenge owing to the complex anatomy of the vertebral column, and variable clinical findings. Osteosclerosis of a pedicle, lamina, articular process is observed. Identification of radiolucent nidus frequently requires special techniques such as conventional tomography or computed tomography. CT scanning has largely replaced conventional tomography in the evaluation of osteoid osteomas. In those cases in which the lesion is small or not readily apparent on conventional radiography, CT may be required. CT is also valuable in a defining osteoid osteomas in the spine, pelvic bones and femoral neck.

The standard treatment for osteoid osteoma is surgical excision of the nidus. This results in rapid, and at times dramatic, relief of the patient's symptoms. Recently, percutaneous removal of nidus of an osteoid osteoma has been introduced as an alternative to open surgery. This method requires precise guidance of drill or other equipment by CT.

Osteoblastoma

Osteoblastoma is histologically similar to osteoid osteoma and is composed of a well vascularized connective tissue stroma in which there occurs active production of osteoid, but which is characterized by its larger size. The age range of occurrence is also similar to that of osteoid osteoma: 75% of osteoblastomas are found in patients in their first., second, or third decade. Although the long bones are frequently involved, the lesion has a predilection for the vertebral column. The radiographic features of osteoblastoma are varied and, in most instances, nondiagnostic. Osteolysis alone, osteosclerosis alone, or a combination of both osteolysis and osteosclerosis may be observed. Radiographically, osteoblastoma has three distinctive presentations [1]. A giant osteoid osteoma which is usually more than 2 cm in diameter and exhibits less reactive sclerosis and a possibly more prominent periosteal response than osteoid osteoma [2]. A blow-up expansion similar to an aneurysmal bone cyst with small radiopacities in the center. This pattern is particularly common in lesions involving the spine [3]. An aggressive lesion simulating a malignant tumor. The major diagnostic problem is differentiating it from osteosarcoma.

Osteosarcoma

Osteosarcoma is primarily a malignant neoplasm with the greatest predilection for the metaphysis, most frequently the distal femur and proximal tibia. Excluding myeloma, it is the most common primary bone tumor and primarily affects older children and young adults. Osteosarcoma is a malignant tumor arising from undifferentiated connective tissue of bone. To qualify as an osteosarcoma, the neoplasm should have proliferating malignant cells that produce either osteoid substance or material histologically indistinguishable from it.

Osteosarcoma is an entity that comprises several subtypes of malignant bone-forming neoplasms, which vary in aggressiveness from the high grade, with a propensity for metastases, to the low grade, usually with potential for local recurrence only. Extensive modification of the classification scheme for osteosarcomas has appeared in recent years. The traditional system using the designations of conventional and parosteal tumors has been replaced owing to the identification of many clinical, radiologic, and histologic varieties of osteosarcoma, although no single method of classification is accepted uniformly. Available systems employ such features as the precise location of the tumor within the bone (intramedullary or central, intracortical, surface, periosteal, or parosteal); the degree of cellular differentiation (high grade or low grade); the histologic composition (osteoblastic, chondroblastic, fibroblastic, fibrohistiocytic, telangiectatic, small cell, clear cell); the number of foci of involvement (single or multicentric).

Radiologic features of conventional osteosarcoma are medullary and corical bone destruction, an aggressive periosteal reaction, a soft tissue mass, and tumor bone either within the destructive lesion or at its periphery including the soft tissue mass. In some instances, an aggressive periosteal reaction determined by conventional means can provide clues as to the correct diagnosis. The most common types of periosteal response encountered with this tumor are the "sunburst" type and Codman triangle. Although additional imaging methods such as scintigraphy, arteriography, CT and MRI have been used in the evaluation of osteosarcoma, the "gold standard" in the specific diagnosis of this tumor remains the conventional radiograph.

CT can provide important evidence of discrete matrix calcification which can significantly narrow the diagnosis and is also useful in assessing the intramedullary and soft tissue extent of the tumor. An increase in the attenuation values of the tissue within the medullary canal is generally indicative of tumor extension or skip metastasis. The presence of edema or hemorrhage in the soft tissue leads to diagnostic difficulties. After the administration of contrast medium, usually well vascularized tumor mass can be distinguished from surrounding soft tissue. In patients receiving chemotherapy, CT is useful for assessing reduction in tumor volume, especially of the soft tissue components, and increase in tumor ossification. However, CT may not show significant changes in the extent or attenuation of marrow lesion, and the active tumor cannot be differentiated from intramedullary necrosis.

References

1. Resnick D (1995) Diagnosis of bone and joint disorders. 3rd ed Philadelphia, Saunders
2. Wegener OH (1992) Whole body computed tomography. 2nd ed Boston, Blackwell Scientific Publications
3. Greenspan A (1992) Orthopedic radiology; a practical approach. 2nd ed, New York, Gower Medical Publishing
4. Assoun J, Railhac JJ, Bonneviale P et al. (1993) Osteoid osteoma; percutaneous resection with CT guidance. Radiology 188:541–7
5. Schlesinger AE, Hernandez RJ (1990) Intracapsular osteoid osteoma of the proximal femur; findings on plain film and CT. Am J Roentgenol 154:1241–4
6. Farmlett EJ, Magid D, Fishman EK (1986) Osteoblastoma of the tibia; CT demonstration. J Compt Assist Tomogr 10:1068–70
7. Schreiman JS, Crass JR, Wick MR et al. (1986) Osteosarcoma: role of CT in limb-sparing treatment. Radiology 161:485–8
8. Seeger LL, Eckardt JJ, Bassett LW (1989) Cross-sectional imaging in the evaluation of osteogenic sarcoma; MRI and CT. Semin Roentgenol 24:174–84
9. Bloem JL, Taminiau AHM, Eulderink F et al. (1988) Radiologic staging of primary bone sarcoma; MR imaging, scintigraphy, angiography, and CT correlated with pathologic examination. Radiology 169:805–10
10. Fletcher BD (1991) Response of osteosarcoma and Ewing sarcoma to chemotherapy; imaging evaluation. Am J Roentgenol 157:825–33

Chapter 27

Computed Tomography in Skeletal Trauma

M. Reiser, A. Stäbler, C. Becker, and N. Holzknecht[1]

For the evaluation of skeletal trauma, plain radiograms are the first diagnostic step. Frequently, however, findings are ambiguous. Using fluoroscopy and spot films, a definite diagnosis can be made in many instances. If not, tomography or computed tomography (CT) is indicated.

Due to its cross-sectional imaging capabilities and high-contrast resolution, CT is able to visualize complex anatomical areas. In addition, coronal, sagittal, and oblique reformations provide superior anatomical display [27]. For three-dimensional (3D) reconstructions, a thin slice thickness and overlap of the slices help to reduce artifacts. Views from arbitrary angles with varying degrees of object transparency can be computed. Shading can be varied in order to show texture and interfaces.

Three-dimensional improves our understanding of the extent of the injury, the fracture components, their orientation, and the degree of displacement. It may have an impact on the surgical approach and the surgical hardware used. Potential surgical procedures can be simulated [6].

In August 1994, a Siemens Somatom Plus 4 Scanner was installed in the Department of Diagnostic Radiology, Klinikum Großhadern. With a scan time of 0.75 s, this is the first subsecond CT scanner. Various features of the Somatom Plus 4 are very useful for the examination of trauma patients. With a scanning volume of more than 1 m, screening for skeletal trauma of large anatomical areas is possible. It allows good access to the patient. Monitoring and intensive care treatment is improved. Shorter acquisition and calculation times allow for better examination of noncooperative and critically ill patients. Moreover, longer spirals allow for improved multiplanar constructions (MPR) and 3D reconstructions.

Pelvis and Hip Joint Injuries

A total of 29% of acetabular fractures are missed on the initial plain film examinations. In up to 40%, plain radiograms will not be adequate for interpretation. This may be due to poor patient positioning, inadequate exposure, or overlaying foreign matter.

One of the obvious advantages of CT is the visualization of the extent of bony, soft tissue, vascular, and visceral injuries in a single examination. In contrast to

[1] Department of Diagnostic Radiology, University of Munich, Germany.

plain film examinations (obturator and ala view) no repositioning and movement of the patient is required in CT. The patient is positioned comfortable on the scanning table and during the same scanning procedure, various anatomical areas of interest, e.g., the brain, the thorax, the abdomen and the pelvis can be examined.

In acetabular fractures, the cause of the fracture lines, displacement of fragments, and stability of the hip joint are clearly assessed using CT [12]. MPR and 3D recontructions allow for superior demonstration of complex injuries [3–5, 13, 14] (Fig. 1). Bony fragments interposed within the joint space and precluding reduction of the fracture are detected with high sensitivity. Femoral head fractures, which are frequently missed in complex hip trauma, are also readily detected.

Sauser et al. [25] discovered that in four out of 13 patients CT significantly influenced the treatment in pelvic fractures.

Using conventional radiography, 30%–70% of sacral and sacroiliac joint injuries remain undetected. CT is ideally suited to evaluate these injuries [2]. Anterior-posterior compression results in disruption of the anterior ligaments and lateral compression in posterior distraction. Vertical shearing forces may cause anterior and posterior sacroiliac ligament disruption with subsequent superior, posterior, or medial displacement. Based upon CT findings, four grades of sacroiliac joint injuries can be differentiated:

- Grade I: vacuum phenomenon
- Grade II: anterior widening
- Grade III: anterior and posterior widening
- Grade IV: complete bilateral rupture with anterior or posterior displacement of the sacrum

Insufficiency fractures of the sacrum are also often difficult to detect with conventional radiography. On radionuclide bone scans, vertical, often bilateral areas of increased uptake are seen. Insufficiency fractures of the sacrum evolve on

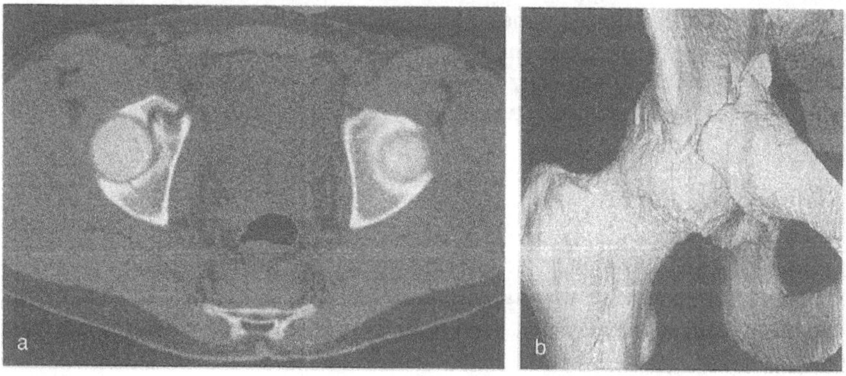

Fig. 1 **a** Fracture of the anterior column of the right acetabulum. In addition, a fracture line without dislocation is seen in the posterior portion of the acetabulum. **b** Three-dimensional reconstruction of an acetabular fracture. The medial wall of the acetabulum is displaced medially

the basis of osteoporosis and prior radiation therapy, rheumatoid arthritis and steroid medication are predisposing factors. On CT, sclerosis of the tabecular bone is seen in the early stages. Later on, fracture lines become evident, which may or may not contain gas [11].

Shoulder Injuries

CT and CT arthrography are very useful for the analysis of post-traumatic shoulder lesions. For the analysis of bony injuries, plain CT is adequate. When soft tissue injuries are suspected, such as labrum or capsule disruptions, CT arthrography should be used. The double-contrast technique with intra-articular administration of 2 ml contrast material and 10–15 ml air gives the best results.

Following glenohumeral luxation, tears of the glenoid labrum, osteochondral lesions of the glenoid rim, detachment of the joint capsule, and Hill-Sachs deformities can be found [22, 26]. These lesions are predisposing factors for recurrent luxation. With CT arthrography, they can be detected with high sensitivity and specificity. The normal glenoid labrum may be triangular of round on the axial CT image [16]. Following glenohumeral luxation, the labrum may be absent, deformed, irregular or fragmented. When the joint capsule is evaluated, variants of insertion of the capsule to the anterior portion of the glenoid process of the scapula have to be borne in mind. Medial insertion of the joint capsule is a predisposing factor to recurrent luxation. Detachment of the joint capsule from the scapula with subsequent dilatation of the joint space may result from prior glenohumeral luxation (Fig. 2). Bony fractures from the anterior and inferior glenoid rim (Bankart lesion) are also readily detected by plain CT.

Hill-Sachs deformaties manifest themselves as an impression fracture of the posterolateral contour of the humeral head at the level of the coracoid process of

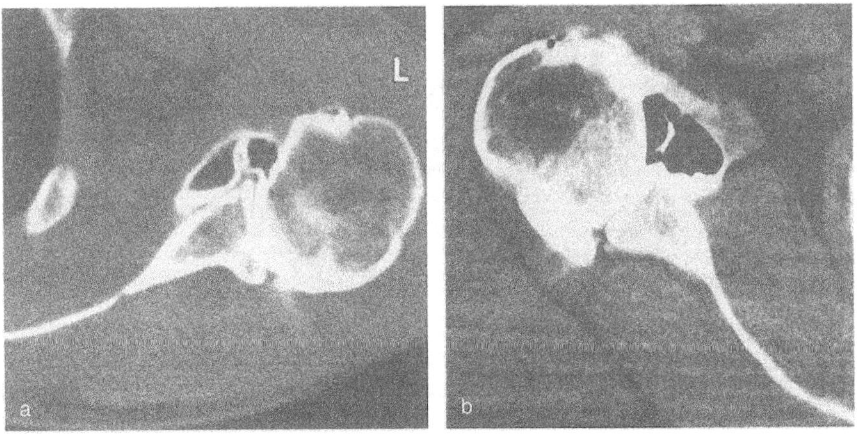

Fig. 2 **a** CT arthrography of the left shoulder. The patient had experienced a shoulder luxation. Detachment of the joint capsule from the anterior surface of the scapula. **b** CT arthrography of the right shoulder. Destruction of the anterior glenoid labrum

the scapula. Depending upon the extension of the humeral head compression fracture, three grades of Hill-Sachs deformity can be differentiated:

- Grade I: small (less than 30°)
- Grade II: moderate (30°–60°)
- Grade III: large (more than 60°)

Posterior shoulder luxation is much less frequent than anterior shoulder luxation (2%–4%) and it is often diagnosed with delay.

In extensive and comminuted humeral head fractures, CT enables a better evaluation of fracture elements [10]. Three-dimensional reconstruction contributes to superior demonstration of the extent of comminution.

Ankle and Foot Injuries

In the majority of cases, ankle fractures are adequately depicted using plain radiography. Subtle or complex osseous injuries of the ankle, however, are best evaluated by axial CT with sagittal and coronal reconstructions [15], which demonstrates the fracture fragments, their alignment, and the integrity of the tibial plafond. Fractures can be subclassified as two-part or three-part fractures. Pylon fractures result from axial compression and include severe distal tibial comminution and involvement of the tibial plafond.

For the precise analysis of calcaneal fractures, CT is extremely useful [7]. A total of 75% of calcaneal fractures are intra-articular, involving the posterior subtalar joint. The degree of calcaneal volume loss, size, and displacement of sustentacular fragments, disruption of the posterior articular facets, and impingement or entrapment of the lateral ankle tendons are detected using CT [23]. Fragments interposed in the joint spaces are also predisposing factors for post-traumatic osteoarthritis and can be detected with CT. The most common long-term complications of hindfoot fractures are subtalar joint arthritis resulting from joint incongruity and peroneal tendon impingement.

The talar dome is a common site of impact fractures resulting from inversion ankle injuries. The medial and lateral aspects of the dome are involved with equal frequency. While osteochondral fractures are clearly visualized on coronal plain CT, intra-articular contrast administration is required for the detection of lesions which are restricted to the hyaline cartilage [8].

Knee Joint

CT arthrography has been widely used for the examination of internal knee joint lesions, such as meniscus, cruciate ligament, hyaline cartilage, and collateral ligament injuries [17, 19, 21]. Following intra-articular injection of air with or without contrast medium, the internal knee structures are precisely depicted when special positioning is employed. When available, however, magnetic resonance imaging (MRI) is preferred because of its noninvasive nature and comprehensive visualization of all internal knee joint structures. With CT arthrography, high sensitivity and specificity for the assessment of cruciate ligament and meniscus tears was obtained [24].

In tibial head fractures or fractures of the femoral condyles, axial CT with MPR and 3D reconstruction allows for precise assessment of fracture elements, depression of the joint surfaces, and congruity of the joint surfaces.

Wrist Injuries

With both direct coronal, sagittal, and oblique scanning [1, 18, 20] and axial scanning with MPR and 3D reconstruction, a superior analysis of complex intraarticular fractures and fracture dislocations of the wrist is possible (Fig. 3). CT should be employed when plain films give ambiguous results. CT allows for precise delineation of fracture elements and entrapment of soft tissue. Ligamentous injuries, however, can only be visualized by arthrography, MRI, and CT arthrography.

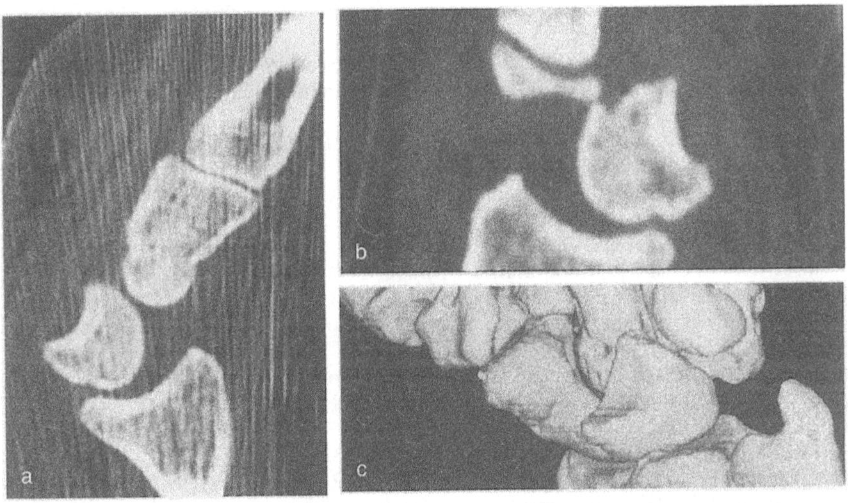

Fig. 3 **a** Direct sagittal imaging of the wrist. Rotation and subluxation of the lunate. **b** Sagittal reconstruction demonstrating the rotation and luxation of the lunate equally well. Streak artifacts are not present. **c** Three-dimensional reconstruction exhibiting dislocation of the lunate

Conclusions

CT is highly useful for the evaluation of musculoskeletal trauma when complex anatomical areas have to be evaluated or when plain film radiography gives ambiguous results. Spiral CT, with its fast image acquisition, allows for short examination times and can also be used in noncooperative and critically ill patients.

Various reports indicate that the use of CT enables better patient management, giving precise information for surgical planning.

However, soft tissue contrast and multiplanar capabilities make MRI a superior method for several indications, e.g., supraspinatus tendon and muscle lesions, chondral and meniscus lesions, and ligament injuries. Bone contusions and occult fractures are better seen on MRI. In daily practice, however, CT is easier to perform, especially when monitoring and intensive care treatment is required.

Plain film radiography remains the primary screening modality in skeletal trauma, and CT can be used as a problem-solving tool whenever further evaluations is needed [9].

References

1. Biondetti PR, Vannier MW, Gilula LA, Knapp P (1987) Wrists: Coronal and transaxial CT scanning. Radiology 163:149–151
2. Fishman EK, Magid D, Brooker AF, Siegelman SS (1988) Fractures of the sacrum and sacroiliac joint: evaluation by computed tomography with multiplanar reconstruction. South Med J 81:171–177
3. Fishman EK, Magid D, Drebin RA, Brooker AF Jr, Scott WW Jr, Lee RH Jr (1989) Advanced three-dimensional evaluation of acetabular trauma: volumetric image processing. J Trauma 29 (2):214–218
4. Scott WW Jr, Magid D, Fishman EK et al. (1987) 3D evaluation of acetabular trauma. Contemp Orthoped 15:17–24
5. Fishman EK, Magid D, Mandelbaum BR et al. (1986) Multiplanar (MPR) imaging of the hip. Radiographics 6 (1):7–53
6. Gerber J, Ney DR, Magid D, Fishman EK (1991) Simulated femoral repositioning with three-dimensional CT. J Comput Assist Tomogr 15 (1):121–125
7. Guyer BH, Levinsohn EM, Fredrickson BE, Bailey GL, Formikell M (1985) Computed tomography of calcaneal fractures: anatomy, pathology, dosimetry, and clinical relevance. AJR 145:911–919
8. Heare MM, Gillespy T, Bittar ES (1988) Direct coronal computed tomography arthrography of osteochondritis dissecans of the talus. Skel Radiol 17:187–189
9. Hindman BW, Kulik WJ, Lee G, Avolio RE (1989) Occult fractures of the carpals and metacarpals: demonstration by CT. AJR 153:529–532
10. Kilcoyne RF, Shuman WP, Atsen FA III, Morris M, Rockwood CA (1990) The Neer classification of displaced proximal humeral fractures – the spectrum of findings on plain radiographs and CT. AJR 154:1029–1033
11. Lourie H (1982) Spontaneous osteoporotic fractures of the sacrum. An unrecognized syndrome in the elderly. JAMA 248:715–717
12. Mack LA, Harley JD, Winquist RA (1982) CT of acetabular fractures: analysis of fracture patterns. AJR 1982:407–412
13. Magid D, Fishman EK, Brooker AF jr, Mandelbaum BR, Siegelman SS (1986) Multiplanar computed tomography of acetabular fractures. J Comput Assist Tomogr 10 (5):773–778
14. Magid D, Fishman EK, Sponseller PD, Griffin PP (1988) 2D and 3D computed tomography of the pediatric hip. Radiographics 8:901–933
15. Magid D, Michelson JD, Ney DR, Fishman EK (1990) Adult ankle fractures: comparison of plain films and interactive two- and three-dimensional CT scans. AJR 154:1017–1023
16. McNiesh LM, Callaghan JJ (1987) CT anthrography of the shoulder: variations of the glenoid labrum. AJR 149:963–966
17. Passariello R, Trecco F, de Paulis F, Masciochhi C, Bonanni G, Beomonte Zobel B (1985) Meniscal lesions of the knee joint: CT diagnosis. Radiology 157:29–34

18. Patel RB (1985) Evaluation of complex carpal trauma; thin-section direct longitudinal computed tomography scanning through plaster cast. J Comput Assist Tomogr 9:107–109
19. Pavlov H, Hirschy JC, Torg JS (1979) Computed tomography of the cruciate ligaments. Radiology 132:389–393
20. Quinn SF, Belsole RJ, Greene TL, Rayhack JM (1989) CT of the wrist for the evaluation of traumatic injuries. Crit Rev Diagn Imag 29:357–380
21. Reiser M, Rupp N, Karpf PM, Feuerbach ST, Anacker H (1981) Evaluation of the cruciate ligaments by CT. Eur J Radiol 1:9–15
22. Ribbons WJ, Mitchell R, Taylor GJ (1990) Computerized arthrotomography of primary anterior dislocation of the shoulder. J Bone Joint Surg (Br) 72-B:181–185
23. Rosenberg ZS, Feldman F, Singson RD, Price GJ (1987) Peroneal tendon injury associated with calcaneal fracutures: CT findings. AJR 149 (1):125–129
24. Sartoris DJ, Kursunoglu S, Pineda C, Kerr R, Pate D, Resnick D (1985) Detection of intraarticular osteochondral bodies in the knee using computed arthrotomography. Radiology 155:447–450
25. Sauser DD, Billimoria PE, Rouse GA, Mudge K (1980) CT evaluation of hip trauma. AJR 135:269–274
26. Singson RD, Feldman F, Bibliani LU, Rosenberg ZS (1987) Recurrent shoulder dislocation after surgical repair: double contrast CT anthrography. Radiology 164:425–428
27. Vannier MW, Totty WG, Stevens WG et al. (1985) Musculoskeletal applications of three dimensional surface reconstructions. Orthoped Clin N Am 16:543–555

CHAPTER 28

Clinical Applications of Spiral Computed Tomography Angiography

Jin Wook Chung and Jae Hyung Park[1]

Spiral computed tomography (CT) angiography (CTA) is a newly developed minimally invasive vascular imaging modality. Several papers have already described that CTA is a promising screening modality for renal artery stenosis [1–2], pulmonary thromboembolism [3] and pulmonary arteriovenous malformations [4]. The value of CTA in carotid artery stenosis has also been evaluated [5–9]. However, there are many other potential fields of clinical application which are currently being investigated.

During the past year, we performed a total of 300 procedures of CTA in 250 patients with diverse vascular diseases including aortic diseases, abnormalities of aortic branches, potential renal donors, postoperative evaluation of aortic surgery or bypass graft, pulmonary thromboembolism, pulmonary arteriovenous malformations, pulmonary sequestration, various venous abnormalities, and pancreas islet cell tumor.

The spiral CT examinations were carried out with Somatom Plus S (Siemens, Erlangen, Germany) scanners with a maximum continuous scanning time of 40 s. The examinations always began with a localizer scan (unenhanced standard CT, 5 mm X-ray beam collimation and 5 mm interslice gap) to screen the nature of the lesion and to determine the range of scan. The length of the lesion to be imaged determines the scanning parameters. As a basic principle, we fixed the nominal slice thickness (X-ray beam collimation) at 3 mm and adjusted the scan volume with a table speed and scanning time. It is generally recommended that the preliminary timing scan be performed with injection of a test dose (10–30 ml) of the contrast material in order to estimate the optimal scan delay time. However, we did not routinely employ it because the optimal scan delay time could be determined empirically according to the age of the patient and the site of the lesion. Only elderly patients or those with cardiac dysfunction were evaluated with timing scan. During the spiral scanning, between 100 and 150 ml of nonionic contrast medium (iopromide, 370 mg iodine per ml) was injected with an automatic power injector. For the evaluation of the thoracic vasculature, we routinely injected contrast material into the peripheral veins of the lower leg or foot. Scans were reconstructed at 2-mm intervals. Multiplanar reformation (MPR), shaded surface display (SSD), and maximum intensity projection (MIP) images were made with commercially available standard scanner software. In some cases, color-encoded three-dimensional (3D) surface reconstruction is more informative. This

[1] Department of Radiology, Seoul National University College of Medicine, Seoul, Korea.

was accomplished on an independent workstation (Allegro; ISG Technologies, Toronto, Ontario).

Aortic diseases

The major vessels of the thorax and abdomen are the best candidates for CTA because of their large luminal diameter. CTA can display the gross morphologic anatomy of the vascular structures, which is useful for surgical planning and is the greatest advantage of CTA to other imaging modalities in the evaluation of aortic diseases. In addition to the 3D display capability of CTA, a thin X-ray beam collimation of 3 mm and maximum vascular enhancement within a single breath-hold period enable accurate delineation of major aortic branches. CTA permits precise measurement of maximum dimension of aortic aneurysms, and demonstrates the extent of aortic aneurysms or dissections in relation to major aortic branches, their 3D morphology, extraluminal pathologies and the relationship to adjacent organs. Furthermore, CTA is the most sensitive technique for detecting and evaluating calcified lesions. Even the hemodynamically unstable patient of impending or acute aneurysm rupture or acute aortic dissection can be examined by CTA because of its short scan time. CTA provides not only the angiographic images reflecting the luminal changes of the aorta or its branches, but also thin high quality axial images that enable the evaluation of mural changes of the aorta. Therefore, mural changes of the aorta caused by atherosclerosis or Takayasu arteritis can be assessed. The diagnosis of aortic dissections, whether the false lumen is thrombosed or not, is no longer a diagnostic problem of CTA. When compared with the conventional CT, CTA provides an overall picture of aortic dissections and much more accurate evaluation of major aortic branch involvement. The site of the entry tear can be visualized in a large proportion of the patients. However, the aortic regurgitation cannot be imaged directly, only the indirect sign of the dilatation of aortic annulus and left ventricle. Highly movable dissection flap and motion artifact at the ascending aorta can obscure or mimic a dissection flap in a few images of a patient. CTA is a promising noninvasive modality for postoperative evaluation of aortic surgery.

Evaluation of Major Aortic Branches

We successfully applied CTA in the evaluation of the stenosis, obstruction or aneurysm of the major aortic branches. Renal artery stenosis and the celiac axis compression by the median arcuate ligament of the diaphragm are well demonstrated by CTA. According to Rubin et al. [2], CTA was 92% sensitive and 83% specific for the detection of high grade stenosis (≥70% stenosis) of the renal artery. CTA not only consistently depicts all main and accessory renal arteries [1–2], but also provides information about renal veins and renal parenchyma. Therefore, in the evaluation of potential renal donors and renal artery stenosis, CTA can be a promising noninvasive alternative to conventional angiography. Cumming and Morrow [5] compared CT angiography with conventional angiography for detecting stenosis at the carotid bifurcation. Results of CT angiography had a high degree of correlation with results of conventional angiography in the evaluation of carotid artery stenosis. CT angiography is multiplanar and allows differentiation of calcified plaque from contrast material, which provides information about plaque calcification, ulceration, and size that cannot be obtained with conventional angiography [5].

Pulmonary Vasculature

Recent papers have already described the clinical utility of spiral CT in the diagnosis of central pulmonary thromboembolism. Remy-Jardin et al. describe that spiral CT can reliably depict thromboemboli in second- to fourth-division pulmonary vessels. Remy et al. have described the clinical utility of unenhanced 3D spiral CT in pretherapy evaluation of the angioarchitecture of pulmonary arteriovenous malformation. In addition, anomalous systemic arteries in pulmonary sequestration and hypertrophied bronchial arteries indenting the bronchial lumen can be evaluated by CTA.

Venous Abnormalities

Spiral CT angiographic technique can also be applied in the evaluation of venous abnormalities. Venous abnormalities can be evaluated with CTA in two different ways. Renal veins, pelvic veins, and portal venous system can be imaged with adequate delay time after antecubital injection of the contrast media. In central or peripheral venous obstruction, diluted contrast media are injected directly into the ipsilateral or bilateral peripheral veins of the hand and foot. This technique achieves strong venous enhancement even with small amounts of the contrast media.

Pancreatic Diseases

We performed spiral CT in six consecutive patients with suspected pancreas islet cell tumor and consistently demonstrated a hypervascular tumor in the pancreas in all patients. Vascular invasion of pancreas cancer and pseudoaneurysm complicating pancreatitis can also be assessed with CTA.

Vascular resolution of CTA largely depends on the voxel size and the degree of vascular enhancement. In the spiral scan with 512×512 matrix, field of view of 25 cm, X-ray beam collimation of 3 mm, and pitch of 1, the voxel size is $0.5 \times 0.5 \times 3.0$ mm. This implies that the z-axis resolution is the limiting factor and the axial projection image has the best vascular resolution. Therefore, one must make an effort to reduce the slice thickness and to utilize the axial projection view adequately. The age, the body weight, and the circulatory status of the patient should be considered in determining the optimal scan delay time and the injection rate of contrast media. In young patients with rapid circulation time, the injection rate of contrast media should be increased. In case of severe valvular regurgitation or left-to-right shunt, the degree of vascular enhancement is markedly decreased. Many other factors affect the quality of CTA images. Cooperation with adequate breath-holding and the body habitus are patient-related factors. Obesity increases the image noise which detracts from the image quality. Anatomic location and the orientation of the vessel are also important. Even the small vessels running perpendicular to the imaging plane can be clearly depicted on CTA. However, a small vessel of oblique or transverse orientation is not clearly seen due to partial volume averaging. For better delineation of these vessels, overlapping reconstruction in thinner intervals may be helpful. CT artifacts around the shoulder and the inflow of the contrast media impairs the delineation of arch vessels.

The value of CTA in vascular imaging can be summarized as follows. It is a noninvasive imaging modality. Although inferior in spatial resolution, it is superior to catheter angiography in contrast resolution. It preserves the advantages of cross-sectional imaging. It depicts mural changes of the major vessels. It displays the gross morphologic anatomy of the vascular structures and their spatial relationship to adjacent organs three-dimensionally. It can demonstrate and specify extrinsic causes of vascular stenosis or obstruction.

References

1. Galanski M, Prokop M, Chavan A, Schaefer CM, Jandeleit K, Nischesky JE (1993) Renal artery stenosis: spiral CT angiography. Radiology 189:185–192
2. Rubin GD, Dake MD, Napel S et al. (1994) Spiral CT of renal artery stenosis: comparison of three-dimensionl rendering techniques. Radiology 190:181–189
3. Remy-Jardin M, Remy J, Wattinne L, Giraud F (1992) Central pulmonary thromboembolism: diagnosis with spiral volumetric CT with the single-breath-hold technique – comparison with pulmonary angiography. Radiology 185:381–387
4. Remy J, Remy-Jardin M, Giraud F, Wattinne L (1994) Angioarchitecture of pulmonary arteriovenous malformations: clinical utility of three-dimensional helical CT. Radiology 191:657–664
5. Cumming MJ, Morrow IM (1994) Carotid artery stenosis: a prospective comparison of CT angiography and conventional angiography. AJR 163:517–523
6. Schwartz RB, Jones KM, Chernoff DM et al. (1992) Common carotid artery bifurcation: evaluation with spiral CT. Radiology 185:513–519
7. Marks MP, Napel S, Jordan JE, Enzmann DR (1993) Diagnosis of carotid artery disease: preliminary experience with maximum-intensity-projection spiral CT angiography. AJR 160:1267–1271
8. Dillon EH, van LeeuwenMS, Fernandez MA, Eikelboom BC, Mali WPTM (1993) CT angiography: application to the evaluation of carotid artery stenosis. Radiology 189:211–219.
9. Castillo M (1993) Diagnosis of disease of the common carotid artery bifurcation: CT angiography vs catheter angiography. AJR 161:395–398

Chapter 29

Contrast Enhancement in Hepatic Computed Tomography

Byung Ihn Choi and Joon Koo Han[1]

Introduction

Although it is generally agreed that intravenous administration of contrast media is necessary for imaging hepatic lesions and that bolus infusion is preferable to drip infusion, a consensus is lacking about the optimal injection protocol. Issues that remain unresolved during hepatic contrast-enhanced computed tomography (CT) include the total volume of contrast material necessary, the rate of injection of contrast material, whether the bolus should be uniphasic or biphasic, and the optimal delay between the onset of injection of contrast material and the beginning of imaging [1, 2].

In this presentation, basic principles and the various techniques available for enhancing the liver during abdominal CT scanning will be reviewed. In addition, controversial issues regarding the most advantageous method of administering intravenous (IV) contrast material for enhancement of the liver will be addressed.

Basic Principles of Contrast Enhancement

Intravenous iodinated contrast material is a fundamental part of abdominal CT examination. If properly administered, contrast medium enhances normal tissue to a greater degree than most infectious and neoplastic processes; determines the course, caliber, and patency of blood vessels; characterizes tissue perfusion patterns; and, in some instances, help to characterize a lesion. When improperly administered, intravenous contrast medium can obscure lesions [3]. Most hepatic abnormalities are identified on CT by visualizing regions of altered hepatic attenuation. Generally, a difference of at least 10 HU between the abnormal and normal regions of liver must be present for accurate detection of liver lesions. Although many of these abnormalities can be detected on non-contrast-enhanced CT, attempts to increase the differences in CT attenuation between normal liver and hepatic abnormalities have been made with various administration techniques of intravenous contrast media [4].

Intravascular administration of contrast medium leads to time-dependent distribution of contrast medium in different tissue compartments. Contrast

[1] Department of Radiology, Seoul National University, College of Medicine, Seoul, Korea.

enhancement is dose dependent on the one hand and, on the other hand, dependent on other pharmacokinetic factors (e.g. hemodynamics, hydrophilia, lipophilia, osmolality, protein binding, etc.).

Water-soluble nonionic contrast media used today are well tolerated, display high renal clearance and low protein binding (< 1%); diffuse from the vessel lumina via the capillary walls to the interstitial space (extracellular contrast media) and are then eliminated from the blood in the kidney and secreted by means of glomerular filtration. Osmosis-related tubular reabsorption of water leads to an increase in the contrast medium concentration in the renal tubules and collecting tubules (urography). High protein binding would prevent rapid glomerular filtration and leads to active uptake of contrast medium into the liver cells (hepatography). In this case, contrast medium is secreted into the bile ducts (choledochography).

Pharmacokinetics

When contrast agents are given intravenously, blood concentrations immediately begin to rise. As soon as the infusion is stopped, blood concentrations will begin to fall rapidly, but at an ever-decreasing rate.

Why does the blood concentration fall and where does the contrast media actually go? This question can be answered simply by naming the three events which account for the fate of the injected contrast media: (1) dilution in the blood, (2) diffusion into the extravascular space, and (3) excretion by the kidneys. The intravascular dilution accounts for only a part of the rapid initial fall in blood concentration. Renal excretion has very little effect on the blood concentrations during the first few minutes after intravenous injection. The fall in blood concentration is largely due to the diffusion of contrast media out of the capillaries into the interstitium, that is, into the extravascular, extracellular fluid spaces (Fig. 1). The rate of diffusion and the amount temporarily accumulated can vary considerably from tissue to tissue, and is affected by pathological processes.

The events occur as follows: contrast media diffuses into the interstitium, beginning even before intravascular dilution has stabilized. In some tissues, such as the liver, heart, lungs, and spleen, this diffusion is very rapid and the concentration-time curves are similar in shape to the blood curve, although lower in magnitude. In some other tissues, such as the skin, fat and skeletal muscle, diffusion is slower and the extravascular accumulation of contrast media is delayed.

As contrast media diffuses into the interstitium of a given tissue, the blood concentration will begin to fall. Renal excretion will contribute to this fall. As the blood concentration gets lower and lower, and the interstitial fluid concentration gets higher and higher, the concentration gradient will continue to fall. Diffusion of contrast media into each interstitial fluid space will eventually stop as the concentration gradient falls to zero. Since the contrast media in the blood is continuously cleared by glomerular filtration, the concentration gradient between blood and interstitium finally reverses. After the reversal of the concentration gradient there will be a net flow of contrast media back into the capillaries. Renal uptake and excretion account for the long-term fall in blood concentration [5].

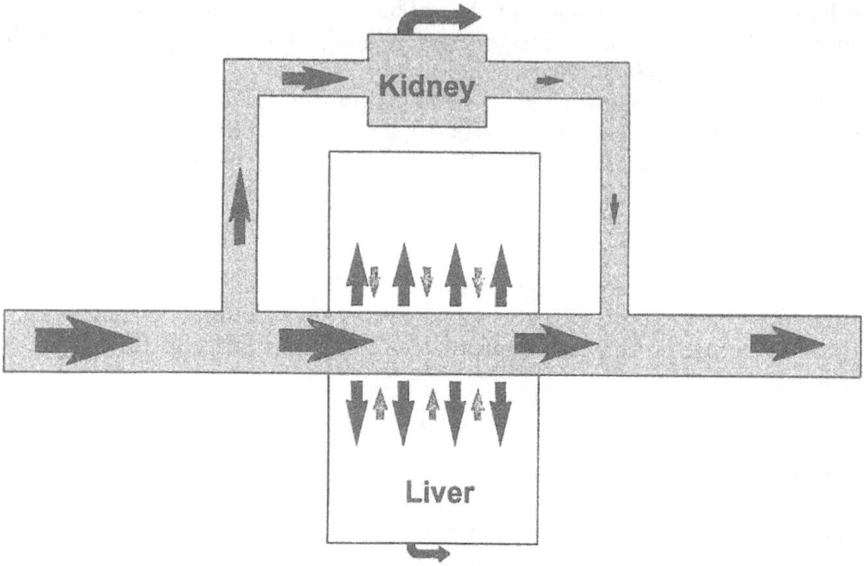

Fig. 1 Distribution of intravascular contrast medium. Contrast injected into the blood stream diffuses into the extracellular space. At the same time, contrast medium is excreted by the kidney. A small amount of the contrast is excreted by the liver. During the early phase, the diffusion of the contrast medium into the interstitial space (extravascular, extracellular space) is the major cause of contrast elimination from circulating blood as well as the contrast enhancement of viscera. As the concentration of the contrast medium in circulating blood decreases because of renal excretion, the contrast medium in the interstitial space diffuses back into the circulating blood

Hepatic Contrast Enhancement

Contrast medium enhancement can be divided into three phases: bolus, nonequilibrium (redistribution), and equilibrium. When aortic enhancement is plotted against time by using either a monophasic or biphasic injection, a characteristic curve with three phases is obtained. Aortic enhancement increases rapidly during the bolus-injection phase. During this bolus phase, the initial circulating contrast material is being replenished by a peripheral intravenous injection. Although processes such as plasma expansion due to osmotic effects and diffusion of contrast material along a concentration gradient into the extravascular spaces will lower aortic enhancement, the replenishment effect of peripherally injected contrast material is dominant. Vascular enhancement increases progressively until the end of injection. Aortic enhancement decreases steeply during the second, "nonequilibrium," or redistribution, phase. During this phase, intravascular contrast material diffuses rapidly into the extravascular space. This diffusion occurs at different time rate constants in different body tissues, but is relatively rapid in the liver and relatively slow in muscle and fat.

The progressive rise in hepatic attenuation that occurs during the bolus and nonequilibrium phases represents both vascular and extravascular contrast material. That hepatic enhancement is maintained near peak late in the nonequilibrium phase even when portal venous enhancement is beginning to fall indicates that most hepatic enhancement at this phase is due to extravascular contrast material. When intravascular and extravascular contrast material equilibrate-the "equilibrium phase"-enhancement slowly declines at a rate determined by means of renal filtration. The onset of the equilibrium phase can be easily determined by means of sequential measurement of aortic and hepatic enhancement. When the two enhancement curves become parallel and decline at an equal rate, equilibrium has been achieved (Fig. 2) [7, 8].

During the bolus phase, an arteriovenous attenuation difference of greater than 30 HU is achieved. In the nonequilibrium phase, the arteriovenous difference falls but is still greater than 10 HU. In the equilibrium phase, the arteriovenous attenuation difference is less than 10 HU. Unfortunately, phase 1 lasts about 60 s and phase 2 persists for only 2 min, although this temporal window depends on various injection parameters of contrast medium.

The importance of scanning the liver only during the bolus and nonequilibrium phases has been well demonstrated [9]. Liver enhancement rises more slowly than that in the aorta, reaches a broad "plateau," and declines slowly. Conspicuity of focal hypovascular hepatic lesions, however, is not equivalent for scanning performed on the upward slope and the downward slope of the hepatic enhancement curve [8].

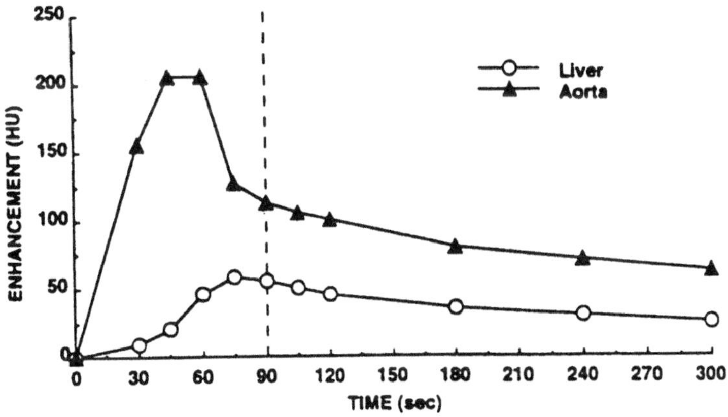

Fig. 2 Determination of "equilibrium phase". The onset of the equilibrium phase occurs when the aortic and hepatic contrast enhancement curve become parallel and decline at the same rate. In this curve, the equilibrium phase begins approximately 90 s after the start of contrast medium injection. (Reprinted from reference [10])

CT Techniques

Incremental Bolus Dynamic Scan

This is the preferred CT technique for routine hepatic evaluation, providing rapid acquisition of axial images using automatic table incrementation during the infusion of a large amount of iodinated contrast medium. In this method, 150–180 ml 60% iodinated contrast material is administered by an automatic power injector. Contrast material is injected in either a monophasic or a biphasic mode. In biphasic mode, 50 ml of contrast material is delivered at 5 ml/s, followed by 130 ml delivered at 1 ml/s (Fig. 3a). The uniphasic technique delivers 150 ml at 2.5 ml/s for 60 s (Fig. 3b). A biphasic injection with a high initial flow rate produces high peak contrast enhancement but delayed onset of equilibrium and thus provides a longer optimal scanning interval (Table 1) [10].

The advantages of a biphasic injection are clear: an earlier, higher hepatic peak enhancement and delayed onset of the equilibrium phase when compared with both slower hepatic peak and short preequilibrium period of monophasic injection [8].

Four to ten images per min should be obtained after the contrast material has had time to circulate into the portal system (approximately 45 s from the start of the bolus). By using automatic table incrementation, an image repetition rate of 10 scans per minute, and a 2-s scan time, the entire liver can be scanned within 2–3 min.

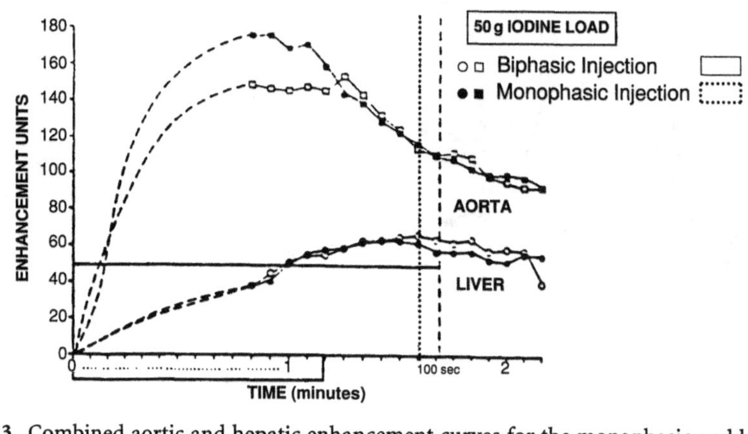

Fig. 3 Combined aortic and hepatic enhancement curves for the monophasic and biphasic injection protocol. The *dotted line* indicates the calculated equilibrium time for the monophasic protocol and the *dashed line* indicates the biphasic protocol. In this study, the monophasic protocol was an injection of 3 ml/s of contrast materials for 60 s; the biphasic protocol was an injection of 5 ml contrast materials for 10 s followed by 2 ml/s for 65 s. With the biphasic protocol, a longer pre-equilibrium period can be achieved. However, the peak enhancement was higher with the monophasic protocol. With helical CT, this slightly longer pre-equilibrium period has minimal impact on the examination. However, with a conventional scanner, the advantage of the biphasic protocol is clear. (Reprinted from [15])

Table 1 Time Intervals [10]

Protocol	Mean time to maximum liver enhancement (s)	Mean time to equilibrium (s)
Biphasic-low flow	106 ± 31[a]	162 ± 11
Biphasic-high flow	87 ± 13	144 ± 11
Uniphasic-low flow	84 ± 14	92 ± 11 (p < 0.03)*
Uniphasic-high flow	71 ± 19	59 ± 11 (p < 0.001)*

Numbers represent mean values ± one standard deviation.
[a] Significantly longer than for the other three protocols ($p < 0.05$).
* p values refer to the difference between each uniphasic protocol and the two biphasic protocols.

Drip Infusion

Slow infusion of contrast medium is the least effective of all possible CT imaging methods. It only mildly enhances the liver tissue and provides time for some lesions to accumulate enough contrast medium to become isodense and obscured. It is actually inferior to noncontrast scans in focal lesion detection [3].

Single-Level Bolus Dynamic Scan

This technique is employed for assessing the contrast enhancement characteristics of a single lesion, such as a hemangioma during the initial vascular phase of enhancement. Again, 150 ml 60% iodinated contrast medium is injected and rapid sequential scans are obtained at the same level.

Delayed High-Dose Contrast CT (Delayed CT)

When the findings of the standard liver CT study are equivocal or negative, delayed images obtained 4–6 h after contrast medium injection may be helpful. The rationale for this technique is based on the fact that normal hepatocytes extract and excrete 1%–2% of the iodine load into the biliary system, whereas focal lesions do not. Contrast medium delivered to a neoplasm during bolus injection has been cleared by this time. The normal liver is enhanced by an average of 20 HU, whereas focal lesions are hypodense. Small lesions that take up contrast medium and become isodense during the bolus phase are missed on dynamic scans but are visible on delayed scans. At least 60 g iodine must be given to the patient to enhance the parenchyma reliably for delayed scanning.

Delayed scanning provides more discrete lesion margination and is useful for patients at high risk for metastases who have normal bolus scans. In one study, delayed scanning was shown to be superior to dynamic CT; however, time and logistic problems limit its routine use [11, 12].

Spiral CT

Spiral CT, because of its relatively short scanning time, overcomes some of the constraints of conventional CT of the liver [13, 14]. With spiral CT, the entire liver can be imaged during the peak of hepatic enhancement without scanning during the equilibrium phase.

For spiral CT of the liver, the optimal scan delay depends on the volume of contrast agent used and the rate at which it is administered. For most IV contrast injection protocols, a scan delay of 60–70 s is appropriate [2, 8]. Another advantage of spiral CT is the ability to scan the liver during both the hepatic arterial and portal venous phases of enhancement to improve detection of vascular hepatic masses. A potential advantage of spiral CT, which remains to be documented, is the possible reduction in the volume of contrast material used for hepatic CT.

Type of Tumor Versus Contrast Enhancement

The visibility of hepatic tumors depends on their enhancement relative to the normal parenchyma. Tumor visibility varies with the vascularity of each tumor and the phase of contrast at the time of CT scanning. Thus, optimization of hepatic tumor detection requires careful timing of scanning to coincide with maximal tumor conspicuity.

Dynamic incremental hepatic CT scanning protocols are designed to optimize imaging during the portal venous predominant phase of enhancement because in Western countries most liver tumors are metastases. Three quarters of hepatic parenchymal blood supply is contributed by the portal vein, whereas tumors derive their blood supply entirely from hepatic artery branches. Hepatic arterial enhancement begins approximately 20 s after bolus initiation, with portal venous enhancement peaking at 70–120 s.

Most metastatic tumors are hypovascular and appear as low-attenuation lesions during much of the bolus and nonequilibrium phases. However, during the latter part of the nonequilibrium phase and into the equilibrium phase, many of the tumors become isodense compared with the liver.

Unlike hypovascular tumors, hypervascular tumors may appear hyperdense relative to the hepatic parenchyma during the early bolus phase and may become isodense compared with the liver in the early nonequilibrium phase. Therefore, such neoplasms are better imaged during the arterial phase of hepatic enhancement.

Conclusion

Although it is universally accepted that the use of IV contrast material improves detection of hepatic and abdominal abnormalities, the method of administration is one of the most hotly debated issues in contemporary radiology. Despite nearly 15 years of research on the subject, it is hard to find more than a handful of radiologists who can agree on what constitutes the optimal method of contrast administration. Most of the controversy surrounds the use of contrast agents for optimizing detection of hepatic tumors [1].

On the other hand, most institutes in Korea use nonspiral CT scan. Therefore, incremental dynamic liver scans with conventional CT is the mainstay for liver imaging. A biphasic injection with a high initial flow rate is recommended for incremental liver scans with conventional CT [10].

Recently, slip-ring scanners with helical scanning capability have been introduced in Korea. Volume helical scanning involving slip-ring systems with table translation, however, offers the prospect of optimizing the "temporal window" for dynamic hepatic CT scanning. Monophasic and biphasic protocols produced equivalent results when tailored for the shorter temporal window of a rapid sequence helical acquisition [15]. Monophasic protocol is better than biphasic protocol in convenience for use. Therefore, a monophasic injection with a moderate flow rate is recommended for the spiral CT.

References

1. Dodd GD, Baron RL (1993) Investigation of contrast enhancement in CT of the liver: the need for improved methods. AJR 160:643–646
2. Walkey MM (1991) Dynamic hepatic CT: how many years will it take 'til we learn? Radiology 181:18–21
3. Gore RM (1994) Liver; normal anatomy and examination techniques. In: Gore RM, Levine MS, Laufer I eds Textbook of gastrointestinal radiology, 1st ed Philadelphia, PA: Saunders, 1801–1804
4. Baron RL, Freeny PC, Moss AA (1992) The liver. In: Moss AA, Gamsu G, Genant HK eds Computed tomography of the body with magnetic resonance imaging. 2nd ed Philadelphia, PA: Saunders, 743–748
5. Wegener OH (1992) contrast media. In: Wegener OH ed Whole body computed tomography. 2nd ed Boston, MA: Blackwell Scientific Publications, 99–105
6. Dean PB, Violante MR, Mahoney BS (1980) Hepatic CT contrast enhancement: effect of dose, duration of infusion, and time elapsed following infusion. Invest Radiol 15:158–161
7. Foley WD, Berland LL, Lawson TL et al. (1983) Contrast enhancement technique for dynamic hepatic computed tomographic scanning. Radiology 147:797–809
8. Cox IH, Foley WD, Hoffman RG (1991) Right window for dynamic hepatic CT. Radiology 181:18–21
9. Burgener FA, Hamlin DJ (1983) Contrast enhancement of hepatic tumors in CT: comparison between bolus and infusion techniques. AJR 140:291–295
10. Heiken JP, Brik JA, McClennan BL, Sagel SS, Forman HP, DiCroce J (1993) Dynamic contrast enhanced CT of the liver: comparison of injection rates and uniphasic and biphasic injection protocols. Radiology 187:327–331
11. Bernardino ME, Erwin BC, Steiberg HV et al. (1986) Delayed hepatic CT scanning: increased confidence and improved detection of hepatic metastases. Radiology 159:71–74
12. Miller DL, Simmons JT, Chang R et al. (1987) Hepatic metastasis detection; comparison of three CT contrast enhancement methods. Radiology 165:787–790
13. Bluemke DA, Fishman EK (1993) Spiral CT of the liver. AJR 160:787–792
14. Heiken JP, Brink JA, Vannier MW (1993) Spiral (helical) CT. Radiology 189:647–656
15. Foley WD, Hoffman RG, Quiroz FA, Kahn CE, Perret RS (1994) Hepatic helical CT: contrast material injection protocol. Radiology 192:367–371

CHAPTER 30

Electron Beam Tomography in Cardiopulmonary Imaging

William Stanford[1]

Indications

At The University of Iowa Hospitals and Clinics, electron beam computed tomography (EBCT) is the imaging modality of choice in evaluating chest and cardiovascular disease. In the chest, most EBCT studies are performed to define lung nodules, masses, infiltrative disease, and interstitial fibrosis. In the heart, EBCT is useful for assessing anatomy as well as cardiac function, including such quantitative indices as ejection fraction (EF), stroke volume (SV), chamber volume, diastolic filling, and myocardial mass determinations. EBCT also has the capability of assessing intracardiac thrombus and wall motion abnormalities as well as the pericardium and great vessels. In the above applications, the short acquisition time of the EBCT scanner allows for the artifact-free assessment of the mediastinum, lung, heart, and major vessels – all of which may be blurred when imaged with scanners with 1 s or longer scan times. This paper will discuss EBCT scanning in cardiopulmonary disease.

Technical Specifications of the EBCT Scanner

The EBCT scanner images at 130 KV with 635 mA. Slice thicknesses of 1.5, 3, 6, and 10 mm are possible in the single-slice mode and 8 mm in the multislice mode. Reconstruction fields of view range from 9 cm to 47.5 cm with image matrices of 256^2, 360^2, and 512^2. Image reconstruction occurs every 0.8 s for 256^2 (50-ms) images and every 3.0 s for 512^2 (100-ms) images.

EBCT incorporates an electromagnetic beam to direct electrons onto four tungsten target rings (Fig. 1). This approach eliminates all scanner mechanical motion and provides image acquisition in less than one tenth of the time required by current CT scanners. Each 210° sweep of the electron beam is accomplished in either 50 or 100 ms, depending on the scanning sequence. The x-rays generated from the target ring pass through the patient onto a double ring of sodium iodide detectors located in the gantry above the patient.

[1] Cardiovascular Imaging, Department of Radiology, University of Iowa, College of Medicine.

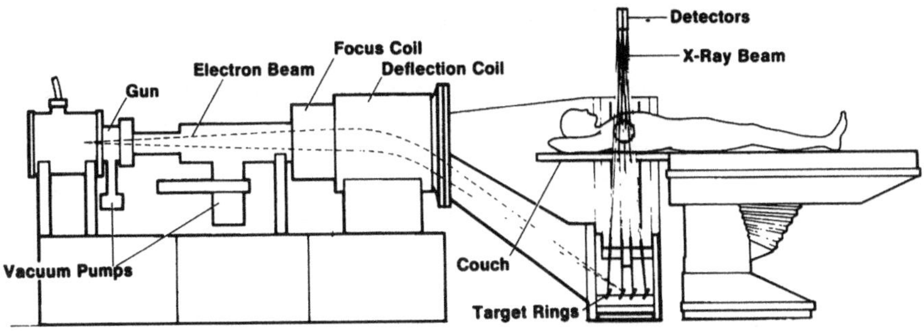

Fig. 1 Cross sectional diagram of the scanner. The electron beam is bent electromagnetically to sweep one of the target rings. The X-rays generated by the sweep of the target ring pass through the patient onto a double ring of detectors located in the gantry above the patient

Modes of Scanning

There are four scanning modes: flow mode, movie mode, step volume scanning (SVS) mode, and continuous volume scanning (CVS) mode.

Flow Mode (Multislice Mode)

In this mode, it is possible to scan 8 cm of the body in 224 ms. The table does not move. These eight slices are acquired from the four target rings through the use of a double detector array. When the 50 ms scans are repeated in rapid succession, the resulting images can be used to analyze contrast arrival time and direction and to assess airway collapse and pulmonary ventilation/perfusion relationships.

Movie Mode (Multislice Mode)

In cardiac imaging, the movie or cine mode is helpful. In the movie sequence, the target rings are swept 17 times per s, with images being acquired every 58 ms. Because of limitations in computer memory, the maximum number of images that can be obtained is 80. Therefore, ten images are normally acquired per level. The target ring sweeps are triggered from the R wave of the electrocardiogram (ECG), and, with this sequence, the image acquisitions are sufficient to encompass an entire ventricular contraction from diastole through systole. By displaying the ten images sequentially, the contracting heart can be viewed in near real-time on a level-by-level basis. Images are generally viewed on a 256 × 256 display matrix, using a 30-cm reconstruction circle. This yields a pixel size of 1.37 mm^2.

Step Volume Scanning Mode (Single-Slice Mode)

In this mode, a single target ring is swept using a 100-ms scan time as the table moves by predetermined increments through the gantry. Longer exposures are accomplished by averaging up to six 100-ms sweeps. The longer scan times increase radiation dose but decrease noise. Scans obtained in 100 ms are usually diagnostic even in patients who cannot breathhold. Scans may be acquired at 1.5-, 3-, 6-, and 10-mm slice thicknesses, and 40 levels can be acquired in 76 s, depending on the number of averages selected.

Continuous Volume Scanning Mode (Single-Slice Mode)

Continuous volume scanning is available in the most recent EBCT scanners. This sequence uses continuous table motion to acquire 40 levels in 16 s. The slice thickness of the continuous scans is adjustable from 6 to 10 mm.

Positional Considerations

Cardiac functional analyses are generally performed on images generated from a short axis study. Short axis positioning is obtained by slewing the scanner couch 25° to the patient's right and placing the table in 15° of downward tilt. This brings the long axis of the heart approximately perpendicular to the scanner gantry. This orientation approximates the parasternal short axis orientation of two-dimensional echocardiography. In this orientation, all wall segments except for the cardiac apex are well visualized.

For better evaluation of the cardiac apex and the lateral and septal walls in a longitudinal orientation, the patient table is slewed 25° to the patient's left. This produces a long axis image, which is comparable to the four-chamber view of echocardiography.

To encompass the entire heart, scanning usually begins at the apex and continues superiorly to include the proximal great vessels. Appropriate slice locations are determined from a scout image. With a slice thickness of 8 mm, it normally requires two eight-level short axis acquisitions to encompass the heart. The long axis study typically requires only eight levels.

Contrast Medium Administration

Quantification of cardiac function requires optimal visualization of the chamber endocardial borders. To ensure optimum chamber enhancement, the patient's circulation time is usually determined. In our institution, a 10-ml bolus of 0.5% magnesium sulfate is injected intravenously, and the interval between the injection and the time the patient experiences a warm salty taste in the mouth is recorded. Alternatively, the circulation time can be determined either by recording the transit time required for a Cardio-green dye bolus to arrive at an ear densitometer or by calculating the elapsed time it takes for a test bolus of contrast material to arrive in the heart.

For functional cardiac measurements, the short axis movie sequence is used, and scanning is delayed for a period equal to the patient's circulation time plus 10 s to allow for optimal chamber contrast enhancement. The contrast dose used is typically 60–90 ml per sequence administered at a rate of 1.5–1.9 ml/s. However, the maximum contrast dose should not exceed 3 ml/kg of body weight.

To ensure optimal chamber opacification in patients with cardiac enlargement, poor cardiac contractility, or long circulation times, the contrast medium administration rate may be increased to 2.2 ml/s. Because it often requires additional sequences to image an enlarged heart, care must be taken not to exceed the contrast limitations. To minimize respiratory motion and further improve resolution, imaging is usually performed during breathholding.

Nonionic contrast material is used for all cardiac function studies because it minimizes the undesirable hemodynamic perturbations that can occur with ionic contrast administration. These perturbations may affect quantitative measurements such as SV by altering heart rate and blood pressure. An additional advantage is that patients experience less discomfort with the use of nonionic material, and this improves patient acceptance.

For lung, mediastinal, and aortic imaging, we use 150 ml of ionic or nonionic 60%–76% iodinated contrast material administered at 1.5 ml/s. and delay scanning for 20 s to allow maximal opacification of the great vessels. In the flow mode sequence, we generally use 40 ml 76% iodinated nonionic contrast material injected at 10 ml/s; for the cine mode, we use 60 ml of 76% iodinated nonionic contrast material injected at 1.5 ml/s. The timing the cardiac sequence is dependent on the circulation time and the type of study performed. For airway and pericardial disease, contrast is not usually administered.

Chest Imaging

Airway Imaging

The use of 100-ms volume mode sequences at 3-, 6-, or 10-mm slice thicknesses provides anatomic definition of fixed or acquired upper airway abnormalities. These abnormalities include soft-tissue masses in the nasal or pharyngeal spaces as well as fixed stenoses of the trachea or bronchi.

The flow mode is used to study nonfixed upper airway disease. In adult patients with sleep apnea, dynamic scanning of the upper airway has shown that small, collapsible oropharyngeal and nasopharyngeal airways plus the posterior displacement of the tongue are the causative mechanisms for the obstruction. EBCT findings also correlate well with the endoscopic findings in laryngomalacia, tracheomalacia, and vocal cord paralysis. Compared with endoscopy, dynamic imaging by EBCT has the advantages of being noninvasive and not requiring sedation. Thus, measurements can be made under more physiologic conditions.

Lung Parenchyma Imaging

High-resolution EBCT scans using 3-mm collimation, 100-ms scan times, and high-resolution reconstruction algorithms have been successfully used to evaluate diseases of the pulmonary parenchyma. Although this technique is associated with increased image noise, the net advantage of EBCT over conventional CT is the marked decrease in motion unsharpness. EBCT accurately displays the anatomy of the secondary pulmonary lobule, which is the basic functional subunit of the lung. Abnormalities of the airway (bronchial wall thickening and bronchiectasis), air space (consolidation), and interstitial septal thickness can be seen on 3- or 6-mm-thick volume mode static images.

Mediastinum Imaging

Volume mode EBCT scans provide excellent anatomic detail of neoplastic, inflammatory, and vascular lesions of the mediastinum. Flow mode sequences can add information about blood flow and the dynamic changes occurring in airway disease.

Pulmonary Embolism Imaging

EBCT has shown promise in diagnosing pulmonary embolism. By virtue of its 100-ms scan time and its ability to encompass the entire chest in 16 s, the EBCT scanner may prove superior to other CT scanners. Teigen et al. [1] reported 86 patients with suspected pulmonary embolism who were studied with EBCT and pulmonary angiography. EBCT detected pulmonary emboli in 39 of these patients. Of this group, 25 patients had angiographic and/or pathologic proof of pulmonary embolism. In this subset, 19 scans showed pulmonary emboli on both EBCT studies and angiography. Four showed no pulmonary emboli on either EBCT or angiography. There was one false-positive and one false-negative examination.

A recent study at the University of Iowa Hospitals and Clinics, investigated the accuracy of EBCT in the detection of pulmonary embolism in the animal model. Eight pigs were scanned with contiguous 3-mm scans from the lung apex to the diaphragm both before and after the introduction of a single 7×15 mm autologous clot into the jugular vein of each pig. To identify the clot, a silk suture was threaded into the center. Opacification of the pulmonary arteries was achieved using 135 ml 76% iodinated contrast material administered via a mechanical injector at 1 ml/s. In the eight animals that received no embolus, no embolus was seen. In six of the eight animals that received an embolus, the embolus was identified on both the EBCT study and autopsy. In six of the animals, the correlation was exact; in one, an embolus was found on the same side, but further distally than at autopsy. In the remaining animal, the clot was not detected by EBCT. (In this instance, a suture with only a few clot fragments was identified at autopsy signifying the shattering of the clot as it was injected.)

Regional Assessment of Lung Ventilation and Perfusion

Regional assessment of lung density changes during inspiration and expiration can provide evidence of the small airway and early interstitial disease.

In addition, we are continuing investigations in correlating ventilation and perfusion measurements with anatomic measurements of rib cage and diaphragm geometry. Other studies have demonstrated that volumetric scanning can be used to determine the exact center lines of airways and vessels including their branch points out to the fifth or sixth generation. This allows investigators to follow a particular lung structure during breathing. Hence, EBCT has the potential of providing anatomic and physiologic information that may supplement other tests of lung function.

High-resolution CT is changing the role of pulmonary imaging. The ability to study airway mechanics and blood flow may soon allow the physician to derive information that is not currently available using our present clinical tools.

Cardiovascular Imaging

Myocardial Contractility

Short axis tomographic images of the beating heart can provide excellent anatomic information relative to global and regional ventricular contractility. The cine display of the heart in near real-time allows the observer to identify areas of hypokinesis, akinesis, and dyskinesis. In addition, these sequences allow for the quantification of ventricular function. If myocardial thinning is present in association with a wall motion abnormality, its presence provides additional documentation of previous myocardial infarction and/or aneurysm formation.

From its early development, EBCT showed promise of being a powerful modality for the qualitative assessment of wall motion abnormalities. An early study by MacMillan and Rees [2] compared EBCT and biplane contrast ventriculography in the evaluation of left ventricular (LV) wall motion abnormalities in patients with ischemic heart disease. These investigators evaluated 84 ventricular segments and found agreement between EBCT and ventriculography in 92%. No wall segment classified as normal by ventriculography was found to be abnormal on EBCT. Similarly, no wall segment that demonstrated abnormal contractility on ventriculography was interpreted as having normal motion on EBCT. Similar findings were described by Bateman et al. [3], who found a 94% agreement between EBCT and cardiac catheterization in characterizing wall motion abnormalities.

Feiring et al. [4] looked at regional wall motion. These investigators found that there was a dyssynchronous pattern of segmental LV contraction in normal subjects. This heterogeneity varied from segment to segment. Specifically, regional contractility was found to be greatest near the apex and decreased in a fairly predictable manner toward the base. These findings have important implications in evaluating ischemic heart disease.

Quantification of Chamber Volumes

Unlike angiography and echocardiography, in which ventricular volumetric measurements are based on geometric assumptions, EBCT measurements are independent of such assumptions. With EBCT, the volumetric analysis of a cardiac chamber is easily performed by tracing the endocardial borders at end-diastole and end-systole. This is performed using a track-ball - assisted cursor tracing and applying a modified Simpson's rule to these data. Pietras et al. [5] found an excellent correlation between EBCT and phantom volumes. These authors also found an excellent correlation between EBCT and biplane cineangiography (*r*, 0.99; SEE, 4.36). Similar results have been shown in the quantification of left atrial cast volumes of dogs.

Stroke Volume

Reiter et al. [6] compared the EBCT quantification of left (LVSV) and right (RVSV) ventricular stroke volumes using thermodilution techniques and electromagnetic flow (EMF) probe measurements in instrumented dogs. In these studies, the EBCT and thermodilution LVSV determinations showed a very good correlation (*r*, 0.99; SEE, 1.47 ml). Correlations between EBCT and EF determinations were almost as impressive (*r*, 0.95; SEE, 1.43 ml).

The quantification of right ventricular (RV) volumes is more difficult, primarily because there are no geometric models that satisfactorily approximate the shape of this ventricle. As a result, accurate RV end-diastolic and end-systolic volumetric measurements using two-dimensional echocardiography and angiography are difficult to achieve. Cross-sectional EBCT imaging, however, permits the reproducible and accurate measurements of RV end-diastolic and end-systolic volumes, as shown in experiments by Ringertz et al. [7] and Mahoney et al. [8].

Regurgitant Volume

Regurgitant volume determinations require measurements of end-systolic and end-diastolic volumes. From these data, it is possible to calculate EF and SV. In healthy individuals, RVSV and LVSV should be nearly identical; therefore, any differences should be the result of valvular insufficiency. Experimentally, good correlations were found between EBCT and EMF measurements of regurgitant volumes in animals with univalvular insufficiency.

Ejection Fraction

EF is the most universally used measure of cardiac performance. The quantitation of EF using EBCT requires planimetry of ventricular end-systolic and end-diastolic volumes at each level. Once the planimetry is accomplished, the EF is computed using the software inherent within the scanner. By applying a modified Simpson's rule to the data, it is possible to calculate the global EF.

Systolic Function

The cross-sectional imaging capability of EBCT readily allows a qualitative assessment of regional wall motion. As mentioned, ventricular contractility varies by location; hence, with EBCT, the regional performance of each individual wall segment can be assessed. With computer assistance, the ventricle at each level can be interrogated by radii, thereby generating data relating to segmental regional performance and EF. By employing either an endocardial or epicardial centroid, regional contractility can also be displayed graphically and numerically calculated. Quantitatively, this form of analysis provides a more specific assessment of ventricular contractility and may be useful in monitoring patients with regional myocardial contraction abnormalities. Similarly, the serial assessment of myocardial contractility by region may prove helpful in following the patient's recovery after myocardial infarction.

Diastolic Function

Myocardial diastolic functional information can also be readily obtained from EBCT imaging. Regional ventricular compliance can vary significantly not only between ventricles but also within each ventricle. From the diastolic filling curve one can calculate time to peak filling fraction and time to peak filling rate.

There are a number of disease processes that can affect diastolic filling, yet have little effect on global systolic function. Specifically, amyloidosis, small vessel coronary disease, and ventricular hypertrophy may all present with abnormal diastolic filling despite a quantitatively normal EF. The assessment of ventricular diastolic filling is particularly applicable in constrictive pericardial disease.

Cardiac Output

Cardiac output (CO) is another measurement of overall cardiac performance. Before the development of EBCT, CO was measured by indicator dilution techniques. Now EBCT has proven to be highly accurate in measuring CO. The time-density software inherent in the EBCT scanner permits these measurements to be performed routinely and simply. Using nonionic contrast material and standard thermodilution techniques, Garrett et al. [9] showed good correlations between UFCT and thermodilution measurements of CO over a wide range of CO (r, 0.92).

Myocardial Mass Quantitation

Ventricular mass is an important measurement in disease processes that produce myocardial hypertrophy. This includes LV outlet obstruction, hypertensive states, and cardiomyopathies. Modalities such as radionuclide ventriculography, thallium imaging, and biplane ventriculography are unable to quantitate ventricular mass. With UFCT, this determination is straightforward and requires only planimetry of the endocardial and epicardial borders.

The EBCT determination of myocardial mass was initially validated by Feiring et al. [10]. These investigators showed an excellent correlation between EBCT and myocardial mass in autopsied dogs (r, 0.99; SEE, 4.1 g). Furthermore, the reproducibility was excellent and there was little intraobserver (r, 0.99) or interobserver variability (r, 0.99). The accuracy of UFCT as compared with that of two-dimensional echocardiography in the estimation of LV mass has also been good (r, 0.89; < 0.002). However, quantification of RV mass by echocardiography and angiography has not been as reliable primarily because these determinations again require geometric assumptions to characterize RV shape. Hajduczok et al. [11] showed that mass measurements using 3-mm thick short axis EBCT images acquired in a volume mode during diastole were reliable and correlated well with autopsy measurements. The authors reported no significant differences in mass when measurements were obtained from thin (3 mm) or thicker (6 mm) slice thicknesses or when calculations were done on contiguous or discontiguous images.

Aortic Aneurysms

EBCT cross-sectional images can define aortic dissection flaps, vessel enlargement, and periaortic tissue abnormalities. These are important in assessing dissections and leaking aneurysms and in evaluating other periaortic pathology. Excellent vessel opacification is possible if the circulation time is first determined.

Measurement Reproducibility

Unlike other imaging modalities, such as echocardiography where results can be influenced by operator performance, EBCT repeatedly has been shown to have little interstudy variability in the calculations of either mass or ventricular volumes. Furthermore, multiple studies over time have shown little interobserver or intraobserver variability.

Disadvantages of EBCT

EBCT has disadvantages that temper its role in functional imaging. Although it may be reasonable to consider EBCT as a noninvasive test, cardiac examinations require contrast enhancement, and this necessitates the placement of an intravenous catheter. The use of contrast material may pose problems for patients with borderline renal function or known allergy to contrast material. Furthermore, the EBCT scanner is not readily available in many medical centers, and the scanner's relatively high price limits its availability. Although there is a negligible whole-body radiation dose for a movie study (0.58 cGy/image), the perceived radiation danger and lack of portability may support a clinician's preference for echocardiography.

Technical problems can also limit image acquisition. Functional quantification cannot be performed unless the scanner is properly triggered from the R wave of the ECG. If mistriggering occurs, the images may not be acquired throughout the entire cardiac cycle. Often, cardiac arrhythmias, particularly atrial fibrillation, are relatively common and may result in improper triggering, thus precluding quantitative analysis.

Electron beam technology has proven to be extremely useful in the qualitative and quantitative analysis of cardiac function. The millisecond image acquisition time, superior spatial resolution, and scanner versatility make EBCT an attractive imaging modality for the determination of cardiac function. High-performance dynamic imaging, coupled with proven measurement accuracy and reliability, characterizes the superiority of EBCT in performing functional cardiac analysis.

References

1. Teigen CL, Maus TP, Sheedy PF II, Johnson CM, Stanson AW, Welch TJ (1993) Pulmonary embolism: Diagnosis with electron beam CT. Radiology 188:839
2. MacMillan RM, Rees MR (1988) Measurement of right and left ventricular volumes in humans by cine computed tomography: Comparison to biplane cineangiography. Am J Cardiac Imaging 2:214
3. Bateman TM, O'Byrne GT, Forrester JS et al. (1986) Global and regional left ventricular function in ischemic heart disease: Accurate evaluation by cine CT (abstr). J Am Coll Cardiol 7:172A
4. Feiring AJ, Rumberger JA, Reiter SJ et al. (1988) Sectional and segmental variability of left ventricular function: Experimental and clinical studies using ultrafast computed tomography. J Am Coll Cardiol 12:415
5. Pietras RJ, Wolfkiel CJ, Veselik K et al. (1991) Validation of ultrafast computed tomographic left ventricular volume measurement. Invest Radiol 26:28
6. Reiter SJ, Rumberger JA, Feiring AJ et al. (1986) Precision of measurements of right and left ventricular volume by cine computed tomography. Circulation 74:890
7. Ringertz HG, Rogers B, Lipton MJ et al. (1985) Assessment of human right ventricular cast volume by CT and angiocardiography. Invest Radiol 20:29
8. Mahoney LT, Smith W, Noel M et al. (1987) Measurement of right ventricular volume using cine computed tomography. Invest Radiol 22:451
9. Garrett JS, Lanzer P, Jaschke W et al. (1985) Measurement of cardiac output by cine computed tomography. Am J Cardiol 56:657
10. Feiring A, Rumberger J, Reiter SJ et al. (1985) Determination of left ventricular mass in dogs with rapid acquisition cardiac computed tomographic scanning. Circulation 6:1355
11. Hajduczok ZD, Weiss RM, Stanford W et al. (1990) Determination of right ventricular mass in humans and dogs with ultrafast cardiac computed tomography. Circulation 82:202

CHAPTER 31

X-Ray Angiography in the Computed Tomography

Dai Jian-ping, and Zhu Ming-wang[1]

X-ray angiography had once been considered as the sole method to evaluate blood vessels, and also is an important examination for intracranial neoplasms. As computed tomography (CT) and magnetic resonance imaging (MRI) is used more extensively, the number of X-ray angiography has been reduced dramatically. CT and MRI can provide more valuable diagnostic information than X-ray angiography about tumor location and nature. However, the persentage of negative cases of X-ray angiography is decreasing, the positive cases is increasing. The role of X-ray angiography changed in the CT era.

MR angiography and CT angiography

MR angiography (MRA), now available in most of MRI system, is sensitive to flowing blood signal and can depress background signal. MRA could be used in evaluating intracranial circulation, aneurysms, vascular malformation, arterial or venous occlusive diseases. But the spatial resolution of MRA is not as good as X-ray angiography, it could not replace X-ray angiography right now. By MRA, patient can be screened in an noninvasive, safe, and convenient way before performing conventional X-ray angiography.

MRA can show all the vessels, include artery and vein, in one acquisition. On its source images, vessels appear as bright signal while brain tissue show moderate singal intensity. The relationship between vessels and brain tissue is displayed nicely. In patient of facial spasm, we can demonstrate the small arterial loop that pulse the facial nerve and cause facial spasm. On MRA images of A-V-M, it also shows the feeding artery, draining vein and malformation vascular nodules as well as hemorrhage. On PC MRA, wen can determine the direction and velocity of blood flow to show the specific vascular structure clearly. MRA can show blood vessels in the three-dimensional (3D) mode, let us observe the vascular structures at many different projections.

CT angiography (CTA) is a newly vascular imaging modality which is very promising in some ways. It not only tells us the morphology of the blood vessels but also its patency. It can demonstrate the calcification of the vessels.

[1] Neuroimaging Center, Beijing Tiantan Hospital, Beijing, China 100050.

X-Ray Angiography

X-ray angiography was an important imaging modality of brain tumors before CT and MRI were widely used. On X-ray angiographs, doctors mainly looked for vascular structures deformation or blood vessels shift, abnormal lumen and abnormal circulation. Upon the X-ray angiographic appearences, doctors decided where the tumor was, what the tumor nature might be, whether or not there was a vascular disease.

After introduction of CT and MRI, we can evaluate the tumor nature and location easily by CT and MRI scan. The excellent spatial resolution and intensity resolution of CT and MRI images can demonstrate the intracranial disease more accurate than ever before. CT and MRI had largely replaced the X-ray angiography in evaluating the tumor location and demonstration the tumore nature. The number of X-ray angiography procedures has been decreased. However, X-ray angiography is the best imaging method for intracranial vascularity. It cannot be replaced completely by CT and MRI. By now, most of X-ray angiography procedures are performed after CT or MRA examination. We do hope angiography can give more diagnostic information about blood vessels which we cannot get from CT or MR scan. So the positive cases of angiography are increased.

On CT or MRI images, we can diagnose the tumor location, possible pathological nature of tumor. We will not perform X-ray angiography for this purpose. To find the relationship between tumor and big vessels, to display abnormal vascularity, to demonstrate the feeding artery and draining vein, we must depend on X-ray angiography to show all these critical details of vascular structures. There is no other imaging methods to show such fine vascular structures.

Based on super-selective X-ray angiography, the interventional radiology developed rapidly. Therapeutic angiography has become a new application field of X-ray angiography.

X-ray angiography is superior to other vascular imaging methods. It can show different blood circulation phases, display vascular lumen of large area with high speed. The most important advantage of X-ray angiography is its spatial resolution, higher than others, and its accuracy and reliablity in clinical diagnosis. However, X-ray angiography is an invasive examination. It cannot show the wall of vessel and surrounding tissue as good as it can be done by CT and MRI.

Conclusion

The number of negative X-ray angiography procedures had been reduced, the percentage of positive cases is increased. Although CT and MRI are widely used, conventional angiography cannot be replaced completely. X-ray angiography is the golden standard of intracranial vessel diseases. X-ray angiography is still a developing imaging technique.

CHAPTER 32

Computed Tomographic Angiography*

M.S. van Leeuwen, L.J. Polman, J. Noordzij, B. Velthuis, and P.F.G.M. van Waes[1]

Introduction

Computed tomographic angiography (CTA) is a vascular imaging technique based on the rapid acquisition of volumetric CT data during the bolus phase of intravenously administered contrast [1–3]. CTA is a recent diagnostic technique and is still under development. Only preliminary studies on its diagnostic value have been performed. In this chapter the technique is described and the clinical experience of various research groups with a number of specific CTA applications is discussed. The latest generation of CT scanners are equiped with slip-ring current and data transfer. This makes it possible to rotate the assembly of X-ray tube and X-ray detectors continuously. During this continuous rotation the patient can be moved at a constant speed through the plane of the X-ray tube and detectors. The simultaneous linear movement of the patient and continuous rotation of the X-ray tube creates a helical path of the X-ray beam relative to the patient's longitudinal axis. From the continuous, helical data acquisition, axial CT slices can be reconstructed at any desired location along the longitudinal axis of the examined volume. Overlapping slices can be reconstructed with no additional radiation to the patient, improving anatomic resolution in the longitudinal direction and enabling image reconstructions to be performed in any desired plane [4, 5]. The quality of these reconstructions is markedly improved from conventional CT due to the continuous helical data acquisition. In conventional CT, data acquisition and subsequent table transport takes 6–12 s for each slice. With helical CT a full rotation usually takes 1 s and, depending on the capacity of the X-ray tube, up to 50 rotations can be acquired in one scan. Therefore, the time needed to image a large number of overlapping slices is dramatically reduced. Vascular detail is optimized because the entire volume of interest is scanned at peak vascular enhancement during a single breath-hold.

* This chapter has been published previously in Lanzer P, Rösch J (1994) Vascular diagnostics. Springer, Berlin Heidelberg New York.

[1] University Hospital Utrecht, Department of Radiotherapy and Nuclear Medicine, Heidelberglaan 100, 3584 CX Utrecht, The Netherlands.

Methods

In order to comprehend the diagnostic scope and technical limitations of CTA, basic knowledge is required of the technical parameters inherent in helical data acquisition, and of different means of image display.

Data Acquisition

As in conventional CT, image quality depends on the combination of contrast and spatial resolution [6, 7]. Contrast and spatial resolution in the transverse plane is defined by the X-ray contrast between anatomic structures, the diameter of the volume of interest, or field of view (FOV), and the reconstruction filter used. Data acquisition during peak vascular enhancement will result in optimal contrast between vascular lumina and surroundings. Consequently, intravenous contrast is administered with a mechanical injector at a high injection rate, and the delay between start of injection and image acquisition is adjusted to the region under study. The size of the FOV is minimized to include only the region of interest, thus further optimizing in-plane resolution. The reconstruction filter is adjusted to optimize the balance between signal-to-noise ratio and in-plane resolution. Spatial resolution along the longitudinal or *z*-axis is limited by the slice thickness, but can be improved by using overlapping reconstructions. Slice thickness itself is the end product of the collimation size, the table speed, and the reconstruction algorithm used to reconstruct axial slices from the helical data.

In any CTA application, helical scanning and contrast parameters have to be adjusted to the anatomy under investigation. For instance, if a large volume has to be investigated, as in CTA of aortic disease, a large number of rotations are required. If aortic dissection is suspected, the entire thoracoabdominal aorta can be imaged in one acquisition if 10 mm/s table speed an 10-mm slice collimation are chosen. Resolution on the *z*-axis will be poor due to volume averaging in thick slices. However, in-plane resolution is not influenced by slice thickness, and intimal tears can be depicted accurately along their entire length. Conversely, if the abdominal aorta is investigated for aneurysmal disease, the presence and location of accessory renal arteries must be assessed. A total of 40–50 rotations with a table speed of 5 mm/s and a collimation of 5 mm will cover the entire abdominal aorta and still yield sufficient resolution on the *z*-axis. In order not to exceed 150 ml of nonionic contrast (iopromide; Ultravist 300, Schering AG), an injection rate of 2–2.5 ml/s, with a scan delay of 30 s, will provide a high intravascular contrast level during the entire acquisition (Tables 1, 2). If CTA is optimized for detection and grading of stenoses in the renal arteries, which are usually located in the transverse plane, resolution on the *z*-axis should be as high as possible and collimation and table speed should preferably be kept at or below 3 mm and 3 mm/s respectively. To optimize spatial resolution intense vascular enhancement at the level of the renal arteries is required. This can be achieved by measuring the transit time between peripheral injection and peak enhancement at the level of the renal arteries after injection of a small amount of contrast. Thus, the scan delay is optimized and the injection rate can be set at 3–5 ml/s to provide maximum contrast and spatial resolution at the desired anatomic level.

Table 1 Data acquisition in spiral volume scanning

Parameter	Value
Number of rotations	50–40
Slice thickness (mm)	10, 5, 3, and 1.5
Pitch (table speed/collimation)	1
Reconstruction index (mm)	5, 2, and 1
Tube voltage (kV)	140–120
Tube current (mA)	250–225 and 125

Table 2 General contrast protocol in computed tomography angiography (CTA)

Parameter	Value
Contrast medium	Iopromide (Ultravist 300, Schering AG)
Volume (ml)	150, 140, or 100
Flow (ml/s)	4.5, 3, 2.5, or 2
Delay (s)	35, 30, 25, or 20

The CTA image display modes used are cine display, multiplanar reformatting (MPR), maximum intensity projection (MIP), and shaded surface display (SSD-3D).

Although the compromise between imaged volume and resolution on the *z*-axis applies to all CTA applications, differences in CT scanners exist. The total amount of rotations with sufficient X-ray power varies between 24 and 50 in one acquisition. Consequently, the scanner with the maximal amount of rotations will be able ot image a longer anatomic region with comparable resolution in the *z*-axis, or an equal anatomic volume with improved resolution along the *z*-axis. At our institute we use a spiral CT scanner (SR 7000. Philips Medical Systems. Best) capable of 50 consecutive rotations with a rotation time of 1 s. A tube voltage of 120 kV and a tube current of 250 mAs is possible, which is relatively high for spiral CT and provides a good signal-to-noise ratio.

To compensate for the limitation in the amount of rotations, a table speed in excess of the collimation can be chosen. For instance, if table speed is increased from 5 to 10 mm/s without an increase in collimation, a twofold increase in imaged volume is achieved. However, the resolution along the *z*-axis will be significantly lower, due to increased volume averaging.

Image Display

Due to the continuous helical data acquisition, overlapping axial slices can be reconstructed at any desired location along the *z*-axis. To minimize partial volume averaging, the distance between the center of the reconstructed slices (reconstruction index) should be approximately half the collimation and table speed [7]. Thus, an acquisition with 5 mm collimation and 5 mm/s table speed should be reconstructed with a reconstruction index of 2 or 3 mm, whereas an acquisition with 10 mm collimation and 10 mm/s table speed should be reconstructed with a reconstruction index of 5 mm.

The reconstructed, overlapping, axial slices can be displayed on film, comparable to conventional CT. However, interpreting vascular anatomy on a series of cross-sectional images on a light box is cumbersome and prone to inaccuracies. The overall geometry of the investigated vascular region is difficult to perceive due to the obliquitiy and tortuosity of the vascular structures relative to the axial slices. For the same reason, detection and grading of stenoses on the axial slices along can be difficult. To overcome these limitations different postprocessing procedures can be performed on the CT operator console or alternatively, off-line, on a dedicated workstation [8].

Cine Display

The entire stack of overlapping axial slices can be loaded into image memory, and can be subsequently displayed in interactive cine mode. Perception of vascular anatomy is more intuitive, and the time needed to examine a large stack of slices in markedly reduced. By tracking the vascular structures in the craniocaudal direction of the data set, focal abnormalities can be searched for, and the optimal level for assessment of disease severity is easily found.

Mulitplanar Reformatting

The stack of overlapping axial slices can be reconstructed along any desired plane by using a multiplanar reformatting (MPR) algorithm. Coronal and sagittal reformations are valuable in displaying longitudinal vascular structures such as the aorta. More recent algorithms allow curved and curved-oblique reformations. Using these algorithms, reformatting along the tortuous course of a vessel results in display of the full extent of the vessel in a single image.

Although informative, some limitations are inherent to MPR. Spatial resolution of the reformations is a resultant of in-plane resolution in the axial slices and longitudinal resolution, defined by collimation, table speed, and reconstruction index. Because in-plane resolution is markedly superior to longitudinal resolution, definition of vascular detail will be low if the course of the vessel deviates significantly from the longitudinal axis. Also, if MPR is used for grading of stenoses, off-axis reformations will result in overestimation of stenoses, while eccentric stenoses can be underestimated by inappropriately chosen reformation planes.

Maximum Intensity Projection

With a maximum intensity projection algorithm (MIP), angiogram-type display is achieved. The entire stack of transverse images is loaded into computer memory and a set of parallel mathematical rays traverses the data volume. Every ray identifies the voxel with the highest CT density (HU or Houndsfield Unit) along its path and displays it on a projection plane perpendicular to the rays. Because a single MIP lacks depth, a cine loop can be created, built op of multiple projections with increasing serial angulation. The resulting display is comparable to that of conventional angiography, but allows an infinite number of projections. In order to be displayed, the vessel of interest should have the highest number of HU along the path of the imaginary projection rays. Consequently, bone or densely enhanced veins can obscure arterial lumina. To solve this problem, bone or veins can be removed from the axial sclices by manual or semiautomatic editing.

The use of MIP to display CTA data has advantages and disadvantages. MIP provides an efficient means of conveying a survey of the anatomic data because all the vascular structures with sufficient density are displayed in the projections. Another advantage of MIP is its relative insensitivity to partial volume averaging.

If a vessel follows a tortuous course, its transverse segments will suffer significantly from volume averaging due to relatively low resolution along the *z*-axis. The HU values in such transverse segments will represent a mixture of luminal contrast and a significant portion of surrounding soft tissue and fat. Conversely, longitudinally oriented segments of the vessel will suffer less from volume averaging, and the HU values will represent luminal contrast, with only a small fraction of surrounding soft tissue and fat. As a result, HU values, equivalent to CT density, can vary greatly among different vessels filled with the same concentration of contrast, depending on their relative size and orientation with respect to the transverse plane. Consequently, MIP display a tortuous vessel with varying densities, higher in its vertical segments and lower in its horizontal segments. Interpretation of MIP of medium-sized and large arteries is not affected by this phenomenon, because the difference in density is not interpreted as a difference in luminal diameter. Only in transverse vessels with a diameter significantly smaller than the collimation and table speed, volume averaging may result in poor or nonvisualization of these vessels on MIP.

A limitation inherent in MIP is the need to remove overlying structures with densities equal to or higher than the vessels of interest. This editing process is time consuming and may result in partial loss of anatomic information.

Shaded Surface Display

Shaded surface display (SSD) is a surface-rendering algorithm, which results in three-dimensional renderings of the surfaces of the structures of interest. In contrast to MIP, an HU threshold is chosen, dividing the continuous scale of HU in a binary data set of values above and below the threshold. All voxels with densities below the threshold will be excluded from the reconstruction, and all voxels with densities above the threshold will be included.

Similar to MIP, SSD vividly display the vascular anatomy in a single image. However, apparent vessel size is strongly dependent on the chosen threshold, creating a significant subjective element in the procedure. Due to volume averaging vertical segments of a vessel will be displayed wider than horizontal parts.

Also, since all anatomic structures with a density above the threshold will be included in the SSD, plaque calcification can be displayed as part of the vessel lumen, resulting in underestimation of stenoses. Manual editing of the axial slices can prevent the inclusion of calcified plaque in the lumen, but such editing is time consuming and adds another subjective element to the resultant surface renderings.

Conclusions

Cine display and MPR are efficient means of presenting the information contained in the axial slices. MIP and SSD are postprocessing algorithms which require operator time and input, and result in overall images of vascular anatomy. An important difference between SSD and MIP is that in the latter no threshold is used: all pixels are shown with a density according to their original HU value. Conversely, in SSD, HU values are reduced to a binary data set in which each pixel either belongs to the volume of interest or is excluded.

Clinical Applications (Tables 3, 4)

CT Angiography in Carotid Artery Disease

Diagnostic Issues

Atherosclerotic carotid artery changes are a major cause of intracranial thromboembolic disease. Detection and quantification of carotid artery disease has gained renewed clinical interest due to the striking sixfold stroke reduction after endarterectomy in comparison with medical treatment alone in patients, which a diameter reduction of 70–99%, as reported in the interim results of the NASCET and ECST studies [9, 10]. The demonstrated beneficial effects of carotid surgery in patients with severe stenoses calls for a vascular imaging technique which is accurate in identifying patients with severe stenoses, and carries minimal risk to the patient.

The standard of reference in grading severity of carotid stenoses is selective angiography. However, this invasive technique carries a risk of permanent neurologic damage, ranging from 0.09% as reported in a nonselected group of patients with cerebral angiography, to 4% as reported in patients with atherosclerotic carotid disease, in whom a stenosis above 30% was suspected on the basis of color Doppler ultrasound axamination [11, 12]. Furthermore, a selective carotid angiogram costs between US $ 3000 and 6000, leading to an estimated annual total in the range of US $ 500 million dollars for the United States health care system (D.E. Strandness, personal communication).

The risk of serious complications and the high cost of carotid angiography have stimulated the development of noninvasive techniques for carotid disease evaluation. Noninvasive carotid imaging will have to answer three questions successfully in order to replace selective angiography: (1) does it identify patients with 70–99%

Table 3 Clinical applications of computed tomography angiography (CTA) and required contrast medium volumes (Ultravist 300)

Application	CTA (ml)	DSA (ml)
Subarachnoid hemorrhage (SAH)	150	200
Carotid artery disease (CAD)	150	150
Dissecting aortic arch aneurysm (DAAA)	140	80
Abdominal aortic aneurysm (AAA)	140	80
Renal artery stenosis (RAS)	140	80
Pulmonary embolism (PE)	140	200
Malignant vascular involvement (MVI)	140	80

DSA, digital subtraction angiography.

Table 4 Protocols for the clinical application of computed tomography angiography

Subarachnoid hemorrhage (SAH)
- Plain CT
- CTA, 6 cm volume in 40 s
- Small focus, 125 mA, 140 kV
- Collimation, 1.5 mm
- Reconstruction index, 1 mm
- Scan delay, 22 s <45 years >27 s

Carotid artery disease (CAD)
- CTA, 15 cm volume in 50 s
- 250 mA, 120 kV
- Collimation, 3 mm
- Reconstruction index, 2 mm
- Scan delay, 25 s

Dissecting aortic arch aneurysm (DAAA) and abdominal aortic aneurysm
- CTA 50 cm and 25 cm volume in 50 s, respectively
- 225 mA, 140 kV
- Collimation, 10 mm and 5 mm, respectively
- Reconstruction index, 5 mm and 2 mm, respectively
- Scan delay, 30 s

Renal artery stenosis (RAS)
- CTA, 9 cm volume in 30 s
- 250 mA, 140 kV
- Collimation, 3 mm
- Reconstruction index, 1 mm
- Scan delay, depending on timing test

Pulmonary embolism (PE)
- CTA, 25 cm volume in 50 s
- 250 mA, 140 kV
- Collimation, 5 mm
- Reconstruction index, 2 mm
- Delay, 20 s

stenosis accurately, (2) does it distinguish complete occlusion from severe stenosis, and (3) does it demonstrate tandem lesions in the carotid circulation? [13].

High sensitivity is required to identify all patients who may benefit from carotid endarterectomy. High specificity is required to prevent exposure of patients with minimal or moderate stenosis to the risk of surgery, for whom benefit from endarterectomy has not yet been proven (in the NASCET study perioperative morbidity in the surgical group was 5.5% compared with 3.3% in the same time interval in the medical group) [9].

The therapeutic implications of coexisting severe stenosis in the intracranial carotid circulation are a controversial matter. Some argue that in the presence of such stenosis surgery should not be performed, while others have not been able to demonstrate disadvantageous outcomes in these patients [13, 14]. The need to demonstrate tandem lesions is to be approached in the context of a low prevalence of such disease; in the NASCET study only seven of 659 patients with severe carotid stenosis demonstrated significant intracranial vascular disease: Four severe stenosis and three aneurysms [9].

Acquisition Technique

Atherosclerotic disease of the carotid arteries is invariably located at the level of the carotid bifurcation and in the proximal internal carotid artery. Disease can be limited to a short segment, and in the presence of more extensive disease the point of maximum stenosis may be short. The existence of a predeliction site of disease allows for a standardized acquisition protocol, whereas detection of short stenosis requires thin slices.

In our hospital the following acquisition technique is used: a lateral scout view identifies the lower border of the sixth cervical vertebral body. From this level upward 50 consecutive rotations are acquired: collimation, 3 mm: table speed, 3 mm/s; reconstruction index, 2 mm, 120 kVp, 250 mAs; FOV 160 mm; matrix, 512. Contrast injection: 150 ml nonionic contrast (300 mg I/ml), injected at 2.5 ml/s; scanning is started after a delay of 25 s. In order to prevent motion artifacts, patients are instructed to breathe quitley and to avoid swallowing. With this protocol a craniocaudal distance of 15 cm is covered, and a survey of the carotid bifurcation and the larger part of the extracranial internal carotid is obtained (Fig. 1). We have recently started experimenting with 1.5 mm collimation, 1.5 mm/s table speed, and a reconstruction index of 1 mm. This technique provides improved depiction of short stenosis: however, a distance of only 7.5 cm can be covered, visualizing only the carotid bifurcation and the most proximal part of the internal carotid.

Display

The reconstructed axial slices can be studied on film on a light box or viewed in interactive cine mode on a workstation, the latter being more efficient, allowing for rapid identification of the carotid bifurcation and the region of maximum luminal reduction. MPR can be created, preferably along the course of the internal carotid.

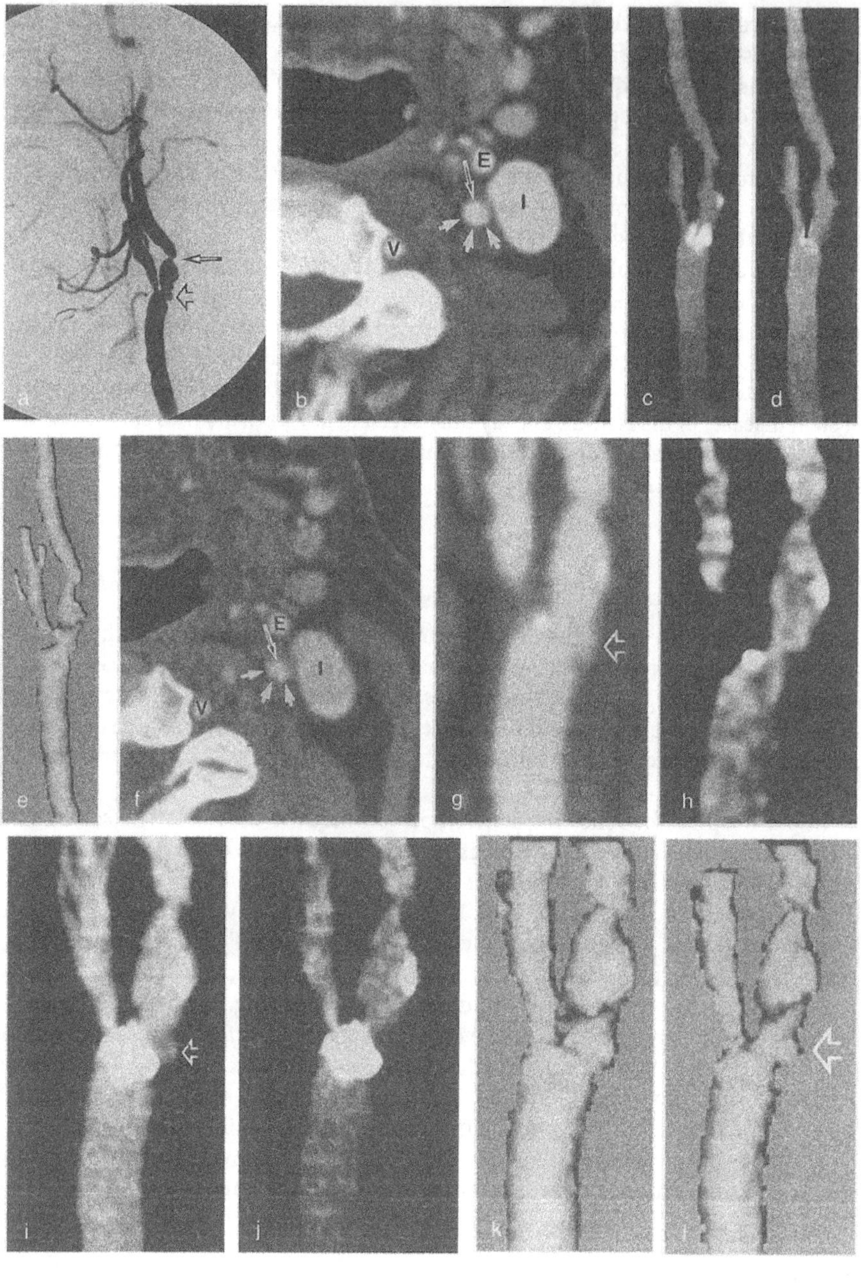
a
b
E
I
V
c
d
e
f
E
I
V
g
h
i
j
k
l

Alternatively, the axial slices can be postprocessed on- or off-line to generate MIP or SSD. Both techniques generate a survey of the carotid circulation in one image, which can be rotated to demonstrate the most severe luminal reduction.

With all techniques difficulties are experienced in assessing the severity of stenosis (Fig. 1). The axial slices are difficult to read if the stenotic carotid segment is oblique with respect to the transverse plane. Also, the window width and window level of the images will affect the diameter of the apparent lumen. MPR along the course of the carotid is very sensitive to proper placement of the reformatting plane, which may result in over- or underestimation of stenosis. MIP readily differentiates calcified plaque from luminal contrast. However, calcified plaque at the site of maximum narrowing may obscure the lumen, preventing accurate assessment of the luminal diameter. The results of SSD rely heavily on the selected threshold value. If too low a threshold is chosen, stenosis will be underestimated, and vice versa. Also, if a single threshold value is used instead of a threshold range, calcified plaque is included in the lumen and stenosis is underestimated. Calcified plaque can be manually removed to improve MIP and SSD reconstructions, but such removal is time consuming and, to some extent, operator dependent.

Fig. 1a–l Selective carotid angiogram and computed tomography angiography (CTA) with 3-mm and 1.5-mm collimation in a patient with severe stenosis in the left internal carotid artery. **a** Angiogram demonstrates ulcerapted plaque in the bifurcation (*open arrow*), stenosis of the external carotid, and, more distally, severe stenosis in the internal carotid (*black and white arrow*). **b** Three-millimeter section of the stenosis in the internal carotid. Averaging due to 3-mm collimation results in a summation of stenosis (*black* and *white arrow*) and distal wider lumen (*short arrows*). *E*, external carotid; *J*, jugular vein; *V*, vertebral artery. **c** Maximum intensity projection (MIP) demonstrates circumferential calcification at the level of the bifurcation, preventing accurate assessment of the lumen. **d** After removal of calcification by manual editing, the lumen is better visualized. On MIP, the stenosis in the internal carotid is underestimated due to averaging. **e** Shaded surface display (SSD) also underestimates the stenosis due to averaging. No image of the 3-mm data demonstrates the ulcer. Two weeks later, the same patient underwent CTA with 1.5-mm collimation, 1.5-mm/s table speed, and 1-mm reconstruction index. **f** Axial slice demonstrates severe stenosis (*black* and *white arrow*) and part of distal, poststenotic internal carotid (*short arrows*) in one image (see Fig. 1b). **g** Curved sagittal multiplanar reformatting (MPR) of the carotid bifurcation demonstrates the stenosis and suggests the ulcer (*open arrow*). **g, h** The severity of stenosis on MPR is affected by the window width and window level, the narrow window (**h**) demonstrating the severity of stenosis more realistically. **i, j** Unedited MIP of the 1.5-mm slices is affected by window width and level in the same manner as MPR. The ulcer is best depicted on the wide window setting (**i**), whereas the severitty of the stenosis is best depicted on the narrow window setting (**j**). **k, l** Two SSD one with a low (**k**) and one with a higher threshold (**l**). The calcification at the bifurcation was removed by manual editing. A higher threshold results in a more severe stenosis. Note that the ulcer (*open arrow*) is best depicted on the high-threshold SSD

Clinical Results

The fist reported studies on CTA of the carotis differ in their methods and conclusion. In two separate studies [15, 16] SSD was used to grade carotid stenosis into four categories: milde, moderate, severe, and occluded. Consensus readings of SSDs and angiograms demonstrated an overall agreement of 92% and 82%, respectively; and no readings differed by more than one category. Schwartz et al. used the attenuation value of the lumen at the level of maximum stenosis to define the threshold, while Dillon et al. derived a threshold by comparing the luminal density of a normal region with the HU value of the sternocleidomastoid muscle, representing the density of unenhanced vessel wall. In a third study, Marks et al. performed MIPs and angiograms on 28 carotids and found overall agreement in grading of stenosis of 89% [17]. All three studies concluded that CTA is a promising noninvasive technique for detecting and grading carotid stenosis.

In contrast to these studies, Castillo reported agreement of only 50% in a study comparing MIPs with angiograms in ten patients [18]. However, his technique was limited by a collimation of 5 mm, a table speed of 5 mm/s, and a very short scan delay of 10 s.

Recently, 5 observers compared interactive crine mode, MIP, and SSD with the same CTA acquisitions (3 mm slice thickness) with selective angiograms in 49 carotids (Polman, unpublished data). Interactive cine mode demonstrated the best overall performance as measured by receiver operating characteristic (ROC) analysis (AUC, 0.82), but also the lowest interobserver agreement (*K*. 062), demonstrating a substantial learning curve. Very short stenosis were consistently underestimated by one category with all three display techniques. These results have prompted us to explore the use of 1.5 mm collimation and 1.5 mm/s table speed to minimize volume averaging in short stenosis, and to further optimize the use of the interactive cine mode.

Circle of Willis CTA

Diagnostic Issues

In 75% of patients with subarachnoid hemorrhage (SAH), a ruptured saccular aneurysm is the cause of bleeding. The disease carries a poor prognosis with a mortality rate of around 50%, half of which die within the first 24 h [19, 20]. A high morbidity characterizes the surviving patients, with only 26%–58% achieving good recovery [19–21]. The leading causes of death and disability, besides the direct effects of the initial hemorrhage, are vasospasm and rebleeding.

Vasospasm occurs in up to 50% of patients [22]. The incidence of vasospasm increases daily in the first 7 days with a maximum in the 4- to 14-day period [21, 22]. However, only minimal vasospasm or none is seen on initial angiography in more than 90% of patients during the first 4 days [21].

Rebleeding occurs in 22% of patients, 70% of which occurs during the first 6 h, and 88% within 24 h [19]. Rebleeding is associated with a very high mortality

(75%) compared with those that do not rebleed (39%). According to Inagawa et al. [19], rebleeding is not related to age or sex of patients, shape or size of eneurysm, or even blood pressure on admission. Angiography increases the risk of rebleeding, especially in the first 6 h [19]. Early surgery (0–3 days), prior to the peak period of vasospasm, will reduce the risk of rebleeding and permit more aggressive treatment of vasospasm with hypertensive and hypervolemic therapy [19, 23]. However, in a large, nonrandomized study early surgery lowered the rate of rebleeding but did not prevent vasospasm [23]. No distinct difference in overall outcome of early surgery (0–3 days) compared with delayed surgery (11–14 days) was found. Only in the intermediate period was the outcome worse. Patients who were alert on admission had the most favorable outcome with early surgery. A smaller, randomized study also showed no significant difference between early and late surgery [24]. Early surgery will become more advantageous if the management of vasospasm becomes more effective. Also, "very early surgery", i.e., within hours after admission, can potentially prevent the large amount of rebleeding which occurs in the first 6 h.

Angiography is still the method of choice for detecting aneurysms. The goals of the examination are: identification of the ruptured aneurysm, location of the neck and parent artery, identification of multiple aneurysms, detection of vasospasm, and assessment of the patency of the circle of Willis. Angiography identifies an aneurysm in approximately 85% of patients [20]. A false-negative angiogram can be due to vasospasm and should be repeated in 1–2 weeks. The majority (78%) of aneurysms are small (<12 mm) [21]. Up to 25% of patients demonstrate multiple aneurysms: therefore three- to four-vessel angiography is needed. Most aneurysms arise from the anterior communicating artery, the internal carotid artery, and the middle cerebral artery. In 4%–10% a vertebrobasilar aneurysm is present.

Computed tomography angiography offers the possibility of a quick and noninvasive examination. Ideally, it should provide an expedient diagnosis, obviating the need for angiography in selected patients, subsequently making earlier surgery possible. Probably, CTA cannot reliably identify vasospasm, however, is absent or only minimally presents in 90% of patients in the first few days.

Acquisition Technique

The vessels which constitute the circle of Willis are small, more or less parallel to the scanning plane, and located close to the bony structures of the skull base and sella turcica. In addition, the size of aneurysms is often in the millimeter range. Therefore, maximal spatial resolution is required and thin slices and optimal contrast enhancement are essential.

We use the following protocol in patients with subarachnoid hemorrhaging (SAH): a lateral scout identifies the dorsum sellae. The circle of Willis is presumed to be located 0.5 cm above the dorsum sellae. A scan plan is set to include the region 3 cm below to 3 cm above the presumed level of the circle of Willis: technique, 40 rotations; collimation, 1.5 mm; table speed, 1.5 mm/s; reconstruction index, 1 mm, 140 kVp, 125 mAs; FOV, 160 mm; matrix, 512. Contrast injection is 180 ml nonionic contrast (300 ml I/ml), injected at 4 ml/s; scanning is started after a delay of 25 s. Patients are instructed to breathe calmly and to avoid swallowing.

Display

The axial slices can be viewed on film, or interactively in cine mode. On the axial slices, identification of the vascular segments is difficult, and cine mode is helpful. Also, differentiation between small vessels, very tortuous vessels, and small aneurysms may be difficult.

A survey of the willisian circulation can be created with MIP or SSD (Fig. 2). The varying obliquity of the vessels in and around the circle will result in different appearances on the MIP and SSD images. On MIP in-plane vessels are less sharply delineated and of lesser density than longitudinally oriented vessels. Also, due to the principle of MIP, wider vessels with resulting high density will obscure thinner vessels with resulting lower density. Superpositioning of surrounding bony structures is to be remedied by manual or semiautomatic editing. SSD images will overestimate the vessel diameter in vertical parts, and simulate spasm due to diminished diameter in the horizontal parts. Adjacent vessels may seem to fuse due to partial volume effects.

Clinical Results

Few studies have described CT as a diagnostic technique for identification of cerebral aneurysms. In 1987, before the introduction of helical CT, Schmid et al. described a study of 102 consecutive patients, with suspected aneurysm of the cerebral arteries [25]. After a noncontrast CT of the skull, 15–20 1.5-mm slices were taken

Fig. 2a–f Computed tomography angiography (CTA) and selective angiography in a patient with suspected aneurysm. **a, b** On the axial slices a large aneurysm (*white arrow*) at the end of the right M1 segment is demonstrated. The left M1 segment demonstrates a small, caudally directed aneurysm (*black* and *white arrow*). **c, d** Maximum intensity projection (MIP) (**c**) and shaded surface display (SSD) (**d**) of the willisian circulation. On the axial slices bone was removed by manual editing. The threshold for SSD was adjusted to demonstrate the circle of Willis optimally. Both aneurysms (*arrows*) are displayed clearly on the MIP and SSD images. Note how partial volume averaging affects the MIP and SSD display of the anterior cerebral arteries. The horizontal A1 segments (*open arrow*) are affected by volume averaging due to their relatively small diameter compared with the 1.5 mm slice thickness. As a result, the A1 segments are depicted less brightly on MIP, and of a smaller diameter on SSD, compared to the vertical A2 segments (*arrowhead*). The closely adjacent, vertical A2 segments appear to be fused on SSD due to in-plane volume averaging, but are clearly separated on MIP. **e, f** Selective right and left carotid angiogram demonstrates the aneurysms (*arrows*), which were both successfully clipped

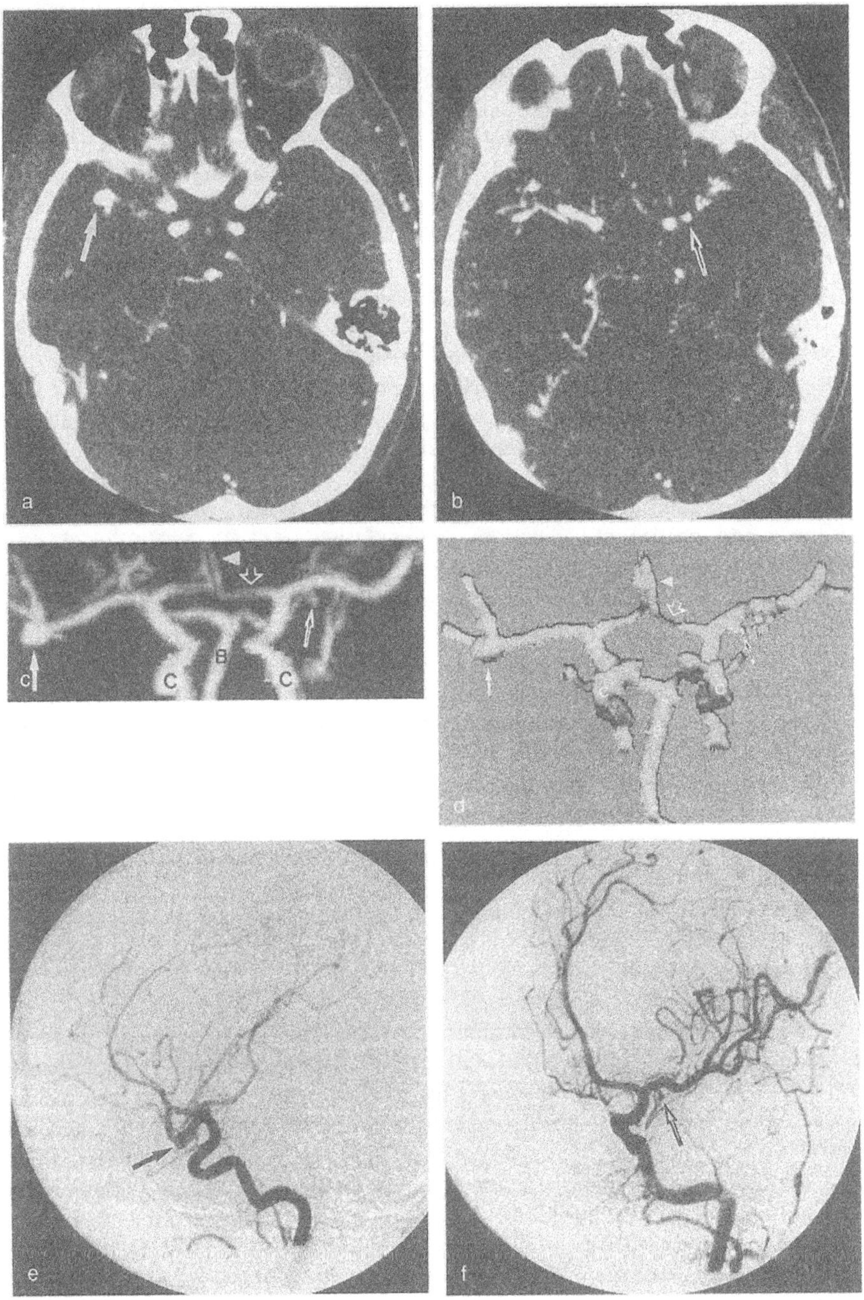
a
b
c
B
C
C
d
e
f

during administration of 100 ml contrast. MPR was used to create sagittal and coronal reconstructions of a possible aneurysm. With this technique the authors were able to visualize 71 of 76 (93.4%) aneurysms prospectively and 74 of 76 (97.4%) retrospectively. In three patients an aneurysm was falsely suspected.

Recently, Aoki et al. used helical CT (1.5-mm collimation and 1.5-mm/s table speed) in 15 patients with clinically suspected cerebral aneurysms [26]. Using a threshold of 100 HU, SSD were constructed, without deleting bone. With this technique they were able to detect all (15 of 15) aneurysms and demonstrate their necks and the parent arteries. In one patient an aneurysm was falsely suspected, at a location where angiography demonstrated a small, tortuous vessel.

Napel et al. [1] used MIP to visualize CTA data from the circle of Willis. They used semiautomatic bone removal and were able to consistently visualize the intracranial part of the internal carotid, including its intracavernous course and the cerebral arteries, beyond the A1 and M1 segments. They argued that MIP is superior to SSD in circle of Willis visualization since it is less susceptible to the effects of volume averaging.

The studies cited agree that CTA of the circle of Willis can be used for early diagnosis and location of cerebral aneurysms in patients with SAH. Schmid et al. describes three conditions where CTA alone is sufficient for preoperative evaluation: (1) adequate identification of the aneurysm, partent vessel, and complete circle of Willis: (2) identification of a temporal hematoma around an aneurysm in the middle cerebral artery in deteriorating patients; and (3) detection of an aneurysm of the posterior communicating artery in patients with oculomotor nerve palsy [25].

With the current helical scanners and the variety of postprocessing algorithms available, it can be expected that, in the near future, a substantial percentage of patients with SAH can be operated upon as soos as CTA, performed on admission, has demonstrated sufficient anatomic information.

CT Angiography in Pulmonary Embolism

Diagnostic Issues

Pulmonary embolism (PE) is a common disease entity with an estimated incidence in, for example, the United States of 630000 cases annually [27]. It is lethal in 30% of untreated patients. Administration of adequate anticoagulant therapy can lower the mortality rate to 8%. However, the estimated complication risk of such therapy totals 32%, 13% being severe bleedings [28]. Consequently, a sensitive and a specific diagnostic test for the detection of PE is needed. In patients with clinically suspected PE, ventilation/perfusion (V/Q) scanning is often used as the screening test. The sensitivity of the perfusion scan is 98% in the detection of PE. Specificity is less: in high-probability V/Q scans. PE is found in only 88% and in indeterminate V/Q scans the prevalence of PE is reported to be 33% [29]. Therefore, pulmonary angiography is often needed to confirm PE in the large group of patients with indeterminate V/Q scans. Pulmonary angiography is reliable in detecting emboli in segmental, lobar, and main pulmonary arteries. However, it is an expensive and invasive test with 2.7% morbidity and 0.2% mortality [30].

The rapid acquisition of helical CT enables direct, noninvasive visualization of pulmonary emboli. Clinical studies indicate that helical CT may be an ideal tool in the diagnosis of PE, preventing the need for V/Q scans and largely replacing pulmonary angiography.

Acquisition and Display Technique

The central part of the pulmonary arterial system is located below the level of the aortic arch and above the domes of the diaphragm. In most patients this region can be covered with 24–30 rotations with the following technique: collimation, 5 mm: table speed, 5 mm/s; reconstruction index, 3 mm. Scans are made during breath-hold or shallow respiration. To prevent streak artifacts a contrast agent with a concentration of 12% iodide can be used, totaling 20 ml, administered at an injection rate of 7 ml/s [31]. In patients with possible pulmonary hypertension or right ventricular failure a contrast agent with a concentration of 30% iodide can be used, totaling 90 ml, injected at a rate of 5 ml/s. Scanning is started 10 s after the beginning of contrast administration.

The overlapping axial slices are best visualized in interactive cine mode. To date, postprocessing algorithms seem to offer no advantage over axial slices.

Clinical Results

Several studies have described the CT appearance of PE [32–41]. However, only recently have attemps been made to define the role of CT in patients with suspected PE, as reported in two studies [31, 42].

Remy-Jardin evaluated 42 patients suspected of PE with contrast-enhanced helical scanning and selective pulmonary angiography [31]. Detection of central PE included analysis of the main, lobar, and segmental pulmonary arteries. Partial filling defects, complete filling defects, and the "railway track" sign (thromboembolic masses surrounded by contrast) were recorded. Overall quality of vascular opacification was insufficient in one case (2%) and good or excellent in 98%. Twenty-two pulmonary arteries in six patients were not interpretable due to their oblique ($n=19$) or parallel course ($n=3$) relative to the scan plane. Central pulmonary thromboembolism was excluded in 23 patients with helical CT, which was confirmed by pulmonary angiography. In 19 patients, CT demonstrated pulmonary embolism which was confirmed angiographically in 18 patients. In the only false-positive CT, angiography demonstrated asymmetry in pulmonary vascular opacification due to increased pulmonary arterial resistance on the left side in a trauma patient with ipsilateral pleural effusion and parenchymal consolidation. Teigen et al. reported 86 patients studied with electronic beam CT [42]. Of all the anatomic zones, visualization was considered adequate in 96%. Among the 86 patients, CT was considered positive for PE in 39 and negative in 47 patients. Pulmonary angiography, V/Q scintigraphy, and surgical or autopsy findings were used as a reference standard. Sensitivity and specificity were not established; yet the authors felt that electron beam CT has the potential to become a primary non-invasive examination for PE.

Precise knowledge of the anatomy of the bronchovascular system is necessary for proper interpretation of CT studies of pulmonary vessels. The presence of intersegmental lymph nodes and apparent filling defects in small pulmonary veins in the upper lobes may mimic the appearance of segmental arterial emboli. Perivascular edema can be misinterpreted as chronic embolic material. Imaging of vessels parallel to the scan plane is problematic due to volume averaging.

It seems logical that CTA might supplant V/Q scintigraphy as the screening tool of choice in suspected pulmonary embolism. Furthermore, CTA seems an attractive imaging technique for follow-up of patients with central thrombo-embolism after anticoagulant or lytic therapy. An important advantage of CTA is that other intrathoracic pathology is accurately depicted on CT.

However, large prospective studies, focussing on patient outcome, are needed to reduce the need for V/Q scanning and pulmonary angiography in patients with clinically suspected PE.

CT Angiography in Aortic Disease

Diagnostic Issues

Suspected aneurysmal disease or aortic dissection are the most frequent indication for aortic imaging. The length and maximal width of the luminal and thrombotic part of the aortic aneurysm and the relationship to renal and visceral arteries constitute the key concern for the surgeon. Furthermore, elongation of the aorta and iliacal vessels, location and extent of mural thrombus, calcification, and coexisting periaortic pathology can influence surgical planning.

In aortic dissections the precise extent of the dissecting hematoma needs to be assessed. The primary laceration is frequently located in the ascending aorta or at the junction of the aortic arch and descending aorta. From the site of primary laceration, the false lumen can extend distally over a varying distance; retrograde extension of the false passage is usually limited. Extension of the dissection into aortic side branches, with possible impairment of blood flow, rupture into the pericardial sac, and aortic insufficiency are the major sequelae of dissection.

Angiography is often used to evaluate aortic disease. Disadvantages are the examination time, relatively high cost, and invasiveness of the procedure, with the risk of complications. The number of possible projections is limited and periaortic pathology is not visualized.

Already, CTA has proved to be very useful in the visualization of the thoracic and abdominal aorta. It is a rapid, minimally invasive diagnostic test, which can be performed as an outpatient procedure and can demonstrate the vast majority of anatomic information needed for patient management (Fig. 3).

Acquisition Technique

The scanning parameters used for CTA of the aorta arte defined by the length of the region of interest. In thoracic scans a collimation of 10 mm and a table speed of 10 mm/s is used with a reconstruction index of 5 mm. If only the ascending aorta, the aortic arch, and the proximal part of the descending aorta need to be visualized, a slice thickness of 5 mm with a reconstruction index of 2 mm is used. Abdominal scans are performed with a slice thickness of 5 mm and a reconstruction index of 2 mm and the FOV is adjusted to include the aneurysm and the kidneys. In all three acquisitions 140 ml of an nonionic contrast agent is injected at a rate of 2 ml/s. Scanning is started 20–30 s after the beginning of contrast injection, depending on whether the thoracic or abdominal aorta ist examined. Patients are instructed to hyperventilate before, and hold their breath during, the acquisition.

One of the issues in CTA of the aorta is the timing of the contrast bolus throughout the entire scanning period. Some institutes assess the individual circulation time with a continuous scan at a single level after infusion of a small amount of contrast (± 20 m) at a flow rate of 3 ml/s. The elapsed time till peak enhancement is measured and the individual scan delay is adjusted accordingly. However, with the protocol used at our institute with a fixed 20- or 30-s scan delay, the thoracic and abdominal aorta and surrounding pathology are well opacified in the vast majority of patients.

Display

Images can be reviewed on a workstation in cine mode, which demonstrates best the advantages of volumetric scanning. The whole extent of the thoracic and abdominal aorta can be displayed smoothly, and aortic branches are easily tracked. In this way most anatomic and pathologic findings, such as extension of the aneurysm, relation to renal arteries, and size of mural thrombus, can be demonstrated. In the presence of dissection, intimal flaps and true and false lumina are displayed well.

Multiplanar reformats with orthogonal and curved reconstructions are of good quality due to the overlapping slices. A curved reconstruction demonstrates a survey of the extent of the aneurysm or dissection, and the relative position of mural thrombus, calcifications, and intimal flaps.

Three-dimensional renderings, such as SSD or MIP, provide the surgeon with anatomic information in a single image, which is important for preoperative planning. SSD demonstrate the opacified aorta and its branches together with bony structures, such as spine and pelvis. Because the threshold is selected by the operator, loss of information is possible. The density of mural thrombus is almost equal to that of soft tissue, which makes automatic reconstruction impossible. To obtain images with mural thrombus in relation to aortic lumen and aortic branches manual editing is necessary, which is time consuming.

In MIP no threshold is used, and lumen and calcifications are easily distinguished. Like SSD, MIP require suppression of bony structures and manual editing is needed to remove them.

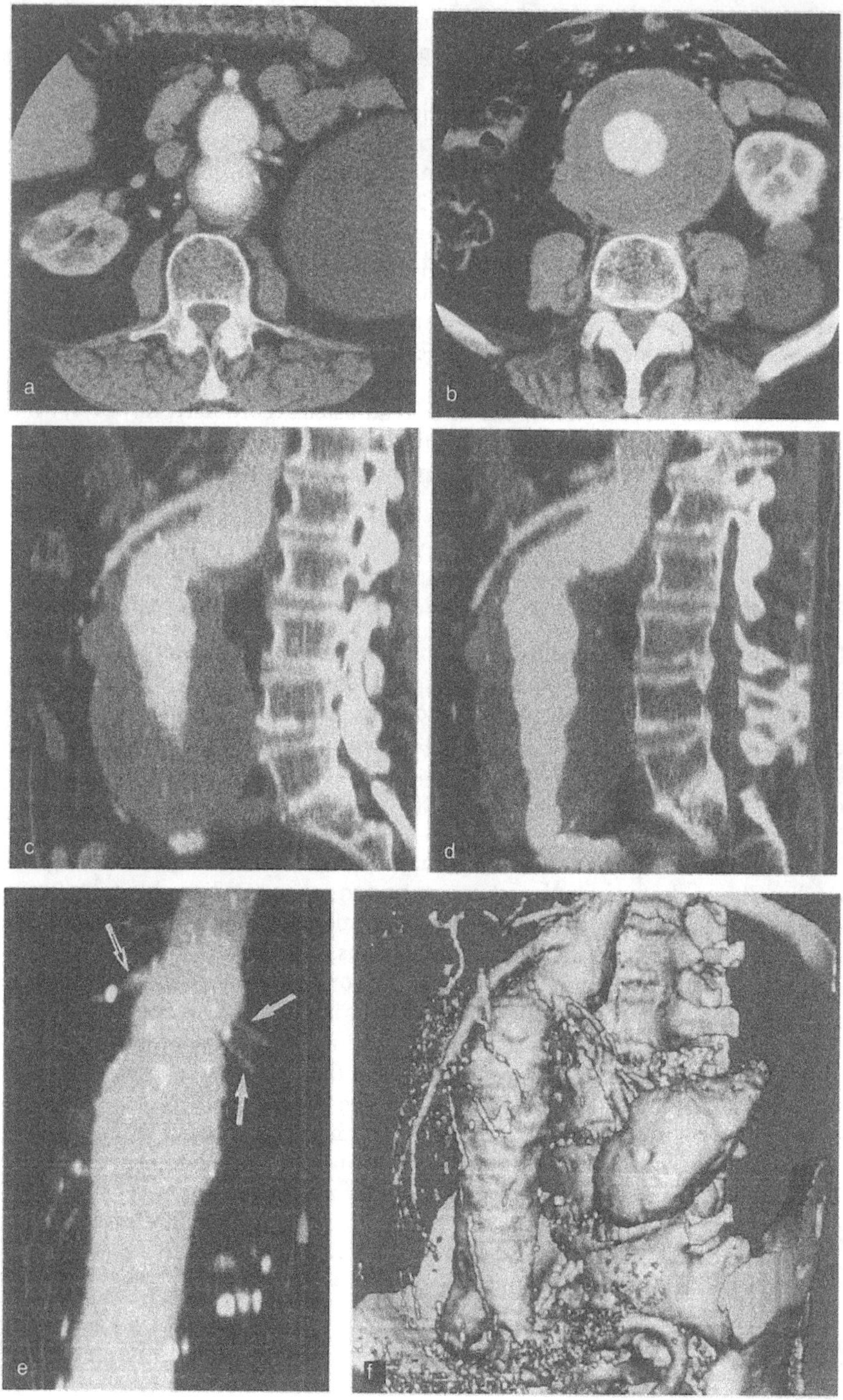
a
b
c
d
e
f

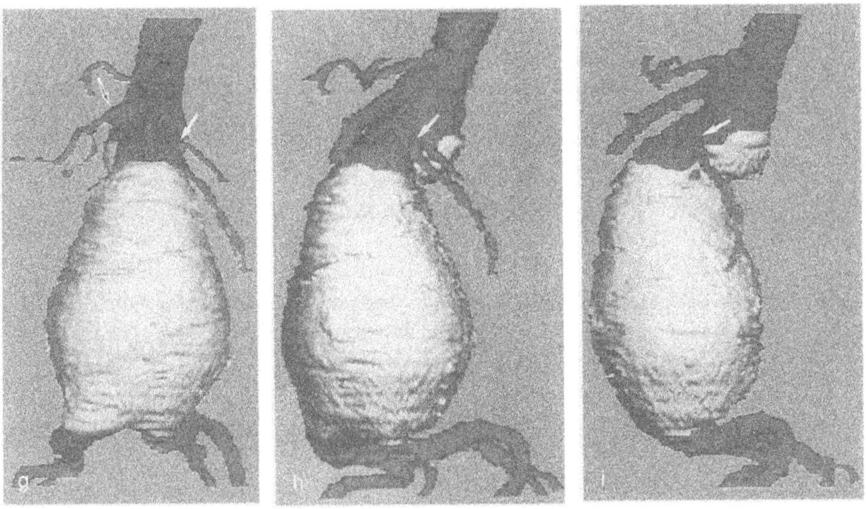

Fig. 3 a–i Preoperative computed tomography angiography (CTA) in a patient with abdominal aneurysm. **a, b** Axial slices at the cranial end and at the level of the largest transverse diameter. **c, d** Sagittal and curved sagittal multiplanar reformatting (MPR). The curved reformat is made along the center of the aortic lumen, which is marked on the orthogonal MPR. The advantage of curved MPR is that it can display the full extent of the aneurysm in one image. **e** MIP is not very useful in aneurysms. Thrombus is not visualized and the origin of the aortic branches is often superimposed on the aortic lumen (*white arrows*, branches of left renal arter; *black* and *white arrow*, right renal artery). **f–i** Different shaded surface displays (SSD) of the aneurysm

f Left anterior oblique (LAO) projection. If no editing is performed, thrombus is not visualized and structures with equal or higher density, like bone and kidney, are all displayed. **g–i** Anteroposterior, LAO, and left lateral projection. After editing, thrombus (*yellow*) and lumen (*red*) can be individually displayed without surrounding structures, allowing assessment of the origins of the right (*black* and *white arrow*) and left (*white arrows*) renal arteries relative to the thrombus and the luminal dilatation. Note the elongation of the iliac arteries

Clinical Results

CT angiography of the aorta can be performed in an outpatient setting, and is less invasive, less costly, much quicker, and often more informative in comparison to conventional angiography. Rubin et al. [2] mentioned consistent imaging of second-to-fourth order aortic branches and good correlation with conventional angiography. All the major aortic branches were clearly demonstrated, except in-plane vessels with severe stenosis.

Costello et al. [43] examined 19 patients with suspected abdominal aneurysmal disease and demonstrated aortic aneurysms in 16 cases. Angiography was available in seven patients, in whom the extent of the aneurysm and the number and location of renal arteries were confirmed. Differential opacification of true and false lumens were also well displayed with CTA, although only a small amount of contrast was used prior to a 24-s thoracic scan [44].

Balm et al. [45] mentioned MPR as a valuable tool for evaluating the craniocaudal appearance of aortic pathology. In complex cases such as supra- and juxtarenal aneurysms, recurrent aneurysms, dissections, and anatomic variants. SSD were more useful.

At our institute CTA has become the examination of choice for abdominal aneurysms and thoracoabdominal dissections. Contrary to conventional angiography, CTA demonstrates mural thrombus, aortic calcifications, and additional abnormalities such as perianeurysmal fibrosis and hematomas. In most cases two-dimensional viewing functions, i.e., cine mode and MPR, are sufficient to obtain the anatomic information the surgeon needs for preoperative evaluation.

CTA provides all the information needed for minimal invasive aneurysmal repair by means of a percutaneously inserted endovascular prosthesis. Accurate measurements of the aortic aneurysm, necessary for a made-to-measure endovascular prosthesis, can be made with a curved multiplanar reformat based on a line positioned centrally in the aorta. Reconstructions parallel and perpendicular to this curve provide projections which best demonstrate the true diameter and length of the aneurysm. SSD are used in case of elongation of the aorta and iliacs and to visualize the extent of luminal dilatation in relation to mural thrombus and aortic branches.

CT Angiography in Renal Artery Stenosis

Diagnostic Issues

Renal artery stenosis (RAS) is a potentially curable cause of hypertension, with a prevalence of less than 5% in patients with arterial hypertension. Stenosis in excess of 50% are considered hemodynamically significant. Due to the large number of patients with hypertension and the small percentage of patients with RAS, a heavy burden is placed on diagnostic workup. A high sensitivity is required to find and subsequently treat all the patients with RAS, and a relatively high specificity is needed to prevent unnecessary invasive procedures in the large group of patients with hypertension. Angiography is not suited as a screening procedure due to its invasiveness and cost. Less invasive procedures such as duplex Doppler and magnetic resonance (MR) angiography have not reached the required high sensitivity and specificity as yet. Captopril renography is a good screening test for RAS, but does not provide anatomic information.

Preliminary studies indicate that CTA of the renal arteries may be sufficiently accurate in the detection and grading of RAS to be used as a screening procedure.

Acquisition Technique

The relatively small size, transverse course, varyable craniocaudal location, and frequent plurality of renal arteries require an optimal scanning technique [46].

The location and number of renal arteries can be appreciated on a noncontrast scan from the level of Th12 downward. Subsequent optimal contrast enhancement requires assessment of the individual transit time at the level of the renal arteries. Galanski et al. report that the measured time from the start of the test injection to peak enhancement should be increased by 5 s to allow for the longer injection time needed for the larger contrast volume. The actual CTA acquisition is started at the origin of the superior mesenteric artery. Between 100 and 150 ml nonionic contrast (300 mg I/ml) is injected 3–5 ml/s. Patients with a body weight above 60 kg receive 150 ml at 3.5 ml/s, and 2.5 ml/kg contrast is given to patients of less than 60 kg body wt. In young patients with a transit time below 15 s, injection rate is increased to 5 ml/s to compensate for the increased dilution caused by their higher cardiac output. Collimation and table speed are kept as low as possible to minimize partial volume averaging. Galanski et al. report good results with a standard 2-mm slice thickness and a reconstruction index of 1 mm. This can be increased to 3 mm slice thickness and a reconstruction index of 2 mm in obese patients and in patients in whom a larger craniocaudal distance has to be scanned because of suspected accessory renal arteries on the noncontrast scan.

Display

Interactive cine mode of the axial slices, MPR, SSD, and MIP can all be used to view the volumetric data. MPR is most informative if a curved reconstruction is made along the often tortuous course of the renal artery. The highest spatial resolution is the in-plane resolution of the axial slices. Consequently, luminal diameter is best judged on these images. However, if the course of the vessel at the point of stenosis is oblique with respect to the scan plane, interpretation is difficult and curved MPR, MIP, or SSD may be useful.

If SSD is used, a threshold has to be chosen, which best fits the individual enhancement level. Due to partial volume effects, small calcifications may be erroneously represented as part of the lumen, leading to underestimation of stenosis. In MIPs, bone has to be removed by manual editing. The enhancing aortic lumen or calcified plaque in aortic plaque may be superimposed on the origins of renal arteries, precluding accurate assessments of luminal diameter.

Clinical Results

Galanski et al. prospectively examined 22 patients with suspected renovascular hypertension with CTA and intraarterial digital subtraction angiography (DSA) [46]. Postprocessing was performed to create MPR, MIP, and SSD. Renal arteries were examined on the axial slices. MPR, MIP, and SSD and each renal artery was graded 0–4: 0, no stenosis; 1, mild stenosis (<50%); 2, moderate stenosis (50%–75%); 3, severe stenosis (76%–99%); and 4, occlusion.

Contrast enhancement was good or excellent in 19 of 22 patients. In five patients 11 accessory arteries were present on DSA and all were detected on CTA.

Twenty-two arteries in 15 patients demonstrated RAS or occlusion of a renal artery on DSA, and all were correctly detected and localized with CTA. In four of 22 stenosis a difference in CTA and DSA grading of stenosis occured. Two stenoses were underestimated (grade 2 on CTA, grade 3 on DSA), one case of fibromuscular hyperplasia was overestimated (grade 3 on CTA, grade 2 on DSA), and one short occlusion with well-developed collateral circulation was graded as grade 3 stenosis.

The authors report that the axial slices are the most important display mode. In 15 of 22 patients the axial slices alone were conclusive. The combination of interactive cine display and curved MPR yielded almost the same results as all four viewing modalities combined. Only one grade 2 ostial stenosis was underestimate as grade 1 and correctly diagnosed as grade 2 with MIP.

The quality of MIP images depended on vessel enhancement, size, course with respect to the scan plane, and differentiation of renal arteries from overlying enhancing veins. In four patients renal arteries were inadequately displayed due to insufficient contrast, and in six patients renal veins prevented accurate assessment of the renal artery. Although grading of stenoses was less accurate than the axial slices in combination with MPR, the authors use MIP as the optimal presentation to document the anatomic findings. Also, MIP may be helpful in the detection and grading of ostial stenoses.

Shaded surface display was only useful in one patient with a kidney transplant and a tortuous renal artery. In most patients the diagnostic value was limited due to merging of lumen and classification, and due to the consistent overestimation of severe stenoses as pseudo-occlusions. Consequently, two short occlusions with good collateral circulation could not be differentiated from the pseudo-occlusion appearance of severe stenoses. The authors conclude that CTA of the renal arteries is an excellent technique for the detection, localization, and grading of renal artery stenoses.

Rubin et al. described 31 patients with suspected RAS, examined with CTA and angiography [47].

The authors compared SSD and MIP with conventional angiography as the standard of reference. The authors did not grade the stenoses on the axial images. Sensitivity for detecting stenoses >70% stenosis was 92% for MIP and 59% for SSD. Accuracy of stenosis grading was 80% for MIP and 55% for SSD.

The lower performance of CTA than in the study of Galanski et al. can be explained by the omission of the axial images and MPRs for grading, and by differences in acquisition technique. In Rubin's study, collimation was always 3 mm and table speed varied between 3 and 6 mm. Consequently, the acquisition technique is more prone to volume averaging compared with the 2–3 mm collimation and 2–3 mm table speed as used by Galanski et al.

Conclusions

Preliminary studies on the diagnostic value of CTA in a number of applications demonstrate good results for the evaluation of aortic disease, pulmonary embolism, and renal artery stenosis. Additionally, CTA seems promising for grading of carotid stenosis and detection of intracerebral aneurysms.

The reported studies stress the need for optimal technique in data acquisition and image display. Technical developments in helical CT will provide more flexibility in scanning parameters, allowing the acquisition to overcome the problems of limited scan length and volume averaging. The actual data acquisition often takes no more than a few minutes. However, several applications are time intensive due to off-line postprocessing. Developments in postprocessing algorithms will result in quicker and more automatic image processing, which is essential for the introduction of these techniques on a larger scale.

The appearance and severity of vascular pathology is dependent on the display technique used. Research is needed to define the optimal display method for each application. The current trend favors the use of nonprocessed axial slices and curved MPR for detection and grading of disease. SSD and MIP are mainly used for survey.

In each developing application, the potential role of CTA must be considered; is it meant to be a screening procedure or a confirmatory test? As soon as acquisition and display techniques are optimized for a specific application, prospective studies will have to examine diagnostic accuracy. Last but not least, CTA reduces production costs by ±50% compared to DSA (see Table 5). Thus, CTA can find its proper place among the other vascular imaging techniques (Table 6).

Table 5 Production costs (in Dfl.) at the University Hospital, Utrecht, Netherlands

Application	DSA	Costs (%)	CTA	Costs (%)
SAH	1525.65	100%	311.27	20%
CAD	1108.82	100%	311.27	28%
DAAA	258.74	100%	328.02	126%
AAA	661.16	100%	469.74	71%
RAS	1076.47	100%	469.74	43%
PE	756.06	100%	328.02	43%
MVI	661.16	100%	469.74	43%

For abbreviations, see Table 3.
DSA requires 2 days in hospital, i.e., Dfl. 1185.00

Table 6 Advantages and disadvantages of computed tomography angiography (CTA)

Advantages	Disadvantages
Fast acquisition time	Postprocessing suboptimal
Straightforward interpretation	Limited number of rotations
Optimal for critically ill patients	Large amounts of contrast medium needed
Reduced production costs ± 50%	
Compared to digital subtraction	
angiography (DSA)	

References

1. Napel S, Marks MP, Rubin GD, Dake MD et al. (1992) CT Angiography with spiral CT and maximum intensity projection. Radiology 185:607–610
2. Rubin GD, Dake MD, Napel SA, McDonnel CH, Jeffrey RB Jr (1993) Three-dimensional spiral CT angiography of the abdomen: initial clinical experience. Radiology 186:147–152
3. Dillon EH, van Leeuwen MS, Fernandez MA, Mali WPTM (1993) Spiral CT angiography. AJR 160:1273–1278
4. Kalender WA, Seissler W, Klotz E, Vock P (1990) Spiral volumetric CT with single-breath-hold technique, continuous transport, and continuous scanner rotation. Radiology 176:181–183
5. Crawford CR, King KF (1990) Computed tomography scanning with simultaneous patient translation. Med Phys 17:967–982
6. Barnes JE (1992) Characteristics and control of contrast in CT. RadioGraphics 12:825–837
7. Polacin A, Kalender WA, Marchal G (1992) Evaluation of section sensitivity profiles and image noise in spiral CT. Radiology 185:29–35
8. Vahlensieck M, Lang Ph, Chan WP, Grampp S, Genant HK (1992) Three-dimensional reconstruction, part I: applications and techniques. Eur Radiol 2:503–507
9. NASCET Collaborators (1991) Beneficial effect of carotid endarterectomy in symptomatic patients with high-grade carotid stenosis. N Engl J Med 325:445–453
10. ECST Collaborators (1991) MRC European Carotid Surgery Trial: interim results for symptomatic patients with severe (70–99%) or with mild (0–29%) carotid stenosis. Lancet 337:1235–1243
11. Grzyska U, Freitag J, Zeumer H (1990) Selective cerebral intraarterial DSA. Neuroradiology 32:296–299
12. Davies KN, Humphrey PR (1993) Complications of cerebral angiography in patients with symptomatic carotid territory ischaemia screened by carotid ultrasound. J Neurol Neurosurg Psychiatry 56:967–972
13. Masaryk TJ, Obuchowsky N (1993) Noninvasive carotid imaging: caveat emptor. Radiology 186:325–328
14. Schuler JJ, Flanigan DP, Lim LT, Keifer T et al. (1982) The effect of carotid siphon stenosis on stroke rate, death, and relief of symptoms following elective carotid endarterectomy. Surgery 92:1058–1067
15. Schwartz RB, Jones KM, Chernoff DM, Mukherji SK et al. (1992) Common carotid bifurcation: evaluation with spiral CT. Radiology 185:513–519
16. Dillon EH, van Leeuwen MS, Fernandez MA, Eikelboom BC, Mali WPTM (1993) CT angiography: application to the evaluation of carotid artery stenosis. Radiology 189:211–219
17. Marks MP, Napel S, Jordan JE, Enzmann DR (1993) Diagnosis of carotid artery disease: preliminary experience with maximum-intensity-projection spiral CT angiography. AJR 160:1267–1271
18. Castillo M (1993) Diagnosis of disease of the common carotid artery bifurcation: CT angiography vs catheter angiography. AJR 161:395–398
19. Inagawa T, Kamiya K, Ogasawara H, Yano T (1987) Rebleeding of ruptured intracranial aneurysms in the acute stage. Surg Neurol 28:93–99
20. Van Gijn J (1992) Subarachnoid haemorrhage. Lancet 339:653–655
21. Kassel NF, Torner JC, Haley EC Jr, Jane JA et al. (1990) The International Cooperative Study on the Timing of Aneurysm Surgery, part 1: overall management results. J Neurosurg 73:18–36
22. Hijdra A, Braakman R, Van Gijn J, Vermeulen M, Van Crevel H (1987) Aneurysmal subarachnoid hemorrhage. Complications and outcome in a hospital population. Stroke 18:1061–1067
23. Kassel NF, Torner JC, Jane JA, Haley EC Jr, Adams HP (1990) The international cooperative study on the timing of aneurysm surgery, part 2: surgical results. J Neurosurg 73:37–47

24. Öhman J, Heiskanen O (1989) Timing of operation for ruptured supratentorial aneurysms: a prospective randomized study. J Neurosurg 70:55-60
25. Schmid UD, Steiger HJ, Huber P (1987) Accuracy of high resolution computed tomography in direct diagnosis of cerebral aneurysms. Neuroradiology 29:152-159
26. Aoki S, Sasaki Y, Machida T, Ohkubo T et al. (1992) Cerebral aneurysms: detection and delineation using 3-D-CT angiography. AJNR 13:1115-1120
27. Dalen JE, Alpert JS (1975) Natural history of pulmonary embolism. Prog Cardiovasc Dis 17:259-270
28. Mant MJ, Thong KL, Birtwhistle RV, O'Brien BD et al. (1977) Haemorrhagic complications of heparin therapy. Lancet I: 1133-1135
29. PIOPED Investigators (1990) Value of the ventilation/perfusion scan in acute pulmonary embolism. Results of the prospective investigation of pulmonary embolism diagnosis (PIOPED). JAMA 263:2753-2759
30. Mills SR, Jackson DC, Older RA, Heaston DK, Moore AV (1980) The incidence, etiologies, and avoidance of complications of pulmonary angiography in a large series. Radiology 136:295-299
31. Remy-Jardin M, Remy J, Wattinne L, Giraud F (1992) Central pulmonary thromboembolism: diagnosis with spiral volumetric CT with the single-breath technique: comparison with pulmonary angiography. Radiology 185:381-387
32. Sinner WN (1987) Computed tomography patterns of pulmonary thromboembolism and infarction. J Comput Assist Tomogr 2:395-399
33. Godwin JD, Webb WR, Gamsu G, Ovenfors C-O (1980) Computed tomography of pulmonary embolism. AJR 135:691-695
34. DCarlo LA Jr, Schiller NB, Herfkens RL, Brundage BH, Lipton MJ (1982) Noninvasive detection of proximal pulmonary artery thrombosis by two-dimensional echocardiography and computerized tomography. Am Heart J 104:879-881
35. Breatnach E, Stanley RJ (1984) CT diagnosis of segmental pulmonary artery embolus. J Comput Assist Tomogr 8:762-764
36. Chintapalli K, Thorsen K, Olson DL, Goodman LR, Gurney J (1988) Computed tomography of pulmonary thromboembolism and infarction. J Comput Assist Tomogr 12:533-559
37. Kälebo P, Wallin J (1989) Computed tomography in massive pulmonary embolism. Acta Radiol [Diag] (Stockh) 30:105-107
38. Ren H, Kuhlman JE, Hruban RH, Fishman EK et al. (1990) CT of inflation-fixed lungs: wedge-shaped density and vascular sign in the diagnosis of infarction. J Comput Assist Tomogr 14:82-86
39. Erol C, Candan I (1993) Non-invasive methods in the diagnosis of chronic major-vessel thromboembolic pulmonary hypertension. Eur Heart J 14:1004-1005
40. Verschakelen JA, Vanwijck E, Bogaert J, Baert AL (1993) Detection of unsuspected central pulmonary embolism with conventional contrast-enhanced CT. Radiology 188:847-850
41. Tardivon AA, Musset D, Maitre S, Brenot F et al. (1993) Role of CT in chronic pulmonary embolism: comparison with pulmonary angiography. J Comput Assist Tomogr 17:345-351
42. Teigen CL, Maus TP, Sheedy PF II, Johnson CM, Stanson AW, Welch TJ (1993) Pulmonary embolism: diagnosis with electron-beam CT. Radiology 188:839-845
43. Costello P, Gaa J (1993) Spiral CT angiography of the abdominal aorta and its branches. Eur Radiol 3:359-365
44. Costello P, Dupuy DE, Ecker CP, Tello R (1992) Spiral CT of the thorax with reduced volume of contrast material: a comparative Study. Radiology 183:663-666
45. Balm R, Eikelboom BC, van Leeuwen MS, Noordzij J Spiral (1994) CT-Angiography of the Aorta Eur J Vasc Surg 8:544-551
46. Galanski M, Prokop M, Chavan A, Schaefer CM et al. (1993) Renal arterial stenoses: spiral CT angiography. Radiology 189:185-192
47. Rubin GD, Dake MD, Napel S, Jeffrey RB Jr et al. (1994) Spiral CT of renal artery stenosis: comparison of three-dimensional rendering of techniques. Radiology 190:181-189

CHAPTER 33

Indications for Magnetic Resonance Angiography

T.J. Vogl, J.O. Balzer, and R. Felix[1]

Introduction

Prior to the availability of computed tomography (CT), Doppler ultrasound (D-US), or magnetic resonance imaging (MRI) and magnetic resonance angiography (MRA), X-ray angiography was commonly the ultimate diagnostic procedure of choice in suspected mass lesions and vascular diseases [1, 4]. Although cut-film and digital subtraction angiography (DSA) – considered together in this chapter as angiography – are the gold standard for the assessment of vascular structures, the invasiveness of these procedures makes them difficult studies to perform, with an essential patient risk of mortality and morbidity resulting from these procedures, especially in neuroradiology.

Recent advances in ultrasound, CT, and magnetic resonance (MR) techniques have in certain settings elevated the role of these new techniques to that of powerful alternatives or even to the method of choice.

The purpose of this chapter is to raise the level of awareness regarding alternative imaging modalities for vascular structures as well as to give overview of current developments on the field of vascular imaging by means of MR techniques.

Techniques of Magnetic Resonance Angiography

Among the noninvasive methods of imaging blood flow, MRA is an attractive alternative. It can be used to evaluate vessel patency, flow magnitude, and flow direction. As an adjunct to conventional MRI studies, MRA can provide information about blood supply and vascular topography of tumors that would otherwise be available only through catheter angiography. MRA exploits the intrinsic properties of flowing blood, thus eliminating the need for catheterization and contrast material. Because of its safety and its noninvasiveness, MRA is playing an increasingly significant role in the work-up of patients suspected of having vascular disease [2, 5]

Nevertheless, MRA is still subject to a number of technical limitations, because of motion-induced artifacts and mainly artifacts caused by alterations in flow

[1] Department of Radiology, University of Berlin, Augustenburger Platz 1, 13353 Berlin, Germany.

behavior through abnormal vessels or tortuous vessel course. Furthermore, it is not yet possible to consistently visualize vessels smaller than 1 mm in diameter [3, 7].

As a result of clinical applications in the past few years, MRA is now regarded as the method of choice in suspected vessel displacement or variation due to mass lesions as well as in thrombosis. MRA is also an alternative to angiography in the evaluation of aneurysms or dissections. In the diagnosis of stenosis, MRA can be performed in addition to D-US, before DSA for evaluation of adjacent soft tissue structures [2, 6–8].

The clinical application of MRA requires an approximate estimation of flow characteristics in the region of interest (ROI) in order to perform an MRA with an excellent depiction of vessel structures. In the following, we will give a brief description of blood flow characteristics with various imaging techniques.

Basic imaging techniques are the spin-echo (SE) technique and the gradient-echo (GE) technique. In conventional SE images, flowing blood appears dark and allows an exact delineation of vessel boundaries to surrounding soft tissue. The SE technique requires 2 RF pulses for imaging. As flowing blood has left the imaging volume by the time the second pulse occurs, it therefore causes a signal void. The advantages of SE sequences with MRA are a higher signal-to-noise ratio, a reduced sensitivity to artifacts caused by higher order motion, and a high spatial resolution of anatomical structures. These sequences allow the differentiation of flowing blood to vessel thrombosis or the exact evaluation of vessel boundary. Evaluation of vessels is possible if the vessel lies within an imaging slice over a longer segment, e.g., in a coronal or sagittal slice orientation [2, 5].

The GE sequence is, in simplified terms, an SE sequence which lacks the second 180° RF pulse so that a single RF pulse produces the MR signal. Therefore, wash-out effects produce negligible signal loss and flowing blood appears bright. Other than in the SE sequence the signal-to-noise ratio depends on the flip angle (α) and the repetition time (TR). Signal reduction or signal void is primarily caused by changes of flow dynamics, e.g., in aneurysms, large field of view or high blood velocities. Special flow-compensated GE sequences used for MRA are the three-dimensional (3D) FISP (fast imaging with steady state precession) and two-dimensional (2D) or 3D FLASH (fast low-angle shot) sequences, which allow vessel visualization in a 3D volume and, after postprocessing with maximum intensity projection (MIP), which display the vessel without soft tissue and permit an MR cineangiography (MTC) [2, 3].

Neuroradiology

MRA in this region is performed using a circular polarized head coil with one to two saturation pulses which are placed appropriately for selective arterial or venous angiograms.

For arterial MRA, usually time-of-flight GE sequences (FISP 3D, TONE, or TONE and MTC) with an axial slice orientation are employed with one or two saturations above the imaging volume. In order to increase spatial resolution, the slice thickness has to be kept as small as possible. In certain settings contrast-

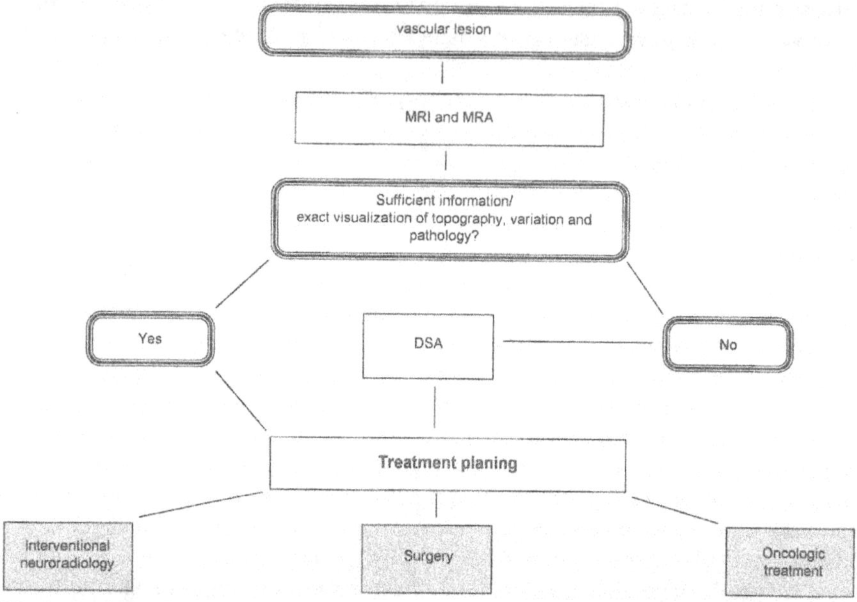

Fig. 1 Angiographic diagnostic strategies in neuroradiology and head and neck. *MRI*, magnetic resonance imaging; *MRA*, magnetic resonance angiography; *DSA*, digital subtraction angiography

enhanced arterial MRA can provide more information with a better delineation of small arteries, although arterial MRA in this region is routinely performed before contrast medium (CM) is administered.

For venous MRA the FLASH 2D sequence is used in the coronal slice orientation and one saturation pulse is placed below the imaging slices. A small overlapping of the imaging slices is required for increased resolution and a higher imaging quality (Fig. 1).

Head and Neck

In the head and neck region, FISP 3D and FLASH 2D sequences are used. Sequence selection depends on the flow velocity in the vessel. MRA is performed with the head coil or the Helmholtz surface coil, which proves to be a limiting factor in the neck due to the coil design.

For selective arterial MRA with fast blood flow, a FISP 3D sequence is used. Slice orientation can be either sagittal with two parallel slabs (each covering one carotid), coronal or axial. The venous flow is eliminated by one or two saturation pulses above the imaging volume. These sequences allow an excellent depiction of the carotid artery with the bifurcation and the intracranial arteries. The advantage of axial slice orientation is its increased resolution and reduced progressive saturation. By using multiple overlapping axial FISP 3D sequences, the whole carotid artery can be scanned. The slower arterial flow in the external carotid artery and its branches are better visualized with the FLASH 2D sequence.

Venous MRA requires the use of sequential flow-compensated FLASH 2D sequences due to the slower blood flow in venous vessels. The slice orientation has to be perpendicular to the vessel in order to avoid signal loss because of increasing saturation of blood within one slice.

Thorax

The appropriate techniques for the evaluation of vascular structures of the thorax vary, as the visualization of the thoracic vasculature is still in clinical evaluation. Vessel depiction is mainly performed by means of TOF MRA with either 3D FISP sequences with first- or second-order motion compensation or for venography with 2D FLASH sequences. Slower flow can be also visualized with rephased/ dephased sequences followed by an internal subtraction technique. So far, the acquisition of conventional SE sequences (black blood angiography) in axial or praxial slice orientation is routinely used in many centers. Additionally, the application of phase-mapping techniques allows quantitative measurements of flow dynamics (Fig. 2) [2, 5].

Abdomen

Several techniques have been suggested to obtain flow information by MRI: these include black blood MRA with SE sequences, TOF MRA with 2D FLASH sequences and bolus-tracking or breath-hold techniques, or phase-contrat techniques, which have been reported to reveal promising results. So far, the most effective and flexible technique is the TOF MRA with 2D FLASH sequences, using the breath-hold technique with appropriately placed saturation pulses (Fig. 2) [5].

Extremities

The evaluation of vascular structures of the extremities has become a standard MR examination in many centers. The visualization of vessels in this region differs to the visualization of vascular structures of the neck as blood flow is not continuous, especially in the lower extremities, but is affected by the cardiac cycle with resulting wave-form blood flow. Routinely 2D TOF with travel saturation or phase-contrast techniques are employed for vessel visualization. For excellent imaging quality, it is also essential that the slice orientation is perpendicular to the main vessel course (Fig. 3) [2, 5].

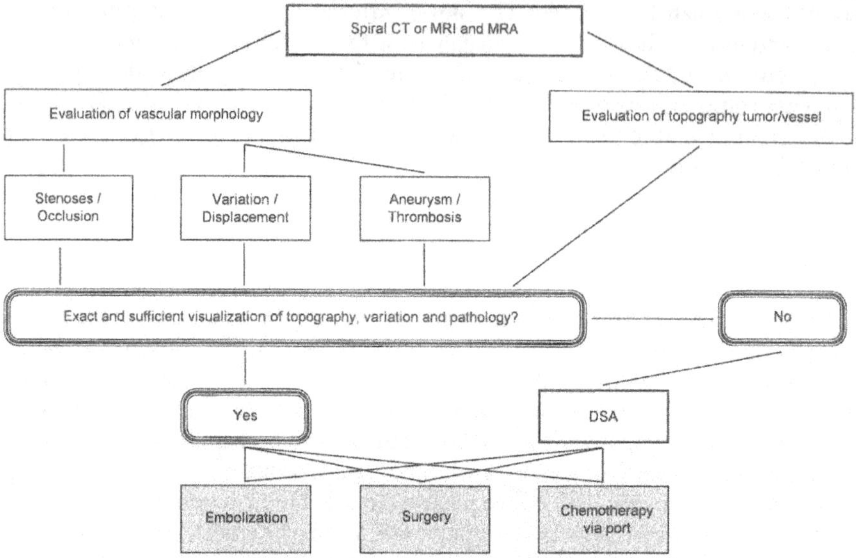

Fig. 2 Angiographic diagnostic strategies in thoracic, abdominal, or pelvic mass lesions. *CT*, computed tomography; *MRI*, magnetic resonance imaging; *MRA*, magnetic resonance angiography; *DSA*, digital subtraction angiography

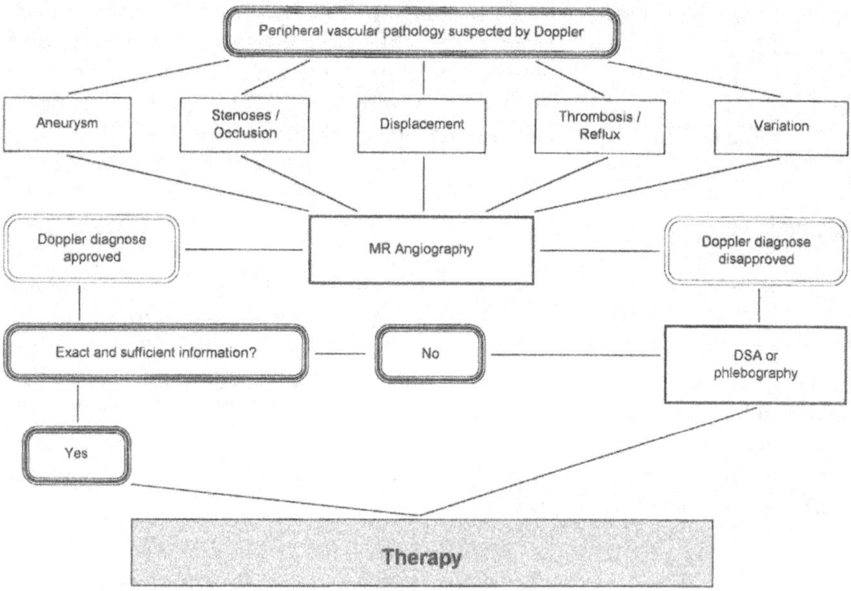

Fig. 3 Angiographic diagnostic strategies in peripheral vascular lesions. *MR*, magnetic resonance; *DSA*, digital subtraction angiography

Indications

Time-of-flight MR angiography is a useful technique for imaging vasculature, although it does have several limitations. Because it depends on the refocusing of inflowing unsaturated spins, it may suffer from increasing saturation within a large imaging volume and incomplete refocusing. Alterations in flow dynamics can cause partial signal loss, because these spins are dephased. Dephasing results from the random, tumbling motion in areas of turbulence and from the increased duration of stay in the measuring slice. Because of signal loss induced by post-stenotic turbulence, grading vessel stenosis appropriately on the basis of MR angiographic findings is rendered difficult with low-grade stenosis. Nevertheless, the grade of stenosis or occlusion as seen on MR angiograms can more accurately be assessed by including conventional MR images and the original data in a review. Another source of error stems from the lack of signal from partially thrombosed aneurysms, which may lead to an underestimation of aneurysm size. However, SE images obtained during the same examination usually provide more information on true size and composition of the aneurysm; indeed, MRA together with conventional MRI may yield more information than DSA alone [7, 8].

A more severe problem is the loss of visualization of small vessels in the process of acquisition and MIP reconstruction. Imaging of small vessels or reduced venous flow in partially thrombosed sinuses requires an increase of in-plane spatial resolution, which can be achieved if the FOV is kept as small as possible. The best achievable in-plane resolution is 1 mm, with a loss of signal from smaller vessels. A further problem arises in image reconstruction. When the vessel size is small compared with the pixel size, small vessels may be lost completely on MIP reconstruction because of partial volume averaging and statistical fluctuations in the background noise. This problem can be overcome by including the original MRA data set in the review, as small vessels or restricted venous flow in partial vessel thrombosis is documented on these images, but eliminated by the MIP algorithm on projection angiograms [8].

Despite the reasonable anatomic correlation of MRA findings with DSA findings, MRA is not likely to be sufficient for the preoperative staging of intracranial aneurysms. In the current state of the art, small vessels arising near an aneurysm, knowledge of which is important in planning surgical strategies, are likely to be missed [2, 5, 8]. In the following, the clinical indications for the use of vascular diagnostic procedures will be presented. Five major areas of interest have to be defined in order to fulfill the requirements for vascular imaging:

- Neuroradiology
- Head and neck
- Thorax
- Abdominal or pelvic mass
- Peripheral vascular pathology

Neuroradiology

Neurovascular MRA is meanwhile widely used for the visualization of normal intracranial vessels (Fig. 4) and the evaluation of vessel displacement, aneurysms, vessel stenosis, AV malformations, and sinus thrombosis, including follow-up (Fig. 5).

So far, primary indications for MRA in this region are regarded to be the visualization of vessel displacement, the diagnosis of sinus thrombosis, and screening for vascular pathologies (Fig. 6). Although MRA reveals advantages in the diagnosis of aneurysms with exact differentiation of thrombosed portions, small vessels arising near the aneurysm can be missed by MRA.

Head and Neck

Indications for arterial MRA of the region of the head and neck are vessel displacement or compression due to expansive tumor growth. Other indications concern vessel pathology itself such as aneurysms, dissections (Fig. 7), stenosis, or carotid body tumors. Changes in intravascular flow behavior (e.g., laminar to turbulent flow) render the exact staging of stenosis grade or aneurysm size difficult. This difficulty can be partially overcome by including the conventional MR images as well as the original MRA data in the review. Indications for venous MRA in the region of the head and neck are thrombosis of the jugular vein or occlusion due to tumors and the detection of glomus tumors of the skull base.

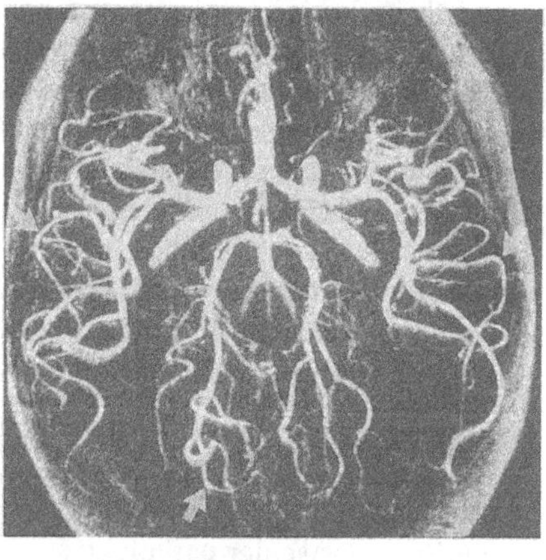

Fig. 4 Normal arterial magnetic resonance angiography (MRA) of the intracranial vasculature. MRA, gradient-echo (GE), TONE, TR/TE=43/8, α=20° plain. The maximum intensity projection (MIP), angiogram reveals an excellent depiction of the intracranial arteries. Note the visualization of the terminal branches of the posterior and middle cerebral arteries (*arrow*)

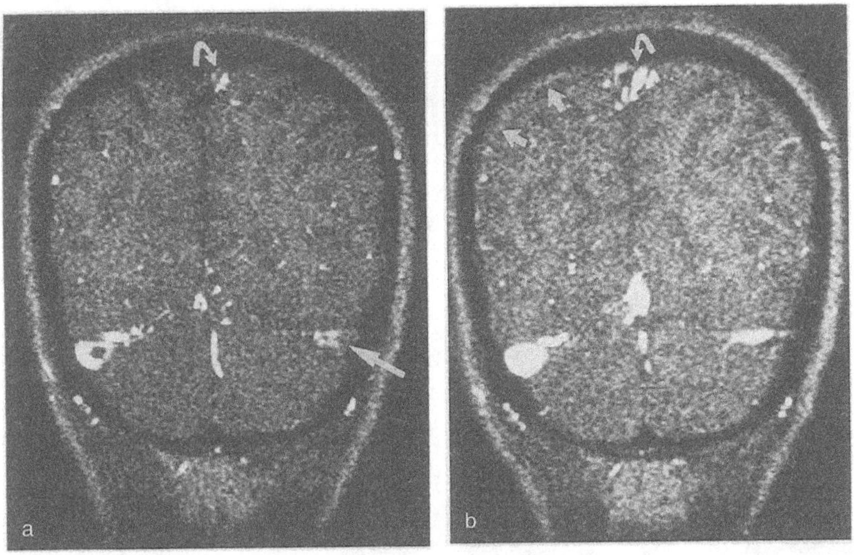

Fig. 5 a, b A 43-year-old male patient with sinus thrombosis before and after therapy. Venous magnetic resonance angiography (MRA), gradient-echo (GE), two-dimensional fast, low-angle shot (FLASH 2D), repetition time (TR)/TE=3610, α=60°, plain. **a** The single-slice images before therapy show the thrombosis of the left transverse (*arrow*) and the superior sagittal sinus (*curved arrow*). These images also allow the verification of rest-perfusion in the occluded left transverse sinus and the detection collateral drainage via cortical veins and the deep venous system. **b** Two months after therapy, a reperfusion of the previously occluded vessels can be observed with the thrombus still evident in the superior sagittal sinus (*curved arrow*) as well as collateral drainage (*arrows*)

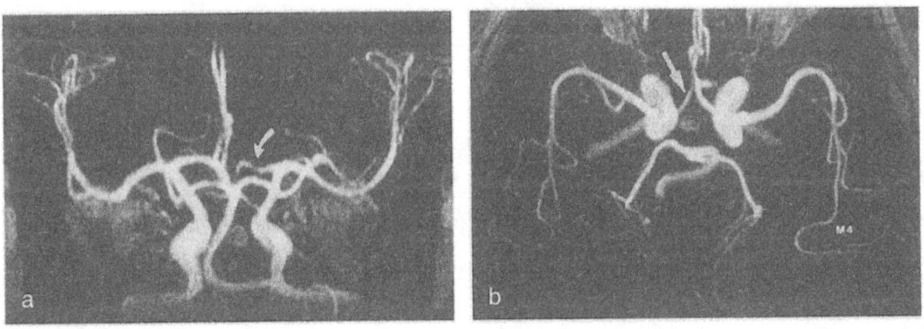

Fig. 6 a, b Arterial magnetic resonance angiography (MRA) in a patient with vasculitis. Gradient-echo (GE), TONE, repetition time (TR)/TE=43/8, α=20°, plain. The maximum intensity projection (MIP) in a coronal view reveals normal perfusion of both internal carotid and the basilar artery. Lower flow signal observed in both middle cerebral arteries and a hypoplastic anterior cerebral artery on the left side (*arrow*). **b** The rotation to a more axial view reveals the reduced vessel perfusion of the middle and posterior cerebral arteries, especially in the terminal branches and the hypoplastic anterior cerebral artery on the left side (*arrow*)

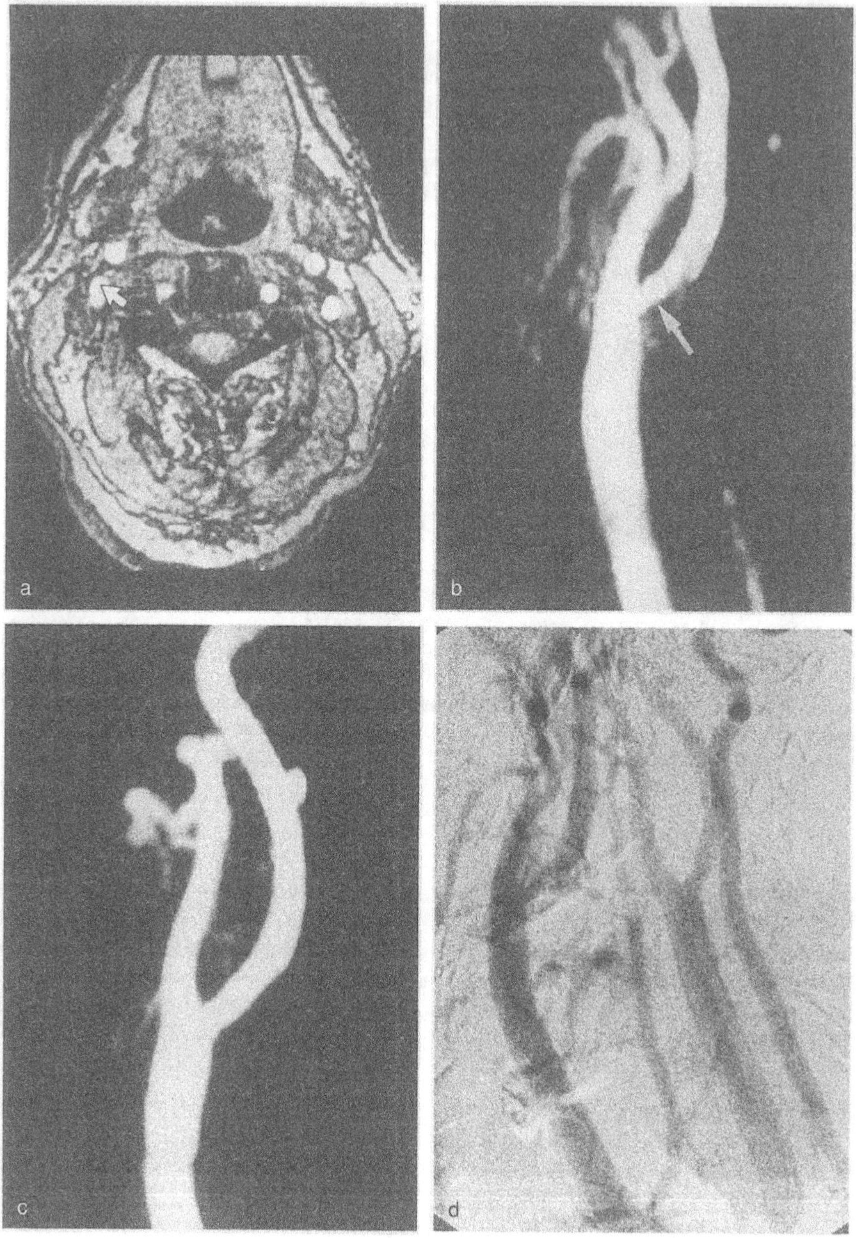

Fig. 7 **a–d** Dissection of the right internal artery. Arterial magnetic resonance angiography (MRA), gradient-echo (GE), three-dimensional fast imaging with steady state precession (FISP 3D), repetition time (TR)/TE=29/7, $\alpha = 15°$, plain. Single slice image of the arterial MRA, visualization of the dissection of the right internal carotid artery (*arrow*) with normal findings in the left internal carotid artery. **b** The maximum intensity projection (MIP) reconstruction of the right internal carotid artery shows the dissection as well as the slight stenosis of this vessel close to the bifurcation (*arrow*). **c** Single MIP reconstruction of the left internal carotid artery with normal finding allows direct comparison with the other side. **d** The additionally performed digital subtraction angiography (DSA) confirms the MRA diagnosis of right-sided internal carotid artery stenosis and dissection

Thorax

MRA of the thoracic vasculature is largely still at the stage of clinical evaluation, and suggested indications for MRA evaluation in this region are currently as follows [5]:

- Congenital aortic anomalies (left pulmonary artery sling, variations of the aortic arch, coarcation, Marfan's syndrome, etc.)
- Acquired aortic diseases (aneurysm, dissection)
- Congenital venous anomalies and thrombosis

Preliminary promising results have been obtained for the visualization of coronary arteries and the depiction of pulmonary artery pathologies.

Abdomen

MRA is routinely used for the evaluation of vascular structures of the abdomen in many centers, and indications for MRA currently include a variety of clinical situations. Standard MRA indications [5] are the visualization of the following:

- Portal venous system
- Hepatic veins
- Renal vasculature
- Abdominal aorta and its major bifurcations
- Portal-systemic communications

MRA can also be used for planning and follow-up of the transjugular placement of a portosystemic stent shunt (TIPS). Further, interventional MRA applications with special catheters are in clinical evaluation.

Extremities

Beside the exclusion of vascular pathologies (Fig. 8), the two major clinical applications for MRA of the extremities are to determine disease distribution and to provide a preoperative road map which, in combination with noninvasive hemodynamic evaluation, could replace routine preoperative angiography. Indications for MRA of the extremities are as follows [5]:

- Vessel thrombosis
- Aneurysms of the popliteal, iliac, or femoral arteries
- Atherosclerotic occlusive disease (Fig. 9).

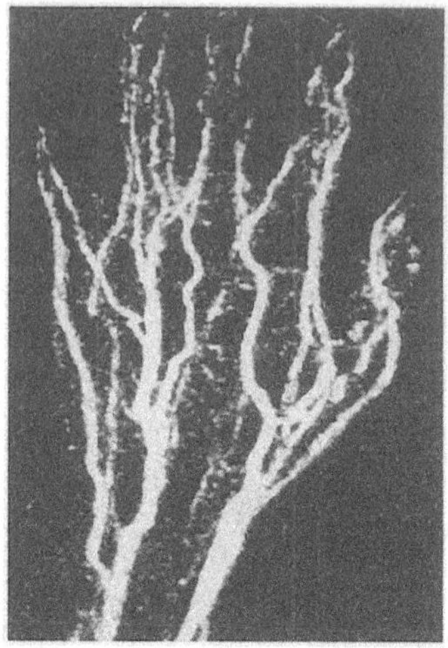

Fig. 8 A 34-year-old patient with suspected traumatic thrombosis of the palmar arteries of the left hand with normal arterial findings in magnetic resonance angiography (MRA). Gradient-echo (GE), three-dimensional fast imaging with steady state precession (FISP 3D), repetition time (TR)/TE=40/7, $\alpha = 20°$, plain. The maximum intensity projection (MIP) reconstruction of the rephased/dephased MRA sequence reveals an excellent depiction of the arterial vessels of the hand with flow inhomogenities in the proper palmar digital arteries without any signs for vessel thrombosis

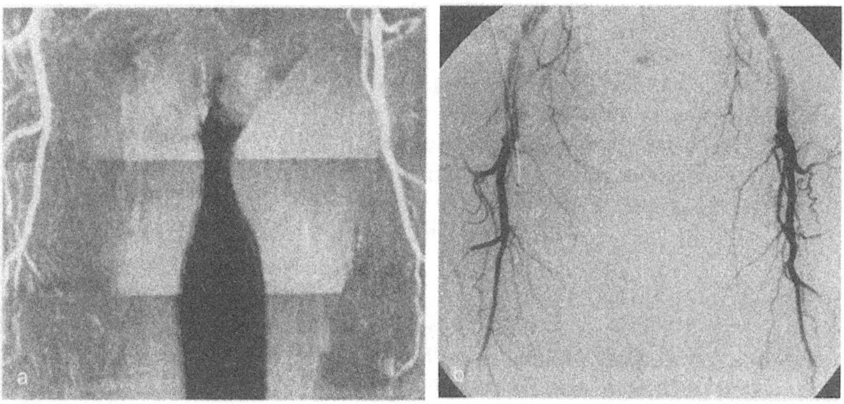

Fig. 9 **a, b** A 50-year-old patient with occlusion of both superficial femoral arteries. Arterial magnetic resonance angiography (MRA), gradient-echo (GE), three-dimensional fast imaging with steady state precession (FISP 3D), repetition time (TR)/TE=29/7, $\alpha = 15°$, plain. **a** The multi-slab maximum intensity projection (MIP) reconstruction of the arterial vessels of the high reveals a total occlusion of both superficial femoral arteries with regular perfusion of the deep femoral arteries. **b** The digital subtraction angiography (DSA) findings confirm the MRA diagnosis and additionally show the collateral vessels

GPSR Compliance
The European Union's (EU) General Product Safety Regulation (GPSR) is a set of rules that requires consumer products to be safe and our obligations to ensure this.

If you have any concerns about our products, you can contact us on

ProductSafety@springernature.com

In case Publisher is established outside the EU, the EU authorized representative is:

Springer Nature Customer Service Center GmbH
Europaplatz 3
69115 Heidelberg, Germany

www.ingramcontent.com/pod-product-compliance
Lightning Source LLC
Chambersburg PA
CBHW071430230926
51846CB00001B/172
9783642798894